618.178   Cooper, Susan,
C   1947-

Choosing   d
reprod   C 618.178   Cooper, Susan,
                                              1947-

$24.95   Choosing assisted
                                              reproduction.

                  $24.95

DATE	BORROWER'S NAME	

BAKER & TAYLOR

CHOOSING

Assisted Reproduction

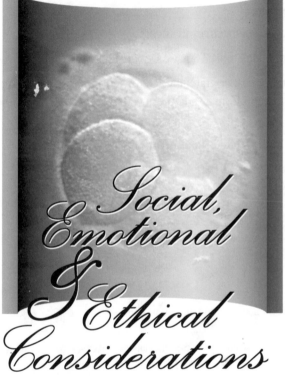

Social, Emotional & Ethical Considerations

Susan Lewis Cooper
Ellen Sarasohn Glazer

Perspectives Press
Indianapolis, IN

Perspectives Press
P.O. Box 90318
Indianapolis, IN 46290-0318
USA
(317) 872-3055
http://www.perspectivespress.com

Book design by Wade Smola, T-Square Design, Fort Wayne, Indiana

The authors and publisher gratefully acknowledge permission to reproduce the cover photograph from a slide produced by Reproductive Science Center-Boston.

Manufactured in the United States of America

Hardcover ISBN 0-944934-19-6
Softcover ISBN 0-944934-22-6

Library of Congress Cataloging in Publication Data:

Cooper, Susan 1947-
  Choosing Assisted Reproduction : social, emotional and ethical considerations / Susan Lewis Cooper, Ellen Sarasohn Glazer.
      p.   cm.
  Includes bibliographic references and index.
  Hardcover, ISBN 0-944934-19-6; Paperback, ISBN 0-944934-22-6
  1. Human reproductive technology — Popular works. 2. Human reproductive technology —Moral and ethical aspects. 3. Human reproductive technology —Psychological aspects. 4. Human reproductive technology — Social aspects. I. Glazer, Ellen Sarasohn. II. Title
  RG1335.5.C673 1998
  818.1'7806—dc21   97-36563
                                                                          CIP

2

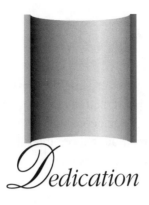

$\mathcal{D}$edication

This book is for Seth and Amanda Cooper and Elizabeth and Mollie Glazer, who have enriched our lives beyond measure.

Ten years ago we dedicated our first book, *Without Child*, to them. At that time they were young children and we thought our time with them was limitless. A short decade later they are teenagers and young adults, having left, or preparing to leave home. Although infertility may not have made us better parents, it provided a valuable perspective during the ups and downs of parenthood—that children are precious gifts, and that neither they, nor the opportunity to parent them, should ever be taken for granted.

Acknowledgments

We begin this book by acknowledging the contributions of the numerous patients with whom we have had the privilege of working for over twenty years. They are wise, courageous, and determined individuals who have taught us an enormous amount about infertility, and specifically about the emotional challenges of assisted reproduction. Their words, their thoughts, and their experiences are reflected throughout this book.

We are fortunate to work with outstanding physicians, nurses, embryologists and others in the field of assisted reproduction. We are especially grateful to our colleagues at the Boston Regional Center for Reproductive Medicine in Stoneham, Massachusetts and the Reproductive Science Center (formerly IVF America) in Waltham, Massachusetts, for their on-going support, care, and comraderie. We admire and deeply appreciate the dedication with which they work to build families.

There were several individuals who graciously answered our questions and responded to our concerns as we prepared this manuscript and we thank them for their help. They include: Joan Barnes of TASC; Dr. Hilary Hanafin; Dr. Natalie Schultz; Dr. Sheryl Kingsberg, and Attorney Susan Crockin. We would also like to acknowledge Susan Levin, LICSW, Jeane Springer, LICSW, and Sharon Steinberg, RN, who helped write the chapter on ovum donation in our previous book, *Beyond Infertility: The New Paths to Parenthood*. Much of that original chapter forms the basis for the current chapter on ovum donation.

We have learned—and continue to learn—so much from our colleagues in the Boston Mental Health Collaborative in Reproductive Medicine and from our colleagues nationwide in the Mental Health Professional Group of the American Society for Reproductive Medicine. Their knowledge, guidance, and wisdom is woven throughout this book.

Finally, and most importantly, we would like to thank our editor and publisher, Pat Johnston, whose enthusiasm, encouragement, guidance, and unsurpassed editing skills made this book possible. Her attention to detail and knowledge of the field shines on every page.

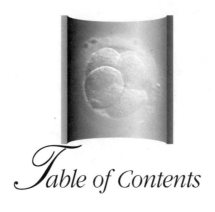

$\mathcal{T}$able of Contents

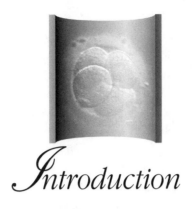

$\mathcal{I}$ntroduction

This book is for individuals and couples who are—or may sometime be—considering assisted reproduction. It is also for professionals—physicians, nurses, mental health clinicians—who work with such couples. The decisions that confront you are difficult and multi-faceted, involving medical, psychological, emotional, financial, ethical, moral, practical and religious questions. Although some may find the decision making process relatively straightforward, many of you will struggle through a complex, unfamiliar and challenging exploration of yourselves and the world around you. We want you to know that your struggle, though painful, will most likely prove valuable in helping you move forward with confidence in the rightness of your decisions.

Many of you have already travelled a long way in your journey through infertility diagnosis and treatment. It must be hard for you to imagine forging onward when the path has already been so tiring. Others, by contrast, are relatively new travellers, having learned through a semen analysis, laparoscopy or other single diagnostic test, that you are candidates for assisted reproductive technology. It is probably difficult to find yourselves so suddenly on the border of this "brave new world" of assisted reproduction. Still others of you are not yet at the point of considering assisted reproduction, but want to look ahead so you can feel more familiar with what may be on the horizon. *Choosing Assisted Reproduction* is for all of you—we hope that it will provide you with a foundation from which you can approach a range of questions and decisions.

Before introducing you to the format, themes and content of *Choosing Assisted Reproduction*, we want to tell you something about how and why this book came about. *Choosing Assisted Reproduction* began as a simple "up-date" of our 1994 book, *Beyond Infertility: The New Paths to Parenthood*. As we noted in the introduction of *Beyond Infertility*, reproductive technology is a rapidly changing field and information is becoming out-dated almost by the time a book on the subject is published. For example, just as this book is going to press we are hearing reports about a birth—the first of its kind—of a baby conceived *in vitro* with cytoplasm from a donor egg, resulting in a child that has both parents' genetic components. This technology is too new, however, to share it with you now, but may ultimately result in significantly fewer (primarily older) women requiring donor eggs in order to conceive. And so we set out, in 1996, to make *Beyond Infertility* more current, believing that new medical information was all that was needed to provide patients with an instructive guide to decision-making regarding assisted reproduction.

The task of updating was fairly easy. However, as we scrutinized each chapter we became aware of how much our own thinking had also become updated and was not reflected in the printed word. In the last few years our thoughts, opinions, and ethical beliefs had become more defined. We also felt more convinced of the soundness of our beliefs and felt more secure about sharing them straightforwardly with patients and with professionals. Thus we decided to expand two important parts of the original book—ethical considerations and disclosure to children—and create two new chapters, the first and last chapters of *Choosing Assisted Reproduction*.

Chapter One, "Ethical Considerations in Assisted Reproduction," is not "easy reading"—it is difficult enough for infertile patients to deal with medical decision making without having to confront serious ethical and psychological concerns. Nevertheless, these concerns exist alongside the array of medical options and it is our hope that by introducing them at the beginning, we provide readers with a framework and reference points to draw upon as they make their way through the medical maze.

The medical process can feel daunting, and yet medical information is essential to sound decision making in infertility treatment. Because we know how overwhelmed patients can feel when they are introduced to an alphabet of ART options—IVF, GIFT, ZIFT, ICSI etc., we have tried to present medical information in a simple—though not simplistic—way. Our hope is that after finishing Chapter Two, readers will feel well versed in the basics of assisted reproduction, knowing what questions to ask their physicians, and knowing how to evaluate their responses.

Although all individuals and couples undergoing assisted reproduction do not become pregnant, many do. We have found that few feel prepared for the stress and the uncertainties of pregnancy after assisted reproduction. For that reason, we have devoted Chapter Three to Pregnancy after ART, including a lengthy section on pregnancy loss. Perhaps more than any other chapter in this book, this chapter attempts to diminish isolation. We want our pregnant readers—and those who have experienced a loss—to know that they are not alone as they make their way through this exceedingly difficult journey.

The first part of *Choosing Assisted Reproduction* concludes with Chapter Four, "Moving Forward: Changing Directions." We include this chapter in recognition of the fact that many of our readers will come to a point at which they must make some extraordinarily difficult decisions regarding ending treatment and moving on to a second choice (and sometimes third choice) path to parenthood. Once the possibility of introducing another person—either as a gamete donor, a gestational carrier, or a surrogate—comes into play, ethical and emotional challenges multiply exponentially.

The second part of *Choosing Assisted Reproduction* is devoted to third party parenting options. Five of these chapters deal with a specific "third party" option: sperm donation, ovum donation, surrogacy, gestational care and embryo donation. We encourage you to read beyond the chapter or chapters that relate directly to your personal situation, as all these options, though different, share common ground. This common ground involves the meaning and relative importance of genetic, generational, gestational and parenting ties. It includes ethical questions involving the best interest of offspring and the rights of people to reproduce.

Choosing Assisted Reproduction ends with what we hope will be a beginning: a strong argument for openness with one's children—i.e. the right to know the truth about one's genetic origins. We also provide some guidelines and suggestions about how to do so. We hope that potential parents—most importantly those who are reproducing with the help of third parties—will enter treatment with the concept of openness as a bottom line. We hope that the foundation offered in Chapter Ten will reassure you that you are not alone and that you, together with other pioneering parents, will be establishing a sound path for future generations.

Choosing Assisted Reproduction was a difficult book to write, and for many it may be a difficult book to read. The first part of the book is difficult because we speak freely and openly about the various challenges associated with undergoing assisted reproduction, as well as pregnancy after assisted reproduction. We do not paint a rosey picture, but rather, acknowledge that there are tough decisions to be made and sometimes, tough experiences to endure. Sadly, all the hard work and wise decisions in the world cannot insure a successful pregnancy, and many people will have to make a second choice regarding family building.

As difficult as the first part of the book is, the second part is probably even more challenging. We know that many would-be parents, regardless of whether they have struggled with infertility, believe strongly that the power of their love can transcend all difficulties. Although love may indeed be the most important ingredient in raising children, it is necessary, but not sufficient for psychological health. Those who pursue third party parenting not only confront a series of financial, medical, social, psychological, and logistical hurdles, but they must also confront the fact that their children will have questions, and possibly unsettling feelings about the way that they entered their families. They must also confront the fact that "keeping it a secret" in hopes of avoiding problems for the child(ren) will most likely lead to even more serious ones for everyone in the family.

Lest we sound too "down," we want to assure our readers that each of us knows countless happy, thriving families who were created by assisted reproduction and by third party parenting. These families are what make our work so satisfying—they are living testimony to the true miracle of creation. Unlike our first book, *Without Child*, this book is not told through personal accounts. However, the words, the smiles and the stories of the families we have known infuse this book. You will not see their names or faces on the pages ahead, but please know that they are in the background, encouraging you onward. Virtually all would tell you that the outcome makes the struggle worthwhile.

Although we have tried to pack a lot into this book, there are some things that are missing. We want to acknowledge them at the outset so that you are not looking for them. First, you will notice that we do not discuss adoption. Nor do we discuss resolving infertility without children. Although both are paths successfully pursued by infertile couples, they are not explored in this book because our focus here is on assisted reproduction. However, our assumption is that some of our readers will move on to one of these options, either because they decide against assisted reproduction and/or third party parenting or because they try one or more of the options discussed here and do not successfully complete their family. We want you to know that we are in no way dismissing either of these options, each of which proves to be the right path for many infertile couples. We encourage couples to read *Adopting After Infertility* by Patricia Irwin Johnston and *Sweet Grapes*, by Jean and Michael Carter.

Second, there are several infertile constituencies that are not addressed directly in this book. Again, we want you to know that this book is for you, but in the interest of space and language we have not included specific discussion of your situations. One such constituency are single women who are pursuing pregnancy without partners. A second group are lesbian couples, and a third group are those who are struggling with secondary infertility. Although members of each group have some unique experiences and concerns, we feel that nearly all of what we have addressed to the presumably childless, heterosexual couple applies to you.

Third, we do not discuss extended family, most importantly, grandparents. Again, this is an issue of space. We are keenly aware of the pain felt by the parents of infertile couples and know that the years spent in pursuit of pregnancy often rob families of precious grandparenting time. All too often, would-be grandparents are older—and perhaps in ill health—by the time their long awaited grandchildren arrive.

In addition to these grandparents, we want also to acknowledge the potential for loss and pain felt by parents of surrogates and gamete donors who may truly feel that they are experiencing the permanent loss of a grandchild or children.

You, our readers, are pioneers. The territory you are exploring—or are about to explore—is still new and the path ahead may sometimes be difficult to find. We hope this book helps you to chart your own course and to identify and follow the paths to parenthood that are right for you.

CHAPTER 1

Emotional and Ethical Considerations of Assisted Reproductive Technology

The book of Samuel in the Old Testament tells the story of Elkanah, a pious man who has two wives, Hannah and Peninnah. Peninnah has many children, but Hannah, his more beloved wife, is barren. Peninnah taunts Hannah, saying that the Lord has closed Hannah's womb. Hannah weeps and cannot eat. Elkanah says, "Hannah, why weepest though? And why eatest thou not? And why is thy heart grieved? Am not I better to thee than ten sons? " Later Hannah prays to the Lord and weeps again, vowing that if the Lord gives her a son, she "will give him unto the Lord all the days of his life..." As Hannah is praying, Eli, the priest, watches her lips moving soundlessly. He assumes that she is drunk and asks her to put away her wine. Hannah speaks intensely: "I am a woman of a sorrowful spirit: I have drunk neither wine nor strong drink, but I poured out my soul before the Lord."

Although the Old Testament is replete with references to infertility, the story of Hannah is especially important because it illustrates the timelessness of the emotions that surround infertility. We see in this short passage the pain of an infertile woman, overcome with despair. She is so saddened by her condition that she is unable to eat, and she cries continuously. Furthermore, she is pained by and jealous of the fecundity of her rival, who appears insensitive to her condition. Her husband, Elkanah, feeling helpless and desperate to make her happier, attempts to use logic to help her feel better. Like many of today's husbands, he cannot understand why his love of her, and the special attention he gives her, is not enough to make her happy.

Today's infertile couples walk in Hannah and Elkanah's shadows. They, like their biblical counterparts, struggle with feelings of isolation, envy, helplessness, and despair. Like Hannah and Elkanah, they may feel misunderstood by their spouses. Like Hannah, infertile women may feel their sense of womanhood mercilessly assaulted. And many turn, as Hannah did, to prayer. Theirs is a centuries old anguish that has been described and re-described throughout history, but was probably best captured in the words of another biblical woman, Rachel, when she exclaimed, "Give me children or I die." Today's infertile couples share the intense longings of Hannah and Elkanah and of Rachel and the many other biblical figures who struggled with infertility.

Yet today's couples travel a very different journey than their counterparts from any prior generation. Even recent generations had few medical interventions to which they could turn. In contrast, today's weary travelers make their way through a complex and confusing medical maze. Although some are fortunate to respond to conservative treatment and bear children along the way and others decide to take different paths to parenthood, many find themselves approaching the unfamiliar terrain of the assisted reproductive technologies. This terrain may necessitate difficult, complicated, and ethically challenging decisions that may even involve third or fourth parties in the parenting experience. In this chapter—and in those that follow—we will take a look at this unexpected journey. We will focus on the emotional burdens and ethical challenges that await couples who consider and/or pursue assisted reproduction.

Today's infertile couples not only experience the emotional burden of infertility, but they must also confront myriad ethical challenges that accompany the new technologies. Because the emotional and ethical dilemmas are entwined, we present them together in this chapter. To do otherwise would be to suggest that they can easily be separated. They cannot. For unlike in biblical times when there were few third party parenting options and there was no medically assisted reproduction, infertile couples today must endure not only the emotional pain of infertility, but they must also grapple with profound ethical dilemmas posed by high tech treatment.

In this chapter we outline the new dilemmas—both ethical and emotional—imposed by the new technologies. We will see that although the feelings infertile men and women experience are timeless, there is also a timeliness to the ways in which these feelings are perceived and resolved. We will see, also, that while advances in reproductive technology have offered new hope to countless couples, these advances have also complicated their experience of infertility, adding new—and perhaps deeper—dimensions to a couple's suffering.

Principles of Medical Ethics

Each of us has a code of ethics that guides us in our daily lives. Most of the time, however, these personal ethical guidelines are not something we think about consciously. Rather, they are there—in the background—for us to draw upon as needed. Occasionally situations arise in all our lives which force us to look more closely at our personal ethics. When this occurs, we become aware of the principles that guide our actions and reactions. We also realize that we each have ethical lines that we are unwilling to cross.

Exploring assisted reproduction prompts most people to confront their personal ethical principles and to ask themselves difficult questions. "Can I do this and if not, why not?" "Can I live with the decision to...?" "Would this decision be 'in the best interests of the child' or would it be a selfish decision?" For many, this questioning is an unfamiliar process and one that they find unsettling. After all, nothing could be more natural and more ethically correct than to want a child: why then, is it so complicated? In fact, the ARTs and certainly, third party reproduction raise profound ethical questions for all of us and force us to carefully consider what it means to create families in new ways.

Although personal ethics cannot necessarily be codified or even described, it can be helpful to know the central principles of medical ethics. This time honored and widely accepted ethical code, which has governed the practice of medicine for centuries, provides each of us with a framework upon which we can examine and understand our reactions to complex ethical questions. We will introduce this code through its three central principles: autonomy, beneficence and justice. Among ethicists, the first principle, autonomy, is frequently determined to be the most important, in the event of a clash between two of the principles.

Autonomy places value on human beings and on their right to make decisions regarding their own welfare, providing that those decisions do not infringe on the rights of others. In medical ethics autonomy refers to an individual's right to receive accurate information about his/her medical condition and the range of treatment possibilities. Furthermore autonomy gives patients the right to refuse or deny treatment that is offered. *Beneficence* refers to the concept of doing good—performing acts of kindness to others. The concept of beneficence also includes a duty to avoid harming a person or to prevent harm from happening to another. The third principle, *justice*, refers to a belief in the equal distribution of society's benefits and burdens, i.e. the concept that everyone should be treated fairly and receive what he/she needs and deserves.

Helping couples to become parents through the use of reproductive technology can be viewed as an effort that supports all three principles. It supports autonomy if couples are given the information pertaining to their situation and the power to make decisions regarding their treatment. It supports beneficence when a long sought-after goal—parenthood—is achieved and a new life is created (a concept that has historically been viewed by ethicists as positive). It supports the concept of justice when all who are in need are able to avail themselves of the technology. (Unfortunately because few states regard infertility as a medical condition, many couples do not have access to necessary treatment due to financial constraints.)

Inevitably there are occasions when the promotion of one principle clashes with the promotion of another. Most commonly this situation arises when autonomy collides with beneficence—when a patient opts for a particular treatment that his/her provider believes may do harm to the patient (or in the case of reproductive technology, to a potential child) and the provider does not wish to offer the treatment. In these situations, one principle must be compromised for the sake of the other. Most frequently, in medical situations, autonomy is granted first. However, as we shall see in this chapter, when the lives of potential children are at stake, it is not clear who should make final or ultimate decisions and what information should influence those decisions.

In this chapter we identify three concepts influencing decision making—the separate components of parenthood, unnatural conception, and avoidance of regret—that pose difficult dilemmas for infertile couples considering assisted reproduction. Although these concepts existed to some degree even before the development of ART, they have become prominent in current times. As we discuss the ways in which the new reproductive technologies have influenced an infertile

16

couple's emotional outlook, we will describe these concepts—and dilemmas—along with the ethical questions that have arisen with them.

The Separate Components of Parenthood

As anyone who has ever experienced infertility can attest, infertility involves multiple losses. From the first moment that an individual or couple realizes that they are having difficulty conceiving or carrying a child, they are confronted with loss. As the experience of infertility continues, many losses come cascading towards them: loss of self-esteem, loss of body integrity, loss of privacy, loss of sexual pleasure, loss of time, loss of money, loss of comfort in friendships and family relationships, and the loss of spontaneous conception. Furthermore, couples—especially those who reaped rewards from hard work and effort—begin to feel they are losing control over their lives. Infertility threatens their ability to plan for the future and to know where they are going.

In addition to the losses mentioned above, today's infertile couples are threatened by the possibility of losses involving basic structures in their lives. These may include threats to the future of their marriage, threats to their relationships with others, threats to their religious faith, and threats to their careers. Managing these primary structures becomes of paramount importance, since the stakes, in each instance, are high.

What's more, infertile couples are threatened with losses that are directly related to reproduction and parenting: the loss of the pregnancy experience, of a genetic connection to one's offspring, of continuity with one's bloodline, of conceiving a child jointly with one's beloved spouse, and of parenting itself. It is these losses that are most distressing to infertile couples and it is also these losses that have been directly impacted by advances in reproductive technology.

For the first time in history, as an outgrowth of *in vitro* fertilization technology and research, the three components of parenthood—the genetic, the gestational, and the nurturant—can be separated, so that the loss of one does not necessarily result in the loss of the others. For a man or woman who may not be able to conceive a child genetically connected to him or her, ovum donation or sperm donation offers the opportunity for gestation and parenting of a child genetically connected to half of the couple. For a woman unable to carry a pregnancy to term, gestational care may be the alternative of choice. For couples who cannot provide egg or sperm, but who wish to experience pregnancy, embryo adoption may be an alternative route to parenthood.

Reproductive choices are not made easily. As couples near the end of their biological options, most contemplate—if only for a split second—what it would be like not to be parents at all. If they decide that raising children is their primary goal, they begin to think about alternative routes to parenthood. The array of adoption and third party parenting options available challenges couples to examine the relative importance to them of gestational vs. genetic connections. Prospective parents must think carefully about what it would mean to them to be a parent without experiencing pregnancy, or a parent with no genetic connection to their child. Others contemplate what it would be like not to be parents at all.

Pregnancy and Childbirth Experience

The observation that women and men experience infertility in different ways is something that has long been known by infertile couples and their caregivers. This phenomena has been studied by several researchers. Women have been found to experience significantly more psychological distress than do their partners, especially in the areas of depression, anxiety, cognitive disturbance and hostility. Researchers suggest that these findings can best be explained by differences in expectations about motherhood and fatherhood.

For women, expectations of motherhood begin with pregnancy. For many, the threatened loss of pregnancy and childbirth represents an immense loss. They report having looked forward for many years to growing a baby inside them—to feeling its movement within their womb and experiencing its birth during labor and delivery. Some find the thought that they might never have this experience unfathomable: it fills them with profound sadness. Thus, for some women pregnancy feels like an essential life event, one that cannot be missed. Without it, many fear that they will feel permanently and powerfully damaged. It is common for women to blame themselves when they learn about their infertility. Those who delayed parenthood, were sexually active, or had abortions may identify these actions as the cause of and the punishment for their infertility. However, even women who cannot remember anything specific they did "wrong," may still blame themselves, fearing that God is punishing them for some unknown transgression.

The threatened loss of the pregnancy experience can be especially difficult and challenging for those couples in which the man is the identified patient. In these instances established gender differences in reactions to infertility are altered. In his 1992 study, Nachtigall[1] found that the gap between men and women's responses to infertility narrows considerably when the man is the identified patient. Although the men in the study spoke of the threatened loss of parenthood, only the men with male factor spoke of a concurrent loss of self esteem. Thus not only do infertile men have to bear the potential loss of being genetically connected to their offspring, and the emotional pain that realization brings, but they invariably feel guilty for depriving their wives of a pregnancy.

Genetic Connection to One's Offspring

Prior to the arrival of assisted reproduction, the loss of the pregnancy experience was inevitably coupled with the loss of genetic continuity. The development of *in vitro* fertilization meant that a woman could become pregnant via an egg from another woman (a donor) or with an embryo donated from another couple, and she could parent the child she gestated. Furthermore, some couples can now parent their genetic children (with the assistance of a gestational carrier) even when they are unable to go through pregnancy and childbirth together. Because genetics can now be separated from gestation, many infertile couples weigh these losses carefully and make choices based on which losses are more tolerable for them.

For a man, whose only connection to his unborn child is a genetic one, this loss may be crucial. For a woman, the loss of a genetic connection to her offspring may or may not seem to be central. A study performed at the University of Chicago asked women if they could only be related to their offspring either genetically or gestationally, which would they choose. Fifty-one percent chose gestation over genetics.[2] In an informal study at Reproductive Science Center, Waltham, Massachusetts, approximately sixty-five percent chose

19

genetics. What is important to note is that many people are guided in their second choice routes to parenthood by their feelings and longings regarding genetic versus gestational ties.

A genetic connection to one's offspring involves two components: the transmission of one's genes and the continuation of one's blood-line. Genes are the building blocks through which traits and characteristics are passed on to one's offspring. Many people fantasize, even prior to conception, about what their children will look and be like. They think about which traits they want to pass on and which traits they hope their offspring will be spared. Couples also think about blending their genes—creating a child who is the combination of the two of them and many see this child as the greatest expression of their love. Couples facing infertility are saddened to think they may not be able to look at their offspring and see parts of themselves reflected back—or parts of their grandparents or greatgrandparents.

For others, genetic connections represent ties to their individual blood lines. These individuals long for genetic offspring to carry on the family line, connecting generations past to generations future. The inability to have genetic children means the loss of this geneaological continuity, and for many couples, especially those whose families were rooted in strong ethnic or religious traditions, this loss is profound.

There is another reason why a genetic connection is important to many people: genes determine a great deal about a person. Although the exact formula of the nature/nurture debate has not been (and may never be) settled, it is increasingly understood that genes play a major role in who we are. Genes are responsible not only for physical traits and talents, but they are also a large determinant of personality and temperament as well as our abilities (or lack of abilities). A predisposition towards mental health (or mental illness) is also thought to be genetically determined, although no one working in the mental health field would dispute that environment is a major factor as well. Many people seek the familiarity and security of having a child who shares their genes.

Parenting Experience

In the past, couples who faced childlessness frequently opted to adopt. Adoption was a means of avoiding the loss of the parenting experience, which to many would have been intolerable. Today, when faced with this same loss, many—perhaps most—couples consider adoption. The decision to adopt, however, has become more complicated with the arrival of third party parenting options and with recent changes in adoption practice, including movement towards greater openness and acknowledgment of birthparents' rights and ties to their birthchildren. Couples who may once have chosen adoption with relative ease, because they knew they wanted to be parents, now move more cautiously. Tempted by third party parenting choices which may appear to offer more control, or frightened by negative media attention to adoption, many would-be parents struggle painfully before deciding to adopt. Their struggle prompts them to carefully examine the relative importance of genetic, gestational, and parenting ties.

The Separate Components of Parenthood: Ethical Considerations

"Just because we can do something, should we do it?" This is a question that has plagued scientists in the last half of the twentieth century. The field of reproductive medicine in particular has faced this question—perhaps more than any other field. The array of parenting options afforded by reproductive technology is staggering. The development of *in vitro* fertilization has made it possible for one child to have as many as five different "parents"—an ovum donor, a sperm donor, a gestational carrier, and two adoptive (rearing) parents. Furthermore, cryopreservation of sperm and of embryos has enabled people to preserve their potential fertility almost indefinitely. Cryopreservation of embryos has even enabled posthumous motherhood to be possible. The new parenting paths—and configurations—raise a profoundly difficult and often disturbing ethical question: Is it in the best interest of children to be created and parented through third, fourth, or even fifth parties?

The Right to Reproduce vs. the Rights/Best Interests of Children

Until recently, a couple's right to procreate has rarely been questioned. However, because of the new reproductive technologies, the question has arisen about whether the right to procreate includes the right to procreate using available technology and/or donor gametes or a host uterus. Many experts in the field, including John Robertson, a U.S. attorney/ethicist specializing in the field of reproductive technology, argue for procreative liberty, asserting that since the United States

21

Constitution affords people the right to procreate coitally, it also gives individuals the right to procreate non-coitally. Robertson believes that having children satisfies basic biologic, social, and psychological drives for many people and that "noncoital reproduction should thus be constitutionally protected to the same extent as is coital reproduction, with the state having the burden of showing severe harm if the practice is unrestricted."[3]

Those who believe in procreative liberty would agree, however, that although the law gives people the right to reproduce, it does not give people the right to parent the children they reproduce if they are deemed unfit. Unfortunately there are many instances in which the State, acting in the best interest of a child, removes that child from its home because the child is determined to be at risk. Furthermore not everyone is eligible to become a parent through adoption. Several states have outlawed private adoptions and require parents to "pass" a homestudy conducted by a licensed social worker before they can legally adopt a child. Thus the purpose of the law is to protect children from harm—both physical and psychological—and the duty of the State is to advocate for the welfare of children. The question here is whether or not someone should be advocating for the rights of children who are not yet born or conceived, and whether we can know—even prior to conception—whether a child will be psychologically harmed as a result of the circumstances of its conception or birth.

There is a great deal of controversy about whether caregivers—from physicians to mental health clinicians—have an obligation to act as gatekeepers for unborn children. Procreative libertarians argue that the role of providers is to offer the technology if it is medically appropriate, rather than to make judgements about who deserves to become a parent or about how children should be created. This group of caregivers believes steadfastly in patient autonomy, in each person's right to choose whether and how to procreate. Others feel strongly that when individuals/couples ask for assistance in procreating, caregivers then have an obligation to protect the interests of children (even if they are not yet born or conceived). They argue that not to do so would be abdicating their responsibility and could even be a violation of beneficence (assuring good and avoiding harm) if the caregiver sincerely believes that harm may be done.

Another ethical question arises from the ability to separate genetic from gestational from rearing parenthood: *Is it is moral to create children from donor gametes when there are already children in the world who have been born and who need homes?* Elizabeth Bartholet, an attorney, adoptive mother, and author of *Family Bonds: Adoption and the Politics of Parenting* (Houghton Mifflin, 1993) is critical of the new reproductive technologies. She believes that ART clinics intentionally attempt to convince couples that reproduction in one form or another is inherently better than adoption and that families created from genetic ties (or partial genetic ties) are stronger and more desirable than those created by adoption. Bartholet argues that what she sees as objective counseling would surely steer more infertile couples away from technological means of reproduction to adoption. In fact many infertile couples do struggle with this issue. Longing for a gestational and/ or genetic (or partial genetic) connection to their offspring, yet aware that too many children in the world need good homes, many prospective parents wonder if this longing to reproduce should take precedence over the right of existing children to have loving homes.

As we will see in Chapter 7, the ability to separate genetic from gestational motherhood means that offspring can be born (and have been born) to women old enough to be grandmothers and greatgrandmothers and who are likely to die before their children reach adulthood. The use of anonymous sperm or egg donation means that children may have several half siblings that they do not know. Furthermore, the separation of genetic and gestational motherhood may mean that a couple who have donated frozen embryos has several biogenetic children who are being raised by different families, and who know nothing about each other's existence. These are but some of the ethical and psycho-social dilemmas brought about by the new reproductive technologies—dilemmas that couples face as they consider their parenting and treatment options.

The Right to Information Regarding One's Genetic Origins

The history of gamete donation in the United States began in the late 1800s. Dr. William Pancoast, who performed the first insemination of donor sperm, claims to have done it secretly, not ever telling his patient that she had been inseminated with a donor's sperm, and not telling her husband until after the fact. Thus began a tradition of secrecy that most donor couples have practiced for almost a century—telling no one (neither the child, the child's physician, nor the extended family, etc.) the circumstances of the conception. Anonymity—the situation in which both donor and recipient couple consent to the process but are unknown (and unidentifiable) to each other—has occurred along with secrecy in donor insemination.

A third concept—privacy—is often confused with secrecy. Privacy refers to the fact that each of us has the right to establish boundaries between ourselves—or our families—and others. When we identify these boundaries we are not being secretive, but rather, we are saying that it is our basic human right to maintain some separateness from those around us. Hence, we are being neither dishonest nor deceptive nor withholding if we do not tell everybody, everything.

The Right to Procreate with Unknown Gametes

Although sperm donation has been occurring for over one hundred years, improved technology, resulting in the ability to separate gestational and genetic motherhood, has paved the way for ovum donation as well. Although few people in the medical and mental health fields have openly questioned the moral acceptability of gamete donation, it does raise an important ethical question: *Is it morally acceptable to bring a child into the world with an unknown genetic parent?*

This issue may be more timely now because our understanding has deepened in recent years about the relative weight of nature versus nurture in determining who a person will ultimately become. Although scientists are not quite ready to map the human genome, more and more information about biological destiny is unfolding on an almost daily basis. Because we now understand that genetics plays a very large role—larger than previously thought—in providing a blueprint for adulthood, the ethics of bringing a child into the world with unknown genetic origins is more questionable today than it was in the past. The concern is whether it may be psychologically or medically harmful to a person to have no information—or little information—about his/her genetic make-up. On the other hand, to deny a would-be parent the right to chose to procreate with donor gametes threatens both the patient's autonomy and his/her reproductive freedom.

The Right to Know the Truth About One's Genetic Origins.

Knowing the truth about one's genetic origins and conception is different from having identifying information about one's genetic parents. As long as the practice of anonymous sperm donation continues in this country and the laws surrounding it do not change, donor offspring will not have access to their donors. Although many sperm banks are currently providing extensive information to parents regarding their donor's medical and psychological history, most couples using DI in this country are still choosing not to tell their children the truth about their origins. In recent years a large body of mental health professionals, including family therapists, have begun to question the ethics of secrecy regarding gamete donation. These clinicians believe that denying people essential information about their identity, especially when it includes their medical history, is morally unacceptable. Furthermore, they cite the literature that comes from family therapy— and from adoption—documenting the negative impact of family secrets on parents and children and on family systems (see Chapter 10).

Separating the various components of parenthood means that individuals and couples can create children who may be deceived about their genetic make-up and possibly (in the case of surrogates or gestational carriers) about who gestated and gave birth to them. As with the previous ethical dilemma—the right to procreate with unknown gametes—questions arise about whether a patient's autonomy—in this case the right to choose not to tell one's offspring the truth—should take precedence over the possible harm done to that offspring if he or she goes through life being duped about his/her identity and conveying a false medical history.

Liberation vs. Exploitation of Women for Reproductive Purposes

Although there are many who believe that the new reproductive technologies are nothing short of miraculous and open up choices to women and to couples that would never have been possible, there are others who believe that they are a curse on families and upon women. Assisted reproductive technology is not without medical side effects or risks (see Chapter 2), and people who are desperate for children may not be in the best position to objectively evaluate these risks to themselves or to third parties. The separation of the various components of motherhood means that some women who are not the intended parents (ovum donors and/or surrogates or gestational carriers) are being subjected to these risks. Many argue that an infertile couple/woman has the right to choose a procedure that involves potential physical harm, but that it is morally unacceptable to subject a young, fertile woman to these same risks when she is not the intended parent.

Furthermore financial incentives may be inducements to third parties to ignore these potential harms. Here we see examples of when concerns about autonomy and beneficence may collide.

A common worry among caregivers and couples opting for known ovum donation, surrogacy, or gestational care (via a friend or relative), is that the physical ordeal may produce short or long term side effects that are harmful. Careful counseling—both medical and psychological—of willing third parties, enables these collaborators to thoroughly consider the risks before deciding to proceed. And many argue that third parties, like infertility patients, are also entitled to autonomy when it comes to decisions regarding their bodies. Others argue, however, that there is always inherent coercion (financial or personal) for donors, surrogates, and carriers that cannot be dismissed and that amounts to exploitation.

Unnatural Conception

Although there are many infertile couples whose intense desire to bear biological children propels them to seek out the most advanced technology available, others are deeply troubled by what they regard as forcing conception. Those who look askance at high tech treatment are not always those who are guided by strong religious beliefs that conception is in God's hands. Many are individuals who simply question the wisdom of creating a child who was not meant to be, and who wonder about the long term medical, social, and psychological effects of creating high tech babies.

Often, however, the question of what is meant to be is closely tied in to a couple's religious or spiritual convictions. There are people of many religious denominations who have a deep and abiding belief in an all-powerful and all-knowing God who makes plans for people. They may even view their infertility as part of that divine plan—or perhaps as a trial imposed by God. The concept of forcing conception when it would otherwise not occur is unacceptable to people holding these convictions and contrary to their spiritual beliefs. Other religious traditions offer a different view of God, one that does not always include a predetermined plan. These traditions offer couples more license to determine their own plan and to take measures—including assisted reproductive technology—to achieve parenthood.

In addition to religious, social, or moral proscriptions against "forcing conception," couples have personal feelings and reactions about what it means for them. The inability to "make" a baby through a natural, loving and intimate sexual union is a loss for most couples who turn to high tech treatment for assistance. The marital bed of an infertile couple already cluttered with temperature charts, thermometers, and ovulation predictor kits, is no longer the place where two people can merge their bodies and create a child from their sacred union. Most couples eventually seem to adjust to this loss and to focus on the pregnancy and baby that will hopefully result, rather than on the means of conception. However, even a miraculous pregnancy does not erase the invasive and painful—often experienced as assaultive —initiation into pregnancy that couples using ART undergo. Margarete Sandelowski and colleagues capture the ART experience in the following words:

> "...pain, not pleasure; struggle, not ease; separation, not unity; public exposure, not intimacy; and artifice, not naturalness, comprised the phenomenology of getting pregnant in infertile couples. In contrast to their fertile counterparts, these couples felt compelled to fight body, nature and convention to achieve conception." [5]

Unnatural Conception: Ethical Considerations

The development of *in vitro* fertilization made it possible for conception to occur outside the human body, and the further development of cryopreservation made it possible for the resulting embryos to be frozen and stored for future use. The ability to create and/or cryopreserve human embryos raises questions about what may be done with them or to them. These questions involve issues regarding freezing, disposition, experimentation, and ownership, and raise even more fundamental questions about what the moral (and legal) status of an embryo is.

The Moral Status of Embryos

There are basically three view points about the moral status of an embryo. One perspective is that an embryo is a human life from the moment of conception. According to the Roman Catholic Church's *Instruction on Respect for Human Life in Its Origin and on the*

Dignity of Procreation (1987), for example, life exists on a continuum, beginning with fertilization and ending with the death of that human being. The Roman Catholic Church believes that because an embryo has the potential to become a human being, it should be treated as such and afforded all the rights and dignities due to a human person. One of those rights is the right to life.

A second point of view—the opposite of the first—is that embryos are akin to property and that those people who "own" embryos should have no limits imposed on them. Thus couples are entitled to do with their embryos as they wish, including disposing of them.

A third point of view, and one that is most commonly held among both patients and providers, is somewhere in the middle—a belief that embryos are neither property nor people, but because they have the potential to become a person under certain conditions, they should be treated with dignity and respect. The Warnock Committee, which was convened in London, supported the last moral perspective. The committee, consisting of physicians, lawyers, researchers, social worker, and theologians, published a report (1984) affirming that embryos have special status due to their human potential, but that they do not have the moral status of a living person.

Couples undergoing *in vitro* fertilization must face the question—and answer it for themselves—of what they believe the moral status of an embryo is, before undergoing treatment. This belief is likely to color many of the decisions they make regarding fertilization, implantation, and cryopreservation of embryos (see Chapter 2).

The Disposition of Extracorporeal Embryos

In an effort to maximize the chances for pregnancy, women undergoing *in vitro* fertilization are prescribed powerful fertility drugs in hopes that they can produce a large cohort of eggs. The more eggs obtained, the more likely the couple is to have several good embryos to transfer and possibly to cryopreserve for future use. All reputable clinics limit the number of embryos they will transfer (usually between three and six, depending on their quality and on the woman's age) in order to maximize the chances of pregnancy and minimize the chances of multiple birth. If the couple opts for cryopreservation, the excess embryos can be transferred to the woman's uterus in another cycle which does not involve the use of powerful fertility drugs or an egg retrieval. Or, if the couple becomes pregnant, the frozen embryos can be stored until the couple is ready to have another child.

Occasionally couples who have embryos in storage feel their family is complete and do not wish to have more children. In other cases, circumstances have intervened and they do not wish to attempt a pregnancy. They must then make a decision regarding the disposition of their cryopreserved embryos.

Because embryos do not have legal rights, most clinics have provisions regarding the disposition of couples' "extra" embryos. These provisions usually permit the couple to donate their embryos to another couple or to discard them. Some states allow research to be performed on embryos under certain conditions and couples who do not wish to have their embryos transferred to themselves or donated to another couple may opt to donate their embryos to research in lieu of discarding them.

Although most couples can reach agreement regarding the disposition of their frozen embryos, occasionally there are disputes, the most well known of which is the *Davis vs. Davis* case. In this much publicized legal battle involving a divorcing couple, Ms. Davis wished to attempt pregnancy with the cryopreserved embryos, while her former husband sought to have them destroyed. Their case involved three trials: in the first trial the lower court found that the embryos were human beings whose best interest was to be brought to life, and so it ruled in favor of Ms. Davis. In the second trial the Tennessee appellate court agreed with Mr. Davis' argument that he should not have to become a father against his will, thus reversing the decision of the lower court. In a final appeal, the Tennessee Supreme Court affirmed the decision of the appellate court, declaring that the burden to Mr. Davis of unwanted reproduction would be greater than the burden to Ms. Davis if the decision were otherwise. (*Davis vs. Davis*, Tennessee Supreme Court, 1992).

The Davis case drew considerable media attention, much of which cast a negative light on reproductive technology. Clearly, an essential question in the case—the moral status of embryos—was never really dealt with in the court of public opinion. However, divergent opinions on the moral status of embryos did form the basis of the legal opinions, with each reflecting a different perspective on this question.

Beyond illustrating different perspectives on the moral status of embryos, *Davis vs. Davis* reveals the need for legal counseling in assisted reproductive technology. Although it is rare for disputes between couples to find their way into a courtroom, there is always potential for disagreement. Legal agreements made at the outset of treatment between couples and any other participants will not prevent all disputes but will clarify intentions and may reduce the potential for conflict.

Before embarking on an IVF cycle, all couples must examine their beliefs regarding the moral status of embryos, and come to some agreement, even if it involves compromise, regarding the disposition of extracorporeal embryos. Many clinics require couples to put this decision in writing before eggs are inseminated. They are, of course, free to change their minds as time unfolds, but their intents must be expressed or noted prior to the beginning of an ART cycle.

Experimentation and Preimplantation Genetics

Questions regarding the moral status of an embryo also bring up questions about what is permissable to do to an embryo and at what stage it is permissible to do it. Because the Catholic Church, for example, believes that an embryo has the status of a human being, the Church does not believe that an embryo should be subjected to experimentation or tampering. The Warnock Committe, recognizing the value of research in order to improve the quality of human life, came up with several recommendations regarding the use of embryos in research. More recently, in the United States, a panel on embryo research convened by the National Institute of Health in 1995 supported research on embryos (referred to as pre-embryos) up to fourteen days post-conception.

Preimplantation genetics is a recent development—an outgrowth of *in vitro* fertilization—in the area of reproductive medicine. This highly technical procedure involves removing one cell from a four cell embryo and examining its chromosomal make-up. Preimplantation genetics is currently offered to couples (who may or may not be infertile) who are carriers of a genetic disease that they do not wish to pass on their offspring. Although not all genetic diseases can be to be detected at the current time, many diseases, such as cystic fibrosis, Tay Sachs, or Huntington's Disease, can be identified. If the embryo in question is found to have the problematic gene, it is discarded at the four cell stage while embryos that do not have the defective gene are then transferred into the woman's uterus.

Many people who do not view embryos as equivalent to human beings are enthusiastic supporters of preimplantation genetics in instances involving genetic disease. The technology, however, gives rise to ethical dilemmas of such complexity that they may soon require King Solomon's wisdom to solve. For example, some diseases that are autosomal dominant (the offspring have a fifty percent chance of inheriting it) such as Huntington's disease, do not appear until mid life so that those who have the disease do have the potential for many years of good quality, relatively normal lives. The parent, who is the potential carrier, may have chosen not to learn whether he/she will inherit the disease, yet requests preimplantation genetic services in case he/she is a carrier! The question is whether such treatment should be granted if it is perceived to be psychologically necessary, though it may or may not be medically necessary.

Although scientists have not yet mapped the entire human genome, it will probably not be too long before they can do so. Soon they will be able to determine physical, intellectual, and perhaps emotional and social characteristics in an embryo. Thus in the not too distant future it will be possible for parents to select some of their offspring's characteristics. And although many people would support the use of preimplantation genetic selection for couples who are carriers of a dreaded disease, many will not support this technology for couples who wish to have a child of a particular sex—or in the future, for a child with blue eyes, or musical talent, or who will be tall.

Pre-implantation genetics, like many other technologies, raises the question of whether, because something can be done, it should be done. Many who believe in procreative liberty may extend that belief even further, asserting that people have a right to "select" the child they want to reproduce. Others, while still believing in the right to reproduce non-coitally, may see inherent dangers in society if couples are allowed to choose the characteristics of their offspring. The dilemma is where to draw the line—if anywhere—on this slippery high technological slope.

Avoidance of Regret

Regret is a powerful and troubling human experience. Regret is similar to sadness, although it encompasses a reflective quality as people look back on decisions they made or actions they took that they wish they had the power to undo. Past abortions, adoption plans, decisions to postpone parenthood, voluntary sterilizations, divorces, and remarriages all provide abundant fuel for the torturous flames of regret. Cursed with the 20/20 vision of hindsight, many infertile people reflect upon their earlier decisions and wonder whether their past "mistakes" are the source of their current pain. In some cases there is an obvious connection—for example, women who had unprotected sex which resulted in pelvic infections, or men who elected to have vasectomies thinking they would never want children. Because no one has a crystal ball, however, and human beings can only do what they believe is best at a given time, mistakes are an inevitable part of life.

Sometimes regret leads to guilt, which unfortunately for many infertile couples is a major component of their experience and figures into the formula with which they attribute meaning to their experience. Thus regret is exacerbated when people torture themselves with self-blame and conclude that they are being punished for their sins. When this anguish occurs, guilt has become the predominant emotion and can prevent the expression of true feelings of sadness and loss.

Knowing the assaultive power of self-blame, many infertile couples go to considerable lengths to absolve themselves of future regrets. Sandelowski, et. al.[6] identifies this phenomenon as "anticipatory intolerance of regret" and describes how people frequently make decisions regarding their infertility treatment based on their efforts to avoid regret. In other words they attempt to discern what they need to do now in order to avoid looking back later with regret about what they did not do. Thus many couples state that if they "try everything" and "do their best" they hope that at the very least they will not have to look back with tortured "if onlys" and "what ifs." Many will go to exhaustive treatment lengths to spare themselves this anticipated regret.

Regret can also run in the opposite direction, and many couples approach it from this different vantage point. They worry that they might regret the enormous amount of time that treatment took away

32

from career, or social life, or relationships with others. They worry that they may regret the enormous financial costs and the personal sacrifices made in order to pursue a pregnancy. Couples may fear the emotional costs as well—including the stress on their relationship if their desires to pursue a pregnancy are not equal. Still others focus on the potential health risks associated with the use of assisted reproduction (see Chapter 2) and worry that they will look back and regret decisions that may have jeopardized their health. Finally, there are couples with secondary infertility, who fear that the time, effort and money they spend on trying to have another child will be spent at the expense of their first. Chapter 4, "Changing Direction" will examine this issue in depth.

Avoidance of Regret: Strategies for Couples

Ultimately all of us learn that regret is part of the human condition. Those who try, who care, who strive to accomplish things all grapple with regret at one time or another. Infertile couples need to remind themselves that they cannot eradicate regret. They must hope that the process of confronting questions squarely, of examining options as best theycan, of trying to make decisions that they can live with will ultimately fortify them against the tyrany of regret.

We encourage couples to conduct an open—and constant— dialogue as they make their way through infertility. The issue of anticipatory regret should be a central part of that dialogue, with both partners trying to keep an eye on "the big picture." They should discuss the ramifications of each of their decisions, not only for the near future but also, for the long run. Are resources of time, energy and money best spent on pursuing this option or that one or might they be wiser to conserve resources for other purposes? They must always remind themselves that just as they run the risk of looking back with regret if they do not pursue another treatment or repeat an as yet unsuccessful one, they also run the risk of regret if they try too much, too long, too often.

Avoidance of Regret: Ethical Considerations

Although avoidance of regret is a consideration for many infertile individuals/ couples in this country, it is a luxury for many others. Those who have the ability to look back and know they did everything humanly and technologically possible to achieve a pregnancy, are only a small percentage of the infertile population. The medical community may have the ability as well as the knowledge to treat most conditions that cause infertility, but unfortunately society is not constructed such that those who have the greatest need will necessarily reap the biggest reward.

Access to Medical Treatment for Infertility

The ethical principle of *justice*—the notion that societal benefits and burdens should be distributed fairly, without discrimination, and that those in need can have their needs met—is frequently overlooked when it comes to treatment for infertility. Unfortunately state laws and/or personal circumstances (age, marital status, and sexual orientation) may dictate how far some people can go in their quest for a biological child. These same circumstances can also determine what adoption avenues are open to some would-be parents. Until legislation or judicial precedent is established, physicians are often forced to make recommendations about treatment according to what their patients can financially afford and according to their personal code of ethics.

Financial Access.

Financial access to any medical treatment is a complicated issue. Because health care dollars are not unlimited, practitioners are often called upon to make determinations about who should be a beneficiary when supplies are short. Traditionally medicine has established systems for prioritizing who should have access to treatment and under what circumstances. For example, not everyone who needs an organ transplant will have one. Age, prognosis, financial constraints, or shortage of donors are all factors that may limit access to life saving treatments.

Infertility is not seen as a medical condition by most health insurance companies; consequently it is not a reimbursable expense for most people. Treatment for infertility has been likened to cosmetic surgery and is often viewed as unnecessary, even frivolous. Currently only ten states in the U.S have insurance mandates either to cover or to offer infertility treatment. In these states, if treatment is offered and not covered, then many people still will not benefit from a mandate because their employers have not opted for a plan that covers infertility. Unfortunately in the remaining forty states—most of the U.S.— there is no coverage. Even those states with mandated benefits do not provide coverage to those who are insured through public programs such as Medicaid. Similarly, in Canada, only one province has mandatory coverage for ART and there it is only for IVF in instances of documented tubal blockage. Thus many infertile individuals/couples who would make excellent parents do not have the option to seek medical care because the financial cost, especially if assisted reproduction is warranted, can be prohibitive.

Many consider this unequal access to treatment to be an injustice. However, the issue of financial access to treatment also raises the ethical question of whether any person/couple—regardless of circumstances—should be able to avail themselves of *any* treatment if another person (or agency) is paying the bill. For example, the odds of a woman delivering a baby from *in vitro* fertilization decrease substantially if she is over forty. After she is forty-five the success rates are almost zero. Other circumstances or diagnoses may lead to equally poor prognoses. The ethical question is whether it is reasonable for private or governmental insurers to cover the costs of an ART procedure—at close to ten thousand dollars a try—when the odds of success are so slim.

Access Based on Personal Criteria.

Physicians have always had the option of refusing to perform a treatment—abortion, for example—when the performance of it would be in violation of their personal ethical code. What is not as clear is whether a physician can refuse to treat a category of individuals based on his/her moral or religious beliefs, and whether refusal to treat is tantamount to discrimination and would therefore be subject to litigation. Many practitioners, for example, struggle with whether to treat single women, lesbian couples, and older women, (especially if their partners are even older than they). The age issue brings up the question of gender discrimination. Because most men are physically able to father children until old age—and many in fact do so—some ethicists and physicians argue that it is discriminating not to offer ovum donation to women who are physically capable of pregnancy.

Some physicians hold deep beliefs that a baby should be born to a married couple and they do not want to actively contribute to an 'out of wedlock' birth. Others do not have trouble in principle with the concept of single women having children as long as the mothers are young enough and well enough to care for the child and they have the financial means to do so. Some situations involving single women present even more complex ethical dilemmas for practitioners, such as when an older single woman presents for ovum donation, or a single woman with a history of cancer, or a history of severe mental illness, wants IVF treatment.

Many clinics refuse to treat lesbian couples; others open their doors providing there is a documented infertility problem; and still others will treat the couple even if all they require is donor insemination. There have been instances in which presumably fertile lesbian couples approached an IVF clinic asking for eggs to be retrieved from one woman, fertilized with donor sperm, and transferred into her partner: that way both women would have a stake in their child's creation — one genetically and one gestationally. Different clinics have reacted differently to that request—some granting it and others refusing it.

Situations involving lesbian couples raise additional questions about access to treatment: whether insurance companies (in states and provinces where treatment is mandated) should be required to pay for treatment when a person is not technically infertile. Some would argue that by definition a lesbian couple is infertile (perhaps they have what might be called gender infertility) because neither has a Y chromosome and they cannot reproduce without medical intervention. Others would argue that infertility must be defined by a diagnosis and if there is no diagnosis there is no infertility.

The issue of age is a recent ethical dilemma for those in ART programs. The development of *in vitro* fertilization which made ovum donation possible now means that a woman can become pregnant at virtually any age. The questions facing medical ethicists, as well as those who treat infertile couples is: how old is too old to bear or to raise a child? The best interest of the unborn offspring comes into question when physicians offer ovum donation to women/couples in their fifties and sixties. Although death can and does occur at any age, it is far more likely that offspring born to women of advanced maternal age may lose one or both parents before they reach adulthood. Or, they may be forced to care for their geriatric parents when they are young adults and not in a position to do so.

There are many practitioners who claim that their responsibility is not to make judgments about how old a woman should or should not be when she gives birth, but rather to treat her if she asks for help in becoming pregnant. Many of these physicians acknowledge having helped women in their late fifties and early sixties bear children. Many other physicians and other practices, however, believe that it is not in the best interest of a child to be born to older parents, and they set age limits—usually forty-five or fifty as that is the very upper limit of natural childbearing—for their patients. Still other physicians agree to offer ovum donation to older women if they have husbands who are much younger, figuring that at least one parent will likely survive the offspring's childhood.

The issue of maternal age highlights the significance—and complexity—of the concept of justice. An important question is whether it is just to offer say, a fifty-five year old woman the same access to ovum donation as a thirty-five year old? Although the answer to this question may seem simple in the abstract, it becomes much more difficult in clinical practice. We have found that when we meet with real people with real reasons for seeking treatment, it is much more difficult to offer treatment to some and to withhold it from others.

The longing for a child is compelling and the losses associated with infertility are profound. In light of these harsh realities, both couples and their caregivers can be tempted to conclude that love and desire to parent are enough. Many tell themselves that if a child is deeply wanted and will be intensely loved, efforts should be made to create that child and to give him/her life. Unfortunately life (and parenting) are not so simple.

We have seen in this chapter that the realities of assisted reproduction are far more complex. The three central pillars of bio-ethics—*autonomy, beneficence*, and *justice*—call upon us to examine carefully our beliefs and assumptions regarding parenthood, identity, and the meaning and value of creating a life. Looking through this lens, we see—albeit sadly—that being wanted and being loved may not be enough. Focusing the lens differently, we see that autonomy, beneficence, and justice collide in this new terrain of assisted reproduction.

Today's infertile couples embark upon a daunting journey. Deeply saddened by loss and exhausted by struggle, few have much energy left to face the ethical challenges that lie ahead. Some are propelled by their longing for a child and forge ahead without thinking too much about future consequences. However, many do find that the dilemmas they face mandate a slower pace and deep reflection. Those who find the patience and the courage to ask the questions are generally rewarded. For although the answers do not come easily, the process alone of soul-searching—of examining the myriad ethical questions in assisted reproduction—offers guidance, and hopefully, wisdom. It is our intention and wish that this book will provide a framework for examing these difficult questions and dilemmas, and for helping those who struggle directly with the unbearable losses of infertility to bear them with courage and hope.

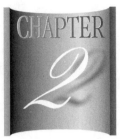

CHAPTER 2

In Vitro Fertilization and the Assisted Reproductive Technologies

In vitro fertilization forms the cornerstone of the new reproductive technologies. When Louise Brown, the world's first IVF baby, was born in 1978, few people, if any, appreciated the range of reproductive possibilities that would result from this new technology. Once eggs could be removed from a woman's body and fertilized outside it, the genetic and gestational components of motherhood could be separated. This separation produced an array of reproductive options: fertile women could provide eggs to infertile women who needed them; women could become gestational carriers for women unable to gestate their genetic offspring; and couples could give embryos they had stored and no longer intended to use to childless couples who would adopt them at the four cell stage. Furthermore, cryopreservation of embryos expanded reproductive possibilities even further, separating conception from pregnancy by months and even years.

Reproductive medicine has indeed come a long way, yet not everyone regards these technologies positively. Ardent feminists, for example, believe that the new technologies dehumanize and degrade women, and religious fundamentalists believe that they are an affront to God. What is clear, however, is that these technologies are here to stay, and they bring with them new dilemmas and decisions about family building.

Couples who begin the process of ART frequently look back and wonder how they got there. If they had been asked early on in their treatment process whether they would ever try IVF, many would have readily said no. Yet months or years later, these same couples find themselves in a new world of high-tech terminology and treatment, investing large sums of money, facing medical risks, and embarking on an even steeper emotional roller coaster than the one from which they recently disembarked. It is important to point out, however, that part of the emotional challenge of ART is that for many it feels like the end of the line—the last possible chance for having a child without third party assistance. For a small group of couples with hopelessly blocked or absent tubes, IVF really is their last medical resort. Yet for many other couples who are ART candidates, trying one or more of the new reproductive options does not mean that they cannot return to less invasive treatments. In fact we have seen couples who have conceived spontaneously after several failed IVF cycles or after a successful IVF pregnancy. Sadly, no one can predict who these couples will be.

In this chapter and the one that follows, we focus on those reproductive technologies in which only the prospective parents' gametes (eggs or sperm) are used in order to be gestated by the woman and raised by the couple. We use the term *assisted reproductive technology* (ART) for the high-tech procedures in which superovulation is usually, but not always, a part of the process. This chapter will continue our discussion of the decision-making process, focusing on practical, medical, and financial considerations.

$\mathcal{T}$he ART Options

Many couples who decide to pursue an ART cycle find themselves bewildered by the various options. Although most lay people are familiar with the term IVF, few would be able to explain the difference between IVF and GIFT or ZIFT or TET or IUI, or any of the other variations of the new reproductive technologies. Some couples, depending on their medical diagnosis, are candidates for all of the procedures; others have only one or two options. Although much of an ART cycle is the same no matter what variation a couple is doing, there are some important differences. What they all share in common is the use of superovulatory medications (except in natural cycle IVF), and all (except IUI) involve an egg retrieval.

In vitro fertilization (IVF), the oldest of the new technologies, involves harvesting oocytes (eggs) from the ovaries (after the woman has undergone a regimen of ovulation inducing drugs) and inseminating each one in a petri dish with approximately 50,000 sperm. (This mixing of eggs and sperm is what is meant by insemination). The sperm are carefully prepared by embryologists so that only the healthiest, most motile sperm are used. Two or three days later (depending on the clinic) the eggs that are fertilized (embryos) are transferred to the woman's uterus. Although there is some variation, most clinics transfer three embryos to women under age 35, four embryos in women 35 to 40 and as many as five or six embryos in women over forty. Decisions about how many embryos to transfer are also influenced by embryo quality; statistically speaking, embryos that are higher quality have a greater implantation rate. If more embryos are transferred, it is more likely that pregnancy will occur, but unfortunately more embryos also increase the chance of a multiple gestation–producing a high risk pregnancy. Among the advantages of IVF are that fertilization can be visually confirmed and the quality of the resulting embryos can be assessed.

Cryopreservation (freezing) was a pivotal development in the field of IVF. Today, virtually all clinics performing IVF have facilities that enable them to cryopreserve extra embryos. Since many women, especially those who are younger, produce many eggs in response to superovulation—often more than a dozen—all the eggs that are retrieved can be inseminated, and the extra fertilized embryos (beyond the ones transferred) can be cryopreserved and used in subsequent cycles. It is important to note, however, that not all embryos qualify to be frozen; many stop dividing before the point at which they can be cryopreserved, or they are too fragmented, or their quality is compromised.

Gamete intrafallopian transfer (GIFT) involves retrieving eggs and placing them directly into the fallopian tubes with large numbers of sperm. The eggs and the sperm are placed into the tubes almost immediately after they are retrieved via a laparoscopic procedure. The primary advantage of GIFT is that fertilization occurs in the tube, its natural site, which is assumed to be a better incubator than a petri dish.

Another advantage of GIFT is that, as with IVF, extra eggs can be inseminated and cryopreserved for later use. When extra eggs from a GIFT cycle fertilize, it is presumed that fertilization occurred in the tube, but this presumption cannot be confirmed unless pregnancy occurs. When extra eggs fail to fertilize, however, one never knows what actually happened in the fallopian tube. It is possible they did fertilize even though the inseminated eggs did not. There are two reasons for this possibility: the best-quality eggs are always selected for the GIFT transfer and are thus more likely to fertilize, and the tube is thought to be more efficient than the petri dish and a more likely site for fertilization to occur.

There are many variations on both IVF and GIFT. ZIFT—*zygote intrafallopian transfer*—is a combination of IVF and GIFT. Eggs are retrieved and inseminated as they are for IVF. Instead of being transferred to the uterus on the second or third day after insemination, however, the zygote (the fertilized egg that has not yet divided) is placed in the fallopian tube approximately one day after insemination. ZIFT has the advantages of both IVF and GIFT: fertilization can be determined and the fallopian tube is used as the incubator. But it also has the disadvantages of both: it is more costly, it involves two days of procedures including a laparoscopy, and although fertilization can be viewed, the embryo quality cannot be determined after only one day. Other variations involve putting eggs, zygotes, or embryos into the uterus or tubes at different points in their development, utilizing different methods of retrieval and transfer.

Intrauterine insemination (IUI) is the simplest of the new reproductive technologies and the least costly, since it involves neither egg retrieval nor zygote or embryo transfer. Despite the fact that it is lower tech than the others, it is considered one of the ARTs because it usually involves superovulation and frequent monitoring in order to determine when ovulation occurs. In IUI when the timing is right, sperm that have been carefully prepared in the embryology laboratory are inserted directly into the uterus. Although fertility drugs are given, they are administered in smaller dosages in hopes of producing no more than three or four eggs. Another advantage of IUI, besides its lower cost and absence of a surgical procedure, is that it may involve less monitoring. Its disadvantages are that fertilization cannot be determined by observation, extra eggs cannot be harvested, inseminated, and the resulting embryos frozen, and, like the other ARTs, a multiple pregnancy may occur.

An IVF cycle in which superovulation is not induced is referred to as a *natural IVF cycle*. These cycles are offered by some programs and are appealing to many couples, particularly those for whom taking drugs is contraindicated by their medical history or those who are worried about long-term side effects. Natural cycles are physically much easier for the woman, and they are much less expensive, but the odds that the one egg is of good quality, that it will fertilize, that the resulting embryo will be of good quality, that it will implant and result in a viable pregnancy, are not as high as in a stimulated cycle in which three to five embryos may be transferred.

In a natural cycle a woman is monitored carefully, so that just before she is about to ovulate on her own, the (usually) one egg she produces is retrieved and inseminated with her husband's sperm, in hopes that it will fertilize. Alternatively, the egg can be combined with the sperm and placed within an intravaginal capsule (in the hopes that fertilization will occur within the capsule). This latter procedure, developed by Dr. Claude Ranoux in collaboration with Dr. Gary Gross, is known as NORIF (natural oocyte retrieval and intravaginal fertilization.

With an alphabet soup of options, it is difficult for many couples to decide which ART treatment to try. Some are guided solely by diagnosis. For example, women whose fallopian tubes are blocked or absent have only IVF available to them. Similarly, couples with male infertility who want to determine whether fertilization can occur are probably best off doing IVF. If there is no fertilization, the couple may have the option to try ICSI (see next section). Women who have one or both fallopian tubes open are theoretically candidates for any of the ARTs as long as adequate numbers of sperm can be obtained from their partner. If the woman has not had a prior laparoscopy to view her pelvic area, GIFT, combined with diagnostic laparoscopy, may be the recommended treatment. This option allows the physician to view her pelvic area while at the same time performing a procedure that may yield a pregnancy. Additionally, if enough eggs are obtained, extra eggs (beyond those put in her tubes) can be inseminated to see if they fertilize.

Different clinics prefer and may become more adept at different procedures. With the exception of conditions involving blocked or absent tubes, in which case the decision is clear-cut (IVF is the only possibility), research is equivocal about what works best for whom. Although physicians make recommendations based on their best judgments, the final decision rests with the couple, who must grapple with their choices. These final decisions may be based on medically minor but individually important issues. For example, a woman who does not tolerate anesthesia well may choose to avoid a GIFT procedure.

Microinsemination (ICSI)

In the early days of *in vitro* fertilization, many IVF laboratories were not able to treat effectively even moderate, let alone severe, male factor infertility. Failed fertilization was common for such couples, who usually then turned toward donor insemination or adoption. Today, however, when a clinic's best efforts still do not result in fertilization, couples can turn to microinsemination.

Microinsemination of eggs and sperm is probably one of the most astounding developments that have arisen from *in vitro* fertilization, and the single most significant advance in the treatment of male infertility.

Simply put, though not simply performed, micromanipulation, commonly referred to as ICSI (Intra Cytoplasmic Sperm Injection), involves injecting a single sperm into an egg—inducing fertilization. Highly trained embryologists inject sperm directly into the cytoplasm of the egg, holding the egg in place with a glass pipette. The procedure is performed under a microscope and involves extremely skillful manipulation. ICSI (and its technological predecessors, Partial Zona Dissection and Subzonal Insemination, which have proved to be less effective and are no longer used) was developed because in many cases of male infertility, even when sperm was placed directly on top of the egg, fertilization failed to occur.

Because just one sperm is injected into an egg, theoretically only very small numbers of viable sperm need to be present in the ejaculate for the technology to work. Hence even men whose numbers are so small that they are considered to be azoospermic—who had no chance of having a biological offspring prior to the development of ICSI—are excellent candidates for this technology. ICSI is also used in cases of severe motility problems, an increased number of abnormally shaped sperm, problems with sperm antibodies, or when sperm do not bind easily to the egg or fail to penetrate it.

Men who have no sperm in their ejaculate due to a blockage in their vas deferens are also prime candidates for ICSI. In these instances men can undergo epididymal sperm aspiration—a surgical procedure in which sperm is extracted from above the blockage in the epididymis. This procedure enables sperm to be obtained and frozen for later fertilization via ICSI in combination with *In Vitro* fertilization.

A final group of men for whom ICSI is being recommended are those who have non-obstructive azoospermia of varying or unknown origins. These men have no obvious blockage of the vas deferens, yet there is no sperm in either their ejaculate or in their epidydemis. In order to obtain sperm a physician performs a testicular biopsy under general anesthesia, removing a piece of testicular tissue. This tissue is examined under a microscope for the presence of sperm, and if any is found, the tissue is frozen for later use during an *in vitro* fertilization procedure involving ICSI.

When ICSI is performed with either fresh sperm or sperm that has been extracted from the epidydemis and frozen, pregnancy rates are generally better than when sperm is obtained via testicular biopsy. In 1996 at Reproductive Science Center-Boston, for example, 230 embryo transfers resulted from 261 inseminations using ICSI procedures with fresh sperm, yielding a 36.5% clinical pregnancy rate per transfer; 36 transfers resulted from 38 inseminations using cryopreserved sperm obtained from epidydimal aspiration, yielding a clinical pregnancy rate per transfer of 41.7%; and 14 transfers resulted from 15 inseminations using sperm obtained from testicular biopsy, yielding a clinical pregnancy rate of 21.4%. Couples needing ICSI should carefully research the programs available to them, as ICSI statistics can vary considerably. It is also critical that they understand the criteria that a program uses for deciding when to use ICSI.

Although the first microinsemination procedure involving human eggs was performed in 1985, it was not until the early 1990's that ICSI was found to be reliable and successful. And it has only been in the last two or three years that many ART clinics have incorporated ICSI into their ART repertoire. Since the technology is so new, accurate statistics are hard to come by. However, it is probably fair to say that reputable clinics with successful ICSI programs are obtaining similar fertilization rates, and hence similar pregnancy rates, as they are for *in vitro* fertilization procedures that do not involve microinsemination. Some clinics may even have higher success rates with ICSI because the women usually do not have infertility problems of their own.

Initial Considerations

Most couples embarking on ART treatment do so after careful consideration, often involving long heart-wrenching discussions. In states that have insurance mandates covering infertility, couples may decide upon ART treatment more quickly, as a major deterrant—money—has been eliminated. Whether the decision has been made rapidly or more gradually, however, there are many issues and considerations over which couples need to mull before they are ready to proceed.

Financial Issues

In the United States and Canada the average cost of an ART cycle in which egg retrieval is involved runs between $6,000 and $10,000, depending on the clinic, the geographical location, and the amount of medication used. Because ART is so expensive, cost is a major factor for many couples in deciding whether to pursue treatment. Frequently couples are forced to decide whether to spend their money on an adoption, a more sure bet, or on one or more IVF cycles, a less certain outcome but a route that might produce their longed-for genetic child.

Unfortunately most U.S. employers which provide health insurance do not cover treatment for infertility, because infertility is not regarded as a 'legitimate' medical condition. Many insurers view treatment for infertility much as they view cosmetic surgery—unnecessary. In 1997, however, ten states have mandates requiring health insurance providers to either offer or cover the costs of infertility treatment. These states are Arkansas, California, Connecticut, Hawaii, Illinois, Maryland, Massachusetts, Rhode Island, New York, and Texas. Couples who live in the other states frequently find that their insurance does pick up a portion of their infertility bill, depending on their diagnosis and treatment. Some causes of infertility, such as endometriosis, are also medical conditions that require treatment and are thus covered by insurance. In Canada neither the government insurance, nor most private plans, cover ART. One exception to this is the government insurance in the province of Ontario, where up to three IVF cycles are covered for women with blocked or absent fallopian tubes.

Couples finance their treatment in various ways: they take out loans, sacrifice expensive purchases, work longer hours, get second jobs, or stay in an unhappy work situation because their insurance covers many of their infertility costs. Others who might choose to undergo high-tech treatment cannot do so because the price is too great. What is relevant here, however, is that for couples who are able to undertake one or more cycles, cost is generally an important consideration. Few couples without health insurance coverage can afford ART without financial sacrifice.

Time Commitment

Another consideration for couples who are thinking about ART is the time commitment. There are three time related factors that are important for couples to keep in mind: the distance to the clinic, the time they will need off from work, and the rigidity of the ART schedule. Depending on where the couple lives, their work schedule, and their life-style, the time involvement can be easily manageable, nearly impossible, or somewhere in between.

Couples who live in or near large metropolitan areas have easier access to ART programs. Although frequent trips for blood and ultrasound monitoring can be inconvenient, most women, even those who have demanding full-time jobs, can manage to meet the requirements of both the program and their jobs, as long as the clinic is within reasonable driving distance of home.

Couples who do not live in areas close to a clinic must put much of their lives aside in order to undergo an ART cycle. Not only do they incur additional expenses of travel, but they must also take time from other aspects of their lives. Some programs allow couples who live a great distance away to have their blood drawn near home and couriered to the clinic; other programs have agreements with hospitals or clinics in different geographic areas to monitor a patient's cycle and fax results back to the home program. But even when much of the monitoring can be done close to home, living a long distance from the ART program complicates the process.

Certain jobs fit better with high-tech treatment than do others. Women who work for themselves, work at home, or work part time have more flexibility than women who are teachers, for example. Women who work full time or whose part-time hours are rigid and conflict with the demands of the clinic feel more pressured by the time commitment.

An egg retrieval and embryo transfer involves two days. But exactly which two days it will be is not known until ovulation is imminent. For couples whose work involves frequent travel or other inflexible time demands, the unpredictability adds significant stress.

The requirements of an ART cycle are rigid. Clinics must carefully monitor each woman's cycle, adjusting her medications according to the results of blood tests and ultrasounds. These tests are performed only once or twice weekly at the start of the cycle, but increase in frequency during the second week. In the three or four days before ovulation approaches, there are daily blood tests and ultrasounds. Injections must be given at the same time each day so that the results accurately reflect how the woman's body is responding to the ovulation induction medications. Thus couples must sacrifice a great deal of spontaneity and adjust their lives according to the demands of the clinic, at least for the few weeks before egg retrieval or ovulation occurs. It is important for couples to know, however, that their social lives do not have to stop altogether. Many are remarkably resourceful during their ART cycles; some have been known to arrange to meet in a bathroom or designated place at a precise hour to do injections, often in the middle of a dinner party or other social engagement. Others have given shots in the back seat of their car or in restaurant parking lots.

Short- and Long-Term Side Effects

The tragic effects of DES (diethylstilbesterol), a drug that was supposed to prevent miscarriage but was later found to cause a high incidence of cervical cancer and other reproductive problems in the offspring of women who took it, has raised the consciousness of both medical personnel and infertile couples about the potential hazards of medications related to reproduction. The need to perform adequate controlled studies that speak to the efficacy and the safety of drugs before they are made available to the public is well recognized. Hence it is understandable that many patients are hesitant to take powerful agents that have a profound and potentially negative impact on their reproductive systems.

The question of whether ovulation-inducing medications can cause or promote the growth of ovarian cancer has been on the minds of infertility patients and their caregivers for many years. Living with the legacy of DES, many have worried and wondered about the long term effects of medically induced hyperstimulation. In 1993, concerns heightened with the publication by Whittemore and colleagues of a study which concluded that women who took fertility medications had an increased incidence of ovarian cancer (between three and 27 fold).[7] The study, however, did not determine whether the medications actually caused the cancer, or whether this group of infertile women was at increased risk for other reasons. Nor did the research identify which medications were taken.

Critics of Whittemore's study claim that her research was flawed. However, even if that is the case, it is still possible that her conclusions are valid. Additional long term research must be done before anyone can know with certainty whether ovulation-inducing drugs may be implicated in ovarian cancer. Nevertheless, the publication of Whittemore's study (and a later study, published in 1994 by Rossing, *et al*, in which women who took clomiphene citrate—Clomid™ or Serophene™—for more than twelve months were also found to have an increased risk of ovarian tumors[8]) marked a significant turning point in the history of reproductive medicine: the long-term effects of taking powerful fertility drugs would now be scrutinized more seriously. This was the good news; the bad news was that many worried that it was too late for them.

Whittemore's study, which received wide publicity in the media, alarmed many infertile couples, as well as their families and friends. Some who were considering the new reproductive technologies changed their minds. Others, who attempted to understand how the study was performed and how the conclusions were drawn, dismissed the findings as being unfounded or premature. The Whittemore study also indicated that women who had had at least one pregnancy either prior to their infertility treatment or subsequent to it were exempt from the group who were more likely to develop ovarian cancer. Women who had used oral contraceptives prior to their infertility were also exempt from that group. This news was reassuring to women who fell into the exempt categories, but devastating to women who had little or no hope for a biological child without using medications which could put them at risk.

This study once again raised the question about whether fertility drugs may cause harmful (in this case life-threatening) side effects. This question is especially difficult for couples who are determined to do whatever is in their power to have a biological child. They wonder whether their perseverance is clouding their judgment. For them and others, the publicity surrounding Whittemore's study may have served an important function: it prompted them to pause in their treatment and question the wisdom of what they were doing.

A review of published data regarding the possible link between fertility medications and ovarian cancer suggests that the correlation does not mean that the association is causal. Since women who have never given birth are at an increased risk for ovarian cancer, it may be that their infertility—and not their use of fertility medications—put them at greater risk. The authors state that:

> "The question of a causal relationship between fertility drugs
> and ovarian cancer can only be addressed adequately by large
> prospective studies with carefully selected control groups.
> Until such data are forthcoming, the need for careful clinical
> evaluation with ultrasound or other imaging techniques cou-
> pled with a high degree of clinical suspicion before, during, and
> after medical treatment of infertility cannot be understated." [9]

There are documented side effects of medications used to treat infertility that are far less ominous than ovarian cancer but are nonetheless troubling. Lupron, a drug commonly prescribed in ART cycles, physiologically puts women into (temporary) menopause; the drug completely suppresses their estrogen levels by suppressing the pituitary hormones that stimulate the ovaries. These women frequently experience headaches and hot flashes. Side effects from ovulation inducing drugs range from headaches to hyperstimulation syndrome in the physical realm, to mood swings, irritability, fatigue, and depression in the emotional realm. On the other hand, it can be difficult to determine whether the depression felt during an ART cycle is due to the medications, the pain of childlessness, or the increased feelings of vulnerability that come with high-tech treatment.)

Hyperstimulation syndrome, when it occurs, is usually mild. However, it can become potentially serious, resulting from ovaries that are extremely responsive to the medications, thereby causing them to become quite large. Hyperstimulation can lead to severe weight gain (from fluid accumulation in the abdomen and low output of urine) and potentially serious changes in blood chemistry. Rarely, a woman experiences such severe hyperstimulation that she must be hospitalized and given intravenous fluids along with having her weight, urine output, and blood chemistry closely monitored.

Multiple gestation is a well known and well documented "side effect" of ART and one that can have a long term impact upon a family. All couples considering ART must be aware of the risks associated with multiple gestation. Not only are these pregnancies physically and emotionally challenging to the mothers (see Chapter 3, Pregnancy After ART), but there are substantial health risks associated with premature birth, something which is very common with multiple gestation. Couples are strongly encouraged to acknowledge that multiple birth is a real possibility for them (unless they transfer only one embryo, thereby limiting their chances for success) and to try to forecast whether they have the physical, financial and emotional resources to handle the challenges involved.

The Physical Ordeal

Couples considering one or more of the ARTs must think about the physical aspects of the procedure. All of the new reproductive technologies use procedures that are physically invasive, time consuming, and (to greater or lesser degrees) painful. Depending on the nature of the ART cycle and the protocols at the specific clinic, all cycles involve several days' worth of injections, daily blood tests as ovulation approaches, and vaginal ultrasound monitoring to determine whether the ovaries are producing follicles. Since eggs grow inside the follicles, it is important that a sufficient number be growing so that several eggs can be retrieved.

Patients undergoing IVF procedures must have an egg retrieval, a minor but invasive and sometimes uncomfortable (depending on what type of sedation is used), surgical procedure performed vaginally via ultrasound guidance. Patients who are undergoing a GIFT procedure also have a vaginal egg retrieval; in addition, they are required to have a laparoscopy in order for the procedure to be performed, because the eggs and sperm are placed directly into the fallopian tube via a catheter. A laparoscopy, which almost always requires general anesthesia, involves two incisions: one just outside the navel and the other lower in the abdomen where a probe is inserted. Although a laparoscopy does not require an overnight stay in the hospital or clinic, recuperation usually takes between two and four days.

The invasive nature of an ART cycle is not taken lightly by most couples. Most often they have already been through several painful tests and treatments, and most women considering one of the ARTs know whether their pain tolerance is high or low. Some women, as part of their previous infertility workup, tolerated procedures such as an endometrial biopsy or a hysterosalpingogram with barely any discomfort; others found them barely tolerable, and when they learn what is involved in ART they become frightened. The amount of pain/discomfort one is able or willing to undergo becomes an important aspect of the decision-making process.

Cryopreservation of Embryos

Once couples have decided to embark on high-tech treatment and have determined, in consultation with their physician, which form it will take, they confront a new set of decisions regarding the freezing (cryopresevation) and disposition of their embryos. Cryopreservation of embryos has been one of the most important developments of the new reproductive technologies, allowing many couples to get far greater "mileage" from a single ART cycle and extending their reproductive possibilities.

There are significant advantages to freezing embryos, as many women produce far more eggs than can be used in any one cycle, and until 1997, no embryologist has been able to freeze eggs. [As this book goes to press we are hearing of the the first births–twins–conceived from cryopreserved ova. This technology probably will not be available to most practitioners, however, for many years.] The extra eggs can be inseminated, and those that fertilize and are of sufficient quality to endure the freezing process can be cryopreserved for later use. If the woman does not conceive in that cycle, the couple can elect to go through a natural cycle in which she is monitored carefully via bloodwork, and when the timing is correct (her uterus is receptive), the embryos are thawed and transferred. Frozen embryo transfer cycles are much easier and less costly for couples than cycles in which fresh embryos are used, as the woman is not required to take fertility drugs (though some clinics do prescribe a hormonal regimen of estrogen and progesterone in order to achieve optimal uterine conditions). Additionally, if a couple does conceive during a fresh cycle and they want more children in the future, they can return and go through a frozen cycle in hopes of achieving another pregnancy. One of the ironies of cryopreservation is that siblings can be conceived at the same time (technically fraternal twins), but born years apart.

Embryos are frozen one to three days after insemination in a cryoprotectant solution, stored in plastic straws or vials, and placed in liquid nitrogen. Depending on when they are frozen and whether they are viable, embryos contain between one and eight cells (occasionally more) when they are frozen. Programs that freeze embryos at an early stage most likely have a greater number of embryos to freeze from any one couple than do programs that freeze at a later stage, as many embryos stop dividing after a day or two (or more). Thus many programs prefer waiting to see if embryos appear viable before cryopreserving them.

Many couples, even those who choose to freeze embryos, worry about the effects of the cryopreservation process on the resulting children. Although there is no evidence that children who are born from frozen embryos have any greater incidence of birth defects or physical or intellectual problems than do other children, the notion of being in suspended animation at the four-cell stage seems bizarre to many people. The oldest children resulting from cryopreserved embryos are still in grade school. Although it looks highly unlikely that any long-term effects will appear, it is impossible to be certain of this for years to come.

Cryopreservation practice in ART clinics usually reflects current legal statutes, which vary from state to state. Some states—Louisiana is one— have strict laws regarding the experimentation and disposition of embryos, implying that physicians who discard embryos can be prosecuted. These statutes may determine how many eggs a clinic is willing to fertilize, should the couple decide against cryopreservation. In other words, if a clinic will transfer only x number of embryos, they will inseminate only x number of eggs if the couple elects not to do cryopreservation.

Couples who cannot accept the idea of freezing extra embryos are at a statistical disadvantage if their clinic will not inseminate more eggs than they are willing to transfer. It is impossible to know ahead of time how many eggs will fertilize. Although approximately 70% of all eggs fertilize in a given cycle in which the sperm quality is normal, sometimes all or almost all will fertilize. Thus, if a clinic inseminated six eggs, in the hope that a couple would have four embryos to transfer, they could end up with five or six embryos, a number that is more than many clinics would transfer, because it puts the woman at too great a risk for multiple birth. Instead, the clinic would inseminate only four eggs, and most likely, even if there is no male factor present, they would end up with two or three good embryos, or possibly one or none. The fewer embryos transferred, the less likely it is that a pregnancy will occur.

Disposition of Embryos

Once couples opt for cryopreservation—and the vast majority do—they are faced with a new set of decisions regarding future disposition of any remaining embryos. It may be that they end up with frozen embryos they do not want to use, as some fortunate couples eventually have the number of children they desire before they have used all their frozen embryos. Others discontinue medical treatment for various reasons, leaving frozen embryos in storage. There are three choices regarding these embryos: donation to another couple, donation to research, or discarding them.

Most clinics require couples to sign consent forms prior to beginning ART treatment that specify whether they will freeze extra embryos, how many they agree to transfer, and how they wish to dispose of any embryos they do not use. Some couples struggle at length with these decisions, attempting to anticipate all possible contingencies. These decisions are not irrevocable; couples are free to change their decision, should they have a future change of heart.

Embryo donation is a relatively new choice that allows a recipient couple to adopt embryos from a donating couple (see Chapter 9, Embryo Adoption). The embryos are genetically unrelated to the recipient couple, though they will be gestated and birthed by the recipient/adopting mother. Donating embryos to research is an option available to couples in some clinics. Couples who donate for research purposes usually do so because they do not want to live with the knowledge that their genetic child was born to and raised by others. These couples, many of whom initially planned to donate any extracorporeal embryos to infertile couples, are finding, in retrospect, that what they had previously thought would be a simple, easy, and altruistic gesture is far more complicated emotionally than they imagined. Donating their embryos to research seems more palatable, as well as more beneficial to society, than merely discarding them.

Many couples do choose to discard their embryos, although some state laws may not allow this option. Couples who opt to discard their embryos may do so themselves or, if the clinic is willing, designate someone to do it for them.

Sometimes even the best-laid plans can go awry. Couples who once agreed about what they wanted to do with their frozen embryos may disagree later, especially if their marriage is dissolving. The case of Mary Sue and Junior Lewis Davis of Tennessee, referred to in Chapter 1, illustrates the legal complications, as well as the emotional pain, that can ensue when divorcing couples disagree about what is to become of their embryos.

At Reproductive Science Center-Boston the majority of couples initially choose to donate unused embryos to infertile couples. This clinic has found, however, that almost all couples who consent, prior to cycling, to donate embryos to infertile couples change their mind years later, when their families are complete, and decide to discard them or donate them to research instead.

ART Statistics

The Society for Assisted Reproductive Technology (SART) is a special interest group of the American Society for Reproductive Medicine. Its membership, though primarily physicians, includes those who have a professional interest in assisted reproductive technology. Most ART clinics in the U.S. elect to be members of SART, which requires that its member clinics report their data to SART. Any interested person can obtain copies of current SART data by contacting the American Society for Reproductive Medicine in Birmingham, Alabama. Although SART membership does not guarantee quality treatment, it does confirm that a program reports its statistical data in a systematic way according to SART guidelines. For this reason we urge all couples considering high-tech treatment to consider only clinics that are members of SART.

In considering whether to do an ART cycle or where to do it, couples must understand the complicated nature of ART statistics. It is not enough to ask a particular clinic what its pregnancy rate is. The response is meaningless without all of the relevant information. Although it is not necessary to be a statistician or mathematician in order to understand what the figures mean, it is necessary to know what questions to ask and how to evaluate the answers. Couples should avoid clinics that do not willingly provide this information. Before discussing how to understand IVF statistics, it is essential to know what the most important determinants of a successful IVF cycle are.

The age of the woman is the most important predictor of a successful pregnantcy. (Until the development of ICSI, sperm quality was equally, if not more, important.) Although the age at which women reach menopause varies (usually between forty and fifty-five), it is understood that due to a decline in egg quality fertility decreases as women get older. Thus for five to ten years prior to menopause, women are considered to be sub-fertile. Although there are some women who have babies at age forty-five, most cannot. Conversely, although most women are fertile at age thirty-five, some women are not. Statistics from all clinics indicate that women under age thirty-five have the best prognosis for ART; after thirty-five, birth rates decline, and after forty they decline rapidly. Given this information, it is fair to assume that clinics that only accept couples if the woman is younger than forty should have higher pregnancy rates than those that accept older women. The Society for Advanced Reproductive Technology requires clinics to break down their statistics and include woman over forty in a separate category.

Some clinics use follicle-stimulating hormone (FSH) levels rather than age as a cutoff for allowing a woman to cycle. FSH is the hormone released by the pituitary, along with luteinizing hormone (LH), that stimulates the ovum as well as the follicle (the sac of fluid that surrounds the ovum) to mature. The lower the FSH level, the more likely it is that the woman will respond well to the medication. FSH levels are most accurate when they are measured on day two or three of the menstrual cycle. (Estradiol levels are also used as indicators in combination with FSH levels. If the estradiol is high it can invalidate a low FSH level.)

Clinics that use FSH levels as a criterion for treatment rather than age have varying cutoff levels that they use to determine whether a woman can cycle (in most programs it must be under fifteen). It is important to note, however, that an FSH level of, say, ten in a forty-year-old woman does not mean that she has the same prognosis as a thirty-year-old woman with the same FSH level. Thus, FSH levels are generally indicative of how well a woman will stimulate on the medication, but they are not in and of themselves a predictor of pregnancy rates.

The Clomid challenge test is another tool that many physicians use to measure ovarian function, believing that it is a more accurate indicator than a day two or three FSH level. The Clomid challenge test involves measuring

FSH levels at the beginning of a woman's cycle. If levels are normal she takes 100 milligrams of clomiphene citrate during cycle days five through nine, and on cycle day ten her FSH level is again measured. If the second level is abnormal then the prognosis is not good. The problem is that clinics do not always agree on the definition of "normal," and different laboratories use different assays which can yield different results. Thus it is important not to assume that a level from Clinic A would be the same as a level from Clinic B, even if performed on the same day.

Sperm quality is another predictor of success rates (but only if the clinic does not offer "state of the art" micromanipulation technology), since IVF is frequently utilized as a treatment for male infertility. When sperm are placed in direct proximity with an egg (as in IVF), the numbers of normal-appearing motile sperm in a sample can be far fewer than they would need to be if the couple were attempting to conceive through coitus. However, even when the embryologist has carefully prepared the sperm for IVF, couples who have male factor infertility have lower fertilization rates than do couples with no identified male problem. The greater the impairment is, the less likely it is that fertilization will occur with conventional IVF. The use of ICSI, however, significantly enhances the possibility of pregnancy for couples with male factor infertility. (Clinics with skilled embryologists who offer ICSI achieve pregnancy rates equal to those of couples with no male factor infertility.)

The question about what percentage of women undergoing ART cycles get pregnant is not a simple one to answer. First, it is important to ask about the type of ART cycle one is considering. In general, IUI pregnancy rates, even with stimulated cycles, are not as good as are GIFT or IVF, with some exceptions depending on age and diagnosis. Worldwide GIFT pregnancy rates tend to be higher than IVF rates, but that may be because women undergoing GIFT tend to have healthier reproductive systems or because not all clinics have the same level of embryology services. Because the eggs and sperm are put back immediately in the fallopian tubes, GIFT procedures do not require the highly scrutinized manipulation and monitoring of eggs, sperm, and embryos as do IVF procedures. Thus, some programs, in particular those that pride themselves on their embryology laboratory, may have better IVF success rates. When couples are comparing statistics from two or more programs, it is important that they compare apples with apples—IVF with IVF, GIFT with GIFT, and so forth.

Once a couple has learned the statistics for the type of ART cycle they are considering, understanding the pregnancy rates can still be confusing.

First, everyone who begins an ART cycle does not undergo an egg retrieval. Not all women stimulate sufficiently, and a cycle may be cancelled prior to retrieval if there is reason to believe that only one or two eggs will be obtained. The older the woman is, the greater the likelihood that her cycle will be cancelled. Programs that accept older women for ART cycles are likely to have higher cancellation rates, as well as lower pregnancy rates, than those that have more stringent age cutoffs.

Second, not all women doing IVF cycles who go through egg retrievals have embryo transfers. Usually only about 70% of eggs that are retrieved fertilize, even when the sperm is optimal. If a program accepts a large percentage of older women who produce only a few eggs and whose eggs are not as viable, fertilization may be very poor or not take place at all. Couples with male factor infertility for whom ICSI is not being performed also have lower fertilization rates and therefore more instances in which fertilization does not occur at all. Couples who do not achieve fertilization obviously do not have an embryo transfer, and those who do not have an embryo transfer are not able to get pregnant (except in the rare instance in which the cycle was cancelled because of poor stimulation, but the woman ovulated and the couple conceived on their own or via an IUI.)

Understanding ART statistics is essential before choosing a program. To illustrate this point with actual numbers, we will use a hypothetical example of 100 couples beginning IVF treatment at XYZ clinic. Because the clinic has a liberal age limit of 45, it attracts more older women than other clinics. Let us say that 15 of these women's cycles were cancelled, so that only 85 women actually went through an egg retrieval. Additionally, ten of the 85 couples did not have fertilization, and therefore only 75 of the original 100 went through an embryo transfer. Fifteen of the 75 women who had embryo transfers had clinical pregnancies. If this clinic tabulates its pregnancy rate based on the original 100 couples who began an IVF cycle, the rate is 15% (15/100). If it derives its rate from the number of couples who went through embryo transfer, the rate will be 20% (15/75). Both statistics are correct, but any comparison of programs must take into account which parameters are being used.

Two more explanations about statistics are important: the definition of pregnancy and the live birth rate. Pregnancy is measured by the amount of human chorionic gonadotropin (HCG) in the bloodstream, measured as the beta subunit of HCG (and therefore also referred to as the beta subunit). The first pregnancy test is given twelve to fourteen days after embryo transfer. In a viable pregnancy, the beta sublevels should double approximately every two days. Most programs require pregnant patients to come back for a second test a week after the first, in order to measure the HCG levels to see how the pregnancy is progressing. They will probably have the patient come back a week or so after the second test as well and will most likely schedule ultrasonography three weeks from the original pregnancy test in order to determine if the embryo is in the uterus (i.e., not ectopic) and has a heartbeat. The patient is considered to have a clinical pregnancy when she has rising beta HCG levels and the presence of one or more intrauterine gestational sac(s) is confirmed by ultrasound. Although most clinical pregnancies result in live births, some do not. Pregnancy loss occurs about 20 to 25% of the time, and its incidence increases with the age of the mother, reaching 40 to 50% if the maternal age is greater than forty.

Although the majority of patients whose initial pregnancy tests are positive go on to have clinical pregnancies, many do not. Sometimes the hormones administered to induce ovulation (HCG) elevate blood levels such that the pregnancy test is unclear. In other cases, the embryo may have implanted for a short time, elevating blood levels slightly, but by the time the patient has a second blood level drawn, the numbers have tapered off. These situations are often referred to as a biochemical pregnancy—a pregnancy that barely got off the ground. It is therefore important to learn how a particular clinic defines its pregnancy rates; biochemical pregnancies should not be included in statistics.

Live birth rates are also important—most consumers feel that they are the only important statistic—especially if there is reason to believe that a program is counting biochemical pregnancies in its success rates. If the difference between clinical pregnancy rates and live birth rates seems to be especially large in a program, it is wise to question these findings. It is important to learn once again, however, whether the live birth rate is calculated from all patients who began an ART cycle or from those who reached the embryo transfer stage.

The various ART clinics reporting to SART generally show consistent clinical pregnancy rates (as well as live birth rates) per cycle. In other words, the percentage of women who get pregnant on their fourth cycle is approximately the same as the percentage who get pregnant on their first cycle. Just as the chance of rolling doubles on one throw of the dice is not nearly as high as it is if one is allowed five throws, the cumulative chance of pregnancy increases if a couple (providing they have embryos to transfer) elects to do additional cycles. It is not clear, for how many cycles the cumulative data hold, but it appears to be true through at least five or six cycles.

It is important for couples to remember that ART is an evolving science and that physicians and biologists are constantly trying to improve upon the techniques that the use. The arrival and widespread use of ICSI in the early-mid 1990's dramatically improved upon IVF success rates, especially with male-factor infertility. Subsequently, the introduction of the Wallace catheter and the Poole medium (a glucose-free culture medium), brought continued improvement in IVF success rates. Since SART statistics are always a year to two years old (because it takes SART that long to assemble, assess and publish information), this information will not always reflect significant new developments.

In order for statistics to be helpful to a couple, they must have a clear understanding about where they fall in terms of age, diagnosis, etc. Once they have all of this objective information, they must make choices that are based also on subjective data, that is, on what *feels* right as well as on what is logical. For example, one couple, upon hearing that they had a five percent chance to become pregnant, might jump at the opportunity to try IVF, understanding that the chances of a pregnancy on their own would otherwise be zero. Another couple, given the same odds, might walk away from a procedure that has such low odds! The point is that couples differ in respect to what odds they feel make it worthwhile for them to proceed with ART treatment. What makes this issue even more confusing is that programs, as well as physicians, differ in the amount of encouragement they offer based on a couple's chance of pregnancy. Some physicians might encourage couples who have a five percent chance to keep trying; many others would strongly encourage them to move on. Each couple must search inside themselves to discover what they need to do—or not do—in order to avoid future regrets.

The ART Process

Couples who undergo ART treatment find themselves in a place that they never expected to be. Few, if any, could have imagined when they set out to have a child together that they would take this intimate process out of their bedroom and into a doctor's office, let alone into an operating room and adjacent IVF laboratory. Even when they accepted their infertility, most hoped that their problem would be resolved long before they faced decisions regarding the new reproductive technologies. Now they find themselves at a crossroads, about to embark upon the complex journey that is ART.

From an emotional perspective, the decision to try ART goes more smoothly for some couples than for others. While some are fortunate to find themselves "in sync"—able to make decisions in harmony—others experience discord. Sometimes this is based on financial pressures, other times on ethical considerations. However, in our experience, most differences involve pacing. Partners move at different paces and may misperceive each other in the process. Although some can resolve the struggles that result from these misperceptions on their own, many will benefit from counseling prior to beginning an ART cycle.

Many programs require or strongly encourage ART couples to have at least one visit with a staff mental health counselor if there is one available. This visit is designed to help couples cope with the multiple challenges of ART. If a particular clinic does not have a mental health clinician available, the couple may want to seek outside consultation to help prepare them for the challenges ahead.

Selecting a Program

Once a couple has decided to try ART treatment, they must select a program. For some, who live in an area where there is only one program, the decision is probably straightforward–they go where treatment is available (some may not see it as so straightforward and may elect to travel some distance–even temporarily relocate–in order to be treated at a facility that offers a better chance of success). However, with the plethora of programs now offering ART, many prospective patients have two or more programs to choose from. In addition to examining statistics, people consider several issues. These include the location and accessibility of the program (is it easy to get to, is there parking, traffic etc.?), the fit with the staff (are people warm and helpful or do they seem over worked, overwhelmed and over-extended?) and insurance coverage (is the program covered by the couple's insurance plan and if not, is another local program under contract?). Some couples make initial appointments at more than one program, hoping to get a sense of their "fit" with physicians and staff, as well as to get a sense of how it feels to be patients in a given program. A visit there inevitably reveals a great deal about the feel and tone of the place, about patient and staff morale and about attitudes towards promptness, phone calls and written communication.

Beginning the Process

Selecting a program is an important milestone, but there are many tasks that follow before a couple can begin a cycle. First, they may have to wait several months—perhaps longer—before they can begin ART treatment. Some programs have waiting lists resulting in a wait as long as a year before a couple is even able to have a consultation, while other programs accept couples almost immediately. The application process may take time to complete; most clinics require that all prior medical records be sent. As a prerequisite to cycling, most programs also require additional testing, which can include various hormonal screens as well as hepatitis and rubella screening and a semen analysis. Most ART clinics also require a test for the presence of human immunodeficiency virus (HIV) antibodies.

Once couples have had a medical consultation and a consultation with a nurse, the woman will probably undergo a complete physical examination, including measurement of uterine size (for IVF patients) so that the physician will know how far to insert the embryos during the transfer. Once all the testing is completed, the woman can begin ART on the appropriate day of the cycle, which is determined by the protocol she is following.

Leaving one's gynecologist and moving on to an infertility clinic can be intimidating. Most patients have built a relationship not only with their physician, but with the nurses and other office staff. They must adjust to a new system and become familiar with new faces, learn new names and understand new routines. Each clinic has its own culture and demands some adjustment. On the other hand, it can be a relief for patients to wait in a room with others going through a similar ordeal, rather than being in the midst of a room full of pregnant women.

It is common for patients to overhear that someone is receiving less medication (or more) than they are, that someone has had far more (or less) follicles on their ultrasound, or better (or worse) quality embryos, and so forth. Some patients appreciate being able to talk to others about their treatment, comparing and contrasting results. Other patients find that it increases their anxiety, especially if they perceive that their chance of success is less than another patient's.

Couples need to make arrangements to fit ART into their schedules, although more often than not it feels as if their lives are being fit into the ART cycle. Many women and men need to rearrange their work schedule, especially if traveling is a job requirement. Hence, couples are also faced with difficult decisions about whom to tell and what to tell them; if they do not tell their employer about their treatment, they may be accused of being lazy or irresponsible if their work attendance falls. However, telling colleagues and/or employers about ART treatment opens them up to questions that can feel intrusive, especially around the time of a pregnancy test.

Couples need to decide whether they will tell family members or friends, or both, that they are attempting IVF. Some couples are private; others tell almost everyone that they are involved in high tech treatment. Having other people to talk to, complain to, and cry with can help make the ART experience less lonely for both husband and wife. The drawback to being open is that everyone who knows wants to know the outcome, and when couples receive bad news, they do not necessarily want to discuss it with others. It can help to make an arrangement such as, "Don't call us, we'll call you if it's good news," with those who know about the ART treatment.

As couples prepare themselves emotionally for ART treatment, it is important that they balance feelings of hope with feelings of caution. Many try IVF in order to feel that they have done everything possible to have a biogenetic child, so that they will not have to look back with regrets. Couples do not want to be overly optimistic about their chances for pregnancy, but at the same time some patients wonder whether there is something to the "mind over matter" theory, and they are that fearful they may "jinx" the cycle if they are too negative.

Most couples do seem to cope with the high emotional stakes inherent in IVF by finding their own adequate balance of optimism and caution. After all, they would not be going through the emotionally exhausting, time-consuming, physically invasive, and financially draining ordeal of ART if they that believed there was no hope that treatment would work. At the same time, couples know—or should know—that the odds, even in the most optimal situations, are against them in any one cycle and are, in fact, still less than 50-50 overall. Most conclude that to have no hope is senseless, but to have too much is also a mistake—one that potentially sets them up for even greater disappointment. It can help—providing a couple is able to make embryos and has the financial and emotional resources to undertake at least a few cycles—to temper long-term optimism with short-term pessimism.

The Mind-Body Connection

Infertility causes great stress in most women, but does stress cause—or contribute—to infertility? This is a question that plagues many infertility patients, especially those whose condition is unexplained. As recently as twenty years ago mental health clinicians and researchers "concluded" that women brought on their infertility, fueled by feelings of hostility towards their mothers, a rejection of their femininity, or other unconscious and unresolved conflicts.

Reproductive medicine has come a long way in the last two decades, identifying many new causes for previously unexplained infertility. Although the etiology of some people's infertility is still unknown, physicians can now diagnose the reasons for most couples' problems. Thus for a while the pendulum swung in the opposite direction. Many involved in treating infertile couples—especially psychotherapists—asserted loudly that infertility caused stress but that stress was not the cause of infertility.

Much has been learned in the last several years about the complex interplay between the brain and the reproductive system. Researchers are beginning to understand that emotions—triggered by stress—may, under some conditions, disrupt the complicated sequence of events necessary for ovulation and, hence, conception to occur. A brief understanding of this biochemical process is important here.

The process of ovulation begins with the hypothalamus, a portion of the brain which in addition to reproduction, regulates mood, appetite, thirst, sleep, and libido. The hypothalamus releases hormones (GnRH–gonadatropin releasing hormone) which signal the pituitary gland to release gonadatropins (FSH—follicle stimulating hormone, and LH—luteinizing hormone), which in turn stimulate the ovaries to release an egg. The hypothalamus—the mood regulator—also produces hormones in response to emotional stress, which can affect gonadatropin release as well. The hypothalamic-pituitary-ovarian loop can affect and be affected by mood, by disrupting the sequence of events necessary for ovulation to occur. There is also speculation about whether stress can cause other reproductive problems—tubal spasm for example.

In recent years several programs that address the mind/body connection have been offered for infertile women. One notable one is in Boston at the Beth Israel Deaconness Hospital. Under the direction of Alice Domar, Ph.D., the Behavioral Medicine Program offers a ten session series which includes instruction in a variety of relaxation and stress reduction techniques. These techniques which focus on the "relaxation response," include diaphragmatic breathing, progressive muscle relaxation, meditation, imagery, and yoga. The program also includes multiple stress management strategies which focus on being good to oneself, eliminating anxiety producing thoughts, reducing negative emotions such as anger and jealousy, and using humor to decrease stress. The ten week program also includes nutritional counseling and exercise.

The Behavioral Medicine Program has a grant from the National Institute of Mental Health to study the effectiveness of mind/body therapy with infertility patients. The intent of this study is to examine both of the following questions: does mind/body therapy reduce stress and depression in infertile patients, and does it improve conception rates? Thus far there are promising findings in relation to both questions.

Dr. Domar and her colleagues studied 110 subjects who attended the program between 1987 and 1989. All participants had documented infertility, with an average duration of over three years. Upon completion of the program, these patients demonstrated significant reductions in anxiety, depression, anger, and fatigue as measured by the Beck Depression Inventory. They also reported significant reductions in such physical symptoms such as insomnia, headache, and premenstrual symptoms. In addition, an average of 34% of the participants conceived within six months of completing the program. Those who underwent IVF treatment either during or immediately after their participation conceived at approximately twice the national rate.[10]

More recent studies of the first 284 patients in the Beth Israel Deaconness Program have further confirmed the efficacy of mind/body treatment for infertility. Of the first 284 patients in the program, 42% were pregnant within six months of completing the program. An especially interesting finding was that the highest pregnancy rate (57% within six months) was found among those who were found to be the most stressed and depressed at the start of the program (as measured by the Beck Depression Inventory).[11] Domar and colleagues speculate that the program may provide the most help to those who are the most stressed by their infertility. However, she is quick to point out that all infertility patients feel stress and anxiety and sometimes even the most anxious women conceive. Domar also is very clear to potential participants that the program may or may not aid in conception—if their only purpose in joining is to become pregnant, they should think twice about it—but that it is a holistic approach to health and overall well-being that will serve them for the rest of their lives.

Rather than indicting themselves for feeling stressed, increasing numbers of infertility patients are becoming aware of the benefits of combining mind/body therapy approaches with medical treatment. Although stress reduction programs like the one at Beth Israel Deaconness Hospital are popular, other non-traditional approaches to wellness, such as acupuncture, Reiki therapy, massage, meditation, and herbal therapy are also appealing and help many infertility patients feel calmer, less depressed, and healthier. Although some patients fear that their physicians will disapprove of these alternative approaches, that is not necessarily the case. We have found that there seems to be a growing respect within the medical community for wholistic approaches to treatment, especially since research is now able to document its benefits.

The Control Factor

Prior to encountering infertility, many people believe that they have some measure of control over their lives—that if they identify realistic goals and work hard to achieve them, they can accomplish almost anything they set out to do. This belief gives them a sense that they are in charge of their lives. The loss of this perception of control (perhaps illusion is a more accurate term) is one of the major losses of infertility. Couples soon learn that hard work does not necessarily ensure success.

By the time couples reach high tech treatment, they feel that they have lost a large measure of control. In many ways, ART reinforces this notion. Undertaking an ART cycle means they must be able to allow others to be in charge; tolerate uncertainty on a daily basis; and endure the agony of waiting, knowing that their best efforts probably will have little to do with the outcome. Couples must wait for test results, ultrasounds, and blood levels.

They must wait to see if fertilization occurs and, if so, once embryos have been transferred, they must endure the wait to see if the pregnancy test is positive.

In vitro fertilization, the most commonly performed ART procedure, paradoxically makes couples feel both more and less in control of conception. On the one hand, a cycle provides important information. A couple learns whether the woman's ovaries produced follicles, how many eggs they produced, and how many cells the embryos divided into before they were transferred to her uterus. They learn whether fertilization has taken place. In addition, they can get a rough estimate of the quality of the embryos transferred, at least from the eye of an embryologist. This is far more information than they have ever before had. On the other hand, the fact that they are so dependent on others to help them get pregnant— something most couples can easily do on their own—promotes a sense of feeling out of control.

In the course of a typical IVF cycle, there are predictable times at which couples feel more or less in control. During the first part of the cycle, patients tend to feel most in control. Although the daily requirements can be grueling and couples must be rigid about following the protocols, there are specific tasks that rest in the couple's hands: injections must be administered at roughly the same time each day; blood must be drawn and ultrasounds performed on schedule; the patient (or partner) must call daily to get instructions about medications; the egg retrieval must be performed at exactly the right time (when the eggs are fully ripe but before the woman ovulates on her own). Most patients make sacrifices (eliminating alcohol, caffeine, and other medications, eating well, resting, exercising mildly) in order to feel in control and reassure themselves that they have made their best effort.

Once the eggs are out of the woman's body and in the embryologist's hands, IVF couples tend to feel a loss of control. Many wonder whether the "right" sperm and the "right" egg were put in the same dish, or whether the "right" embryos were transferred. It is a time when couples may be especially fearful, perhaps remembering the case of Julia Skolnick, who in 1986 gave birth to a child of a mixed race, presumably because of a mixup in the laboratory (sperm got switched). They may recall a more recently publicized case of a European couple who gave birth to twins after an intrauterine insemination; one twin was caucasian and the other bi-racial. A similar situation occurred in Florida in 1996: a bi-racial couple gave birth to caucasian twins, claiming a laboratory mix-up.

In reality most clinics have extremely high standards. Eggs, sperm, and embryos are labeled and relabeled, checked and double-checked. It is understandable that couples might worry about mistakes in the laboratory, but of everything that could go wrong in a cycle, using the "wrong" gametes or transferring the "wrong" embryo is probably the last thing about which couples should have concerns.

The "mix-ups" referred to above were human errors that presumably could have been avoided. Unfortunately, however, in the spring of 1995 a scandal occurred at an ART clinic affiliated with the University of California—Irvine that stunned practitioners of reproductive medicine and their patients. The charges involved three physicians who were accused of allegedly "stealing" eggs from IVF patients without their consent and inseminating them with sperm from either the recipient's partner or from an unknown (and unconsenting) "donor." The recipient couples were told that the donors had voluntarily donated their eggs. To date, over one hundred lawsuits have been filed by patients claiming their eggs (or embryos) were misused and donated to other couples or used for unauthorized research. In response to these shocking allegations, the state of California quickly enacted both civil and criminal legislation imposing strict penalties for such actions.

Because trust is an issue for many couples, especially following the criminal activity at the Irvine clinic, they may find it reassuring to meet the embryologists who will be handling their gametes and their embryos. Usually laboratory staff is all too happy to have direct patient contact and to talk with people about the work that they do.

Following embryo transfer, women typically struggle with attempting to regain control. Perhaps because they have felt so out of control, some go to extraordinary efforts to take charge of their bodies: they meditate, take naps, or refrain from rigorous exercise to decrease stress or tension. If nothing else, they know these actions will prevent, or at least reduce, self-blame, making it harder to look back and be critical about what they did not do to nurture the embryos. Yet despite their best efforts, most do not get pregnant, at least in a given cycle. Commonly those whose cycles have failed feel intense disappointment and sadness.

Waiting is a fact of life throughout the entire ART experience, and it enforces a sense of not being in control. Much of the waiting actually involves brief time periods—for example, waiting to get the results of daily blood drawings or ultrasounds to see if the medications are working. Other waiting periods are longer—waiting to see if there are enough eggs to retrieve or awaiting the results of fertilization. However, the wait that feels endless is that leading up to the pregnancy test: with fewer tasks to focus on, and fewer protocols to follow, hours and days crawl by. Even if the news is disappointing, receiving it provides relief from the suspense and restores some sense of control.

Stimulation and Monitoring: The Daily Ordeal

Although the specifics of a medication protocol vary by program and patient, all ART cycles (with the exception of natural cycle IVF or GIFT) involve several days of medications that are given by injection. The injections must be timed precisely (generally in the evening) and are administered daily (in some cases twice a day), most often by husbands or partners. Alternatively friends or neighbors help out, or women inject themselves.

For many couples, the daily injections are a central stress of IVF treatment. Sometimes the stress is focused on the needles themselves. Men are troubled that instead of conceiving a baby in pleasure, they are forced to inflict pain on the woman they love. Men with male factor infertility, whose partners are undergoing IVF solely because of the male factor, have a particularly difficult time "hurting" their mates and watching them suffer as a result of "their" problem. Although they initially worry that they will cause real physical harm—hitting a vein or a vital organ—most realize soon enough that it is not a complicated task, and they develop confidence in their ability to do the job.

Two main medications are used in the stimulation phase of an IVF cycle. The first is Lupron (a GnRH agonist) which suppresses the ovaries by shutting down the body's normal production of LH and FSH, hormones essential in triggering ovulation. In the early days of IVF, before Lupron was used, cycles were frequently cancelled when one follicle became dominant. Because follicles grow at a constant rate, if one becomes dominant the others cannot catch up in order to produce a cohort of follicles maturing together. Another frequent cause of cancellation, before Lupron suppression was commonly used, was a premature surge of the woman's LH, which can trigger premature ovulation. Lupron is given by injection and administered subcutaneously (just under the surface of the skin) and is generally not experienced by patients as being very painful. Lupron shuts down the ovaries completely, so that when ovulation induction drugs are introduced, follicles will mature evenly.

The second type of medication used during the stimulation phase are gonadatropins which consist of either pure FSH (follicle stimulating hormone) or FSH in combination with LH (luteinizing hormone). These hormones are given by injection to stimulate the ovaries to produce eggs in a controlled but hyper-stimulated manner. Physicians strive for the dosage that will produce the most number of good quality eggs without unduly increasing the risk of hyperstimulation syndrome.

Until the fall of 1996, ovulation induction drugs (Pergonal™, Metrodin™, Humegon™) were always administered by injection intramuscularly (usually in the buttocks). In 1996, Serono, the drug company that manufacturers Pergonal and Metrodin, developed a purified form of Metrodin called Fertinex™ that is injected subcutaneously using a small needle. In the fall of 1997 Serono introduced Gonal-F™, and Organon, another large manufacturer of fertility drugs, introduced Follistim™—both are recombinant forms of pure FSH made from cell cultures. These subcutaneous forms of ovulation inducers will soon become universal, replacing the intramuscular injections altogether.

Some medication protocols (those referred to as *down regulation*) require that Lupron begin in the luteal phase (second half) of the previous menstrual cycle. The gonadatropins are begun on day one of the next cycle. Although down regulation extends the number of days in which medication is given, many physicians feel that it yields the best results in the majority of women. In other protocols (referred to as *flare-up*), Lupron is begun almost simultaneously with Pergonal, on the first day of the cycle in which IVF (or GIFT) is being performed. Most programs also prescribe progesterone–a hormone that is secreted naturally during pregnancy—to women post transfer (during the luteal phase of their cycle). Although progesterone comes in different forms, many physicians prefer that it be injected intramuscularly for best absorption. If the woman is not pregnant, she discontinues the medication. If she is pregnant, she usually continues it for several weeks (a small price to pay at that point.)

The injections described above are not the only instances in which a woman encounters needles during her ART cycle. In order to have her blood levels checked (which will determine whether she is being properly stimulated and whether her medication dosage needs to be changed), she must make several trips to the clinic to have blood drawn. Programs differ in the number and frequency of blood tests, but most programs insist on daily monitoring of the cycle in the week prior to egg retrieval.

Although most women say that they get used to needles, the process is still painful. A small but significant percentage have a longstanding fear of needles, which makes the injection process even more difficult. For other women, especially those with small veins or veins that are difficult to find, the blood drawing is one of the most upsetting aspects of treatment. Relaxation or hypnosis can be helpful tools for coping with injections or blood draws in such instances.

In the first part of an ART cycle, couples are involved in an ongoing drama that centers around the question of how they are responding to the medications. Since eggs mature inside follicles, patients must have frequent ultrasound monitoring in order to determine whether the medications are doing their part and causing a good number of follicles to grow. For some women this monitoring is comforting since it provides them with up-dates on the progress of their cycle. However, for others the ultrasound—performed by a vaginal probe—is an upsetting experience. Some find it invasive and embarrassing, but most report that these feelings diminish overtime. Some women who have experienced sexual trauma, including abuse and/or rape have reported substantial difficulties with this procedure and may benefit from counseling to help them cope with it.

Follicles are carefully measured by the ultrasonographer because size is one of the gauges, along with blood levels, used in determining when the eggs will be retrieved. Although not all enlarged follicles contain an egg, most do. The process of seeing them grow can have an emotional impact: some couples regard their follicles as the beginning of their children. Thus feelings of attachment can actually precede conception.

No matter which ART protocol a woman is involved in, the same questions are crucial: How large are the follicles? How many are there? and When will the eggs be ready for retrieval? Tension builds as the couple nervously awaits news of how the cycle is progressing. They may even have irrational thoughts, such as "maybe all the follicles disappeared" or "perhaps they shrunk." It is also tempting (though not necessarily helpful) to compare one's progress with the progress of other women who are cycling at the same time. Since each woman's body is unique, and since age and FSH levels vary greatly from woman to woman, one IVF patient may have twenty "ripe" follicles, while her compatriot in the waiting room may only have a few, or perhaps none.

Although women undergo frequent blood tests and ultrasounds, with most medication protocols couples must wait several days before they know how well their cycle is progressing. Not all cycles go smoothly, and some must be cancelled because the woman's ovaries did not stimulate sufficiently. However, this situation can often be corrected in a subsequent cycle by employing a different drug protocol. Sadly, if a woman is clearly peri-menopausal, no amount of medication will induce her follicles to mature.

Egg Retrieval, Insemination, and Embryo Transfer

The egg retrieval and subsequent embryo transfer are the focal points of an IVF cycle. Couples, especially those undergoing their first cycle, approach those events with anticipation and anxiety. They wonder when the retrieval will be, which physician (in the case of larger programs) will do the procedure, and how many eggs will be obtained.

Although the egg retrieval is a source of anxiety, especially for women, it is a brief and relatively simple procedure from a medical standpoint. Most women discover, to their relief, that it is not nearly as uncomfortable as they had imagined. They are given sedation and some form of anesthesia to help them relax and dull the pain (general anesthesia can be used but is rarely necessary nor advised). This medication, together with the gentle support and encouragement of IVF nurses, goes a long way towards helping women cope with the discomforts of the procedure.

Depending upon how many follicles there are—and upon other factors—an egg retrieval takes anywhere from thirty minutes to an hour. Guided by ultrasound, the physician places a probe, on which a needle is attached, into the woman's vagina. The needle pierces the vaginal wall and is inserted into each ripened follicle. The physician removes the follicular fluid and gives it directly to an embryologist who examines it under a microscope, and hopefully finds an egg. Depending upon the woman's age, the stimulation protocol, and other factors, a retrieval may yield anywhere from one or two to a few dozen eggs.

GIFT differs from IVF in that a woman must undergo a laparoscopy so that the eggs and sperm can be placed directly into her fallopian tubes. The procedure is done under general anesthesia and requires two small incisions, one just outside the navel and the other deep in her abdomen, where a probe is inserted. An overnight stay in the hospital is not required, but recuperation usually takes two to three days.

Another source of anxiety is semen collection. Although most men have had numerous experiences producing a semen sample prior to the ART procedure, many acknowledge that they never truly get used to it. Moreover, the drama of IVF, and the emotional buildup leading to the retrieval, can cause even the most easygoing men to feel anxious about producing on demand. How devastating—and humiliating—it would be to have the cycle cancelled because no sperm could be obtained! However, the pressure is more imagined than real, as sperm does not need to be collected as soon as eggs are retrieved. Furthermore, sperm can live several hours before being inseminated, and eggs can be inseminated up to ten hours after they have been retrieved. Nonetheless, there are couples who are comforted by alternative arrangements–retrieving sperm in advance and freezing it, collecting at home if they live nearby, or agreeing to collect it in the privacy of a hotel room.

Although eggs are inseminated the day they are retrieved, the couple must wait one more day to find out if fertilization occurred. This time also passes slowly, especially for couples with male factor infertility, or for couples who have never had a pregnancy together, and therefore do not know if fertilization is possible. If only a small percentage of eggs fertilize or the embryo quality is poor, couples are understandably upset because their likelihood of pregnancy is greatly reduced.

If fertilization does not occur with standard IVF procedures, it is devastating, even for couples with male factor infertility who may have been prepared, at least intellectually, for this outcome. However, if a couple has the means to pursue another cycle using microinsemination (ICSI) they should have very different results. ICSI, with its growing success rate, is truly one of the wonders of reproductive medicine in the nineties, making biological parenthood possible for couples with previously "hopeless" male infertility!

The embryo transfer is the high point of the IVF drama for couples who have achieved fertilization, especially if they have many embryos to transfer and/or freeze. Embryologists rate the embryos according to the number of cells into which they have divided, their uniformity, and the degree of fragmentation. However, each laboratory has different standards, and to a great extent the ratings are subjective; two embryologists may disagree about the quality of a particular embryo.

Having excellent-looking embryos does not guarantee a pregnancy. An embryo may appear perfect forty-eight hours after fertilization, but there is no way of knowing whether it will ultimately survive. Conversely, an embryo may get off to a slow start, or appear to be of marginal quality, but later transform into a viable fetus. Hence, embryo quality is only one measure of a couple's chances for pregnancy.

A dilemma for many couples involves how many embryos to transfer. All ART couples are alerted to the chance of multiple gestation, and are told by their physicians that efforts must be made to minimize this risk. Because most ART couples feel quite barren—and cannot imagine having one, let alone two or more babies—many are confused by this cautious approach.

As we noted earlier, many programs offer—or mandate—counseling prior to ART. One of the central roles of the counselor is to help couples make an informed decision about how many embryos to transfer. In order to do so, couples must be able to reconcile their feelings of pessimism about even one embryo attaching with the fact that if they transfer more than two or more embryos, they will promote the *possibility* of a multiple gestation. Counseling can help couples make decisions that are guided by reason, as well as emotion.

Programs differ about the minimum/maximum number of embryos they will transfer. Since pregnancy rates generally increase when more embryos are transferred, most physicians are reluctant to transfer fewer than three embryos (if that many are available). However, since the incidence of multiples increases with each embryo transferred, most cautious physicians also set an upper limit of four or possibly five embryos. Beyond those general guidelines, decisions are made on an individual basis, taking a woman's age, embryo quality, and treatment history into consideration. If a woman has had several failed cycles, for example, the physician might elect to transfer more embryos in a subsequent cycle. Although unlikely, she may become pregnant with a high level multiple gestation and face the challenges associated with carrying—or reducing—this pregnancy (see Chapter 3, Pregnancy After ART).

From a medical standpoint, the embryo transfer is a relatively painless procedure, similar to an IUI, a treatment many women experience prior to undergoing IVF. A thin catheter containing the embryos is inserted through the woman's cervix, and the embryos are placed into her uterus. This seemingly simple procedure must be done with great care. The introduction, in 1996, of the Wallace catheter—a very thin, smooth edged and flexible instrument—has made embryo transfer much easier for both physicians and patients and appears to have greatly improved the pregnancy rate per embryo transfer.

Following embryo transfer, women are instructed to lie still for one to four hours. Although there are some physicians who recommend that their patients rest at home for three or four days afterwards, most do not. Instead they suggest that women resume normal activities, but avoid heavy lifting, strenuous exercise, and hot baths. Most patients are only too happy to follow these recommendations, and many add prescriptions of their own, trying to eliminate any activity that might jeopardize a pregnancy, or that might cause them to look back guiltily if they are not pregnant.

The Endless Wait

The twelve- to fourteen-day wait for pregnancy results is a test of emotional endurance. During this time many women feel distracted, preoccupied, and anxious. Unlike the days before embryo transfer, which were filled with specific tasks and which included daily contact with caregivers, this is a time when they are left on their own, trying to cope with the slow passage of time. Many women focus on trying to ensure the well-being of the embryos. Some talk to them; others play quiet music, avoid conflict or seek solace in prayer. Others find it helpful to try to maintain life as usual, modifying strenuous activities, but otherwise trying not to focus on what may—or may not—be happening inside them.

Women typically try to figure out whether the embryos attached to their uterus. Unfortunately, the medications and hormones that are given to stimulate egg production or to support a presumed pregnancy often mimic the signs and symptoms of pregnancy. Hence, women have no accurate clues to follow. Although they may dutifully remind themselves that ART patients can *feel* pregnant and not *be* pregnant (and of course, the converse is true), it is often difficult to prevent fantasies of pregnancy from taking over.

The pregnancy test is done twelve to fourteen days after the embryo transfer. As it approaches, tension mounts. Women wonder how they will ever manage to get through the actual day of the test and how they and their partners will await and receive the call. As devastated as they are if they begin to bleed a day or so before the test, they may also appreciate this "advanced warning." It is crucial, however, that women not decide to skip the pregnancy test if they believe they are menstruating, for sometimes women do bleed even though they have a healthy pregnancy.

When the Pregnancy Test Is Positive

For fertile couples the reality of pregnancy begins when the chemical solution in their home pregnancy test changes color. From that moment on they are expecting. And although couples who planned their pregnancies are usually thrilled and find a way to celebrate, they are not surprised—they merely did "what comes naturally." ART couples, by contrast, have no such moment. For them pregnancy begins tentatively, and it is never quite clear when they can safely believe it—when the blood levels appear high enough, when they see a fetal heartbeat, or at the end of the first trimester? (see Chapter 3)

The roller coaster journey of infertility never completely prepares anyone for the even steeper ride they may encounter during early pregnancy. Although thrilled, many feel overwhelmed by questions and fears. Will this hard earned pregnancy end in loss? (Those who have suffered prior miscarriages will focus on this worry.) Is the pregnancy in my uterus? (Those who have gone through a previous ectopic pregnancy will dwell on that concern.) Others (especially those whose early numbers were high) may focus on whether there are too many embryos in their uterus, and if so, what they would decide to do. These worries loom large to couples pregnant after ART. And although some percentage of couples will face their worst fears, the large majority of women whose first test is positive will bring babies home eight-and-a-half months later.

Couples are often confused by the process of testing for pregnancy. Unlike their fertile friends, who enjoy the ease of a home pregnancy test, ART couples undergo a series of blood tests that measure beta subunits, estradiol and progesterone levels. Those whose initial levels are strong will probably be told to come back in a week for a second test to make sure that the pregnancy is progressing normally. Others, with more questionable inital tests, may be monitored more frequently.

ART patients undergo an ultrasound at week six or seven of the pregnancy (which is five weeks after the embryo transfer). An ultrasound can determine whether there is a sac located in the uterus and whether it has a fetal heartbeat. Although confirmation of a heartbeat bodes well for the pregnancy—and many couples allow themselves to feel excitement at that point—there is still a possibility of a miscarriage, especially in women over age thirty-five.

Like other pregnant women, those pregnant after ART treatment usually have some symptoms: morning sickness, frequent urination, fatigue, or sore breasts. Most are grateful to have these pregnancy signs, reassuring themselves that all is going well. However, any lessening of these symptoms, however slight, can be frightening. In fact, when symptoms do disappear suddenly in the first trimester, it may be a sign that the pregnancy is in jeopardy.

As unpleasant or as inconvenient as the symptoms of pregnancy are, women who do not experience them, even if their pregnancy is perfectly healthy, worry that it is not viable. They may require extra monitoring via blood tests or ultrasounds, depending on how far along the pregnancy is. The monitoring can be reassuring to them, in the way that side effects are to those who have them, that all is well within their womb.

As thrilled as they are to be pregnant, women who are pregnant after high-tech treatment can also feel cheated. They cannot be normal, pregnant women. Their feelings of disbelief, confusion, anxiety, and even isolation are unique to their experience. And although many are able to relax to some degree after their first trimester, most remain vigilant throughout their pregnancies.

Most clinics follow ART patients through their ultrasound, and if everything is normal, the couple moves on to their obstetrician. The transition from infertility patient to obstetrical patient is not an easy one. Women are most keenly aware of this when they make the actual move. Although it is a "graduation" they worked hard for and are delighted to have accomplished, the leave taking can feel bittersweet and the arrival can feel awkward and uncomfortable. After all, the staff of the infertility practice have accompanied them on a long, difficult, and still incomplete journey. Many patients fear that their new physician will consider them "just another pregnant woman," having no understanding of what is at stake for them.

When the Pregnancy Test Is Negative

There is no good way to give bad news, and unfortunately someone has to give it. Most often the burden falls on the nursing staff, the very people who have worked closely with patients throughout the cycle. Many say that being the "bearers of bad tidings" is the one part of their job that they dread. When the test is negative, it is hard to know what to say to a woman or man who has invested so much to become pregnant. Some patients prefer a straightforward, matter-of-fact response when they call for the results; others appreciate consolation. Knowing the patient helps to determine how best to deliver the bad news.

When infertile couples attempt any new treatment, they usually have a great deal of hope that it will be the "magic formula." that will produce their longed-for child. That is especially true with ART: even couples who faced repeated disapointments with other treatments hold out high hopes that ART will be different. When IVF or GIFT fails, it is usually devastating.

All ART couples, even those who are "ideal candidates," and who participate in the most successful programs, have the odds stacked against them in any given cycle. Most are probably aware of their chances of pregnancy before beginning an ART cycle, and are also aware that another cycle can yield very different results. Yet even this awareness barely mitigates their feelings. For many couples an embryo transfer has brought them as close as they have ever come to being pregnant, and for those who viewed their embryos as potential children, it can feel as if they had a miscarriage.

Why a Cycle Fails

When normal, healthy-appearing embryos are transferred and pregnancy does not occur, couples and physicians wonder what went wrong. In many instances everything seems to have gone right: the stimulation went well, the sperm quality was good, and the embryos looked excellent—but the pregnancy test was negative. And although ART staff know very well that the odds in any cycle are always against a pregnancy occurring, they find themselves perplexed at how often the test results are negative.

Although the reasons why a particular cycle failed will never be known for sure, there are two possible and probably obvious explanations: the embryos stopped dividing or there was a problem with implantation. In these situations, there is every reason to hope that another cycle will yield a pregnancy. Although this information can be consoling to some couples, it is frustrating to others who cannot afford more ART treatment or who found the protocols too rigorous.

Physicians review ART cycles that fail and try to determine what went wrong. Poor stimulation or poor embryo quality are common explanations for a failed cycle, especially in older women. In some instances a change in the medication protocol may yield different results. However, in many instances physicians can provide no explanation nor optimistic new plan, leaving couples as confused as they are disappointed.

There are some couples who consider the first cycle a "trial run." These couples anticipate repeated ART cycles, recognizing that the medication protocol may not be optimal in the first or even the second cycle. However, if repeated cycles do not yield success, they, too, are left with confusion and profound disappointment.

What Next?

When an ART cycle fails, couples consider what to do next. This decision is based on a series of questions that they ask themselves and their physician:
- Was their treatment a good option for them that simply did not work the first time?
- Would another treatment be better—or at least as good—and perhaps less expensive?
- Can they afford (financially, emotionally and physically) to try again?

Assuming that finances are not a deterrent, some may decide to try the same treatment, coming to the conclusion that one failed cycle is by no means an indication of future failures. Other couples will try something different because of financial considerations, stress, the desire to try something new, or their physician's recommendation.

If the woman has one or more fallopian tubes open, her physician may recommend switching to another type of ART cycle. Some couples who tried IVF in part to learn whether fertilization could occur, might decide if it did to attempt GIFT next, believing it might work because the fallopian tube is a better incubator. Or they may opt for IUI, avoiding an egg retrieval, as well as reducing their expenses. On the other hand, couples who began high tech with GIFT and did not become pregnant may be advised to attempt an IVF cycle next, in order to be certain that fertilization is possible. Still other couples may elect to try ZIFT, which involves more physical effort and more expense than the others but offers the benefits of both GIFT and IVF. The high-tech possibilities are numerous, and couples frequently feel overwhelmed by their choices. Some physicians are more vocal about what they feel a couple should do; others prefer the couple themselves make the final determination if more than one option appears to be a good choice.

Different programs specialize in different treatments. One clinic may believe GIFT is the treatment of choice as long as at least one tube is open. Other clinics, priding themselves on their embryology laboratories, may believe strongly in IVF as the treatment that yields the most information and the best results. Researchers and clinicians are constantly debating the

78

question of what is the most effective treatment, comparing and contrasting all the possibilities. The point is that each couple's medical situation is different, and in the absence of definitive data, couples, in consultation with their physician, must choose the treatment that seems right for them.

When only a small portion of eggs are fertilized, or none at all, ICSI will most likely be recommended. In many cases, the clinic that has already been treating them can offer it. Because ICSI is such a highly technical procedure requiring extremely skilled embryologists, couples need to be very careful before proceeding. As we have mentioned previously in this chapter, it is important to be able to evaluate a program's clinical pregnancy rates using ICSI procedures, before deciding where to go for treatment.

When to End ART Treatment

It would be much easier emotionally for couples if it was the case that ART either worked or did not work on the first cycle. As upsetting as it would be to get the bad news, couples would be able to grieve their disappointment and loss and move on, without wasting more time, money, and energy chasing a dream that could never be. But because a couple's chances of pregnancy, assuming they reach the embryo transfer stage, are consistent through several cycles, it is impossible to know whether the next cycle will be the one to work.

Since ART treatment is covered by medical insurance in only a few states, many couples know that they can afford only one cycle. Others know that they can afford two or perhaps three cycles. Still other couples, regardless of their economic situation, decide at the outset that they wish to try only one time.

Most couples who have health insurance or can afford to pay for extended treatment) do decide to continue ART treatment. In Massachusetts, where infertility treatment (including ART) is a mandated insurance benefit, couples do an average of two and a half ART cycles. It is important to remember, however, that this average includes all couples who begin an ART cycle regardless of whether they get as far as embryo transfer, and those couples who become pregnant on a first or second cycle but would have continued had they not been pregnant.

Most women have an easier time managing ART than they anticipated, although there are a few who have extreme reactions to the medications or some of the procedures and decide to end treatment after a single cycle rather than put themselves through another endurance test. Most ART couples set a number—commonly between three and six cycles—at which point they will stop if they have not achieved pregnancy. Unless given definitive reasons why additional cycles would not be fruitful, they feel inclined to continue, hoping to avoid looking back with regret. It is important, however, for all couples to remember that continuing or ending treatment is an individual decision and that they must decide for themselves when they are truly ready to stop.

Although most couples can find a reasonable end point to treatment, a few cannot. They continue to undertake ART cycles long after it seems unlikely that treatment will work. They include women who adjust to the protocols and regimes quite easily, who claim that the injections do not hurt, the blood drawings are no problem, and they have become used to the drive to the clinic. Also included in this group are those who appear unable to grieve, those who cannot—or will not—pursue a second choice, and those who disagree with their spouses about what to do next. For them, ART has become a way of life. Although physicians may have advised them after six or more cycles that their chances of getting pregnant are probably miniscule, they refuse to give up. One patient made the following declaration to the social worker at her clinic: "I've decided to stop counting and just do cycles. I'll keep cycling and cycling as long as I can until it either works or I'm in menopause."

Sometimes a pregnancy that ends in miscarriage makes a couple rethink their plan to discontinue treatment. For instance, if they were planning to try four cycles but a pregnancy loss occurs after a third or fourth attempt, they may be understandably tempted to try additional times. After all, since ART "worked" once, there is reason to believe it might work again, this time with a better outcome. A pregnancy that ends in miscarriage can be like a carrot that is held out. At the same time, however, it is a tragic reminder that things can go wrong, even after an ART "success."

There are couples who want to try ART within a limited time frame. Their plan is to undergo consecutive cycles for an identified period of time and then move on. Because most programs require a month of rest between stimulated cycles, such couples can do as many as six ART cycles in a year. Although this is a rigorous schedule, it enables them to actively confront ART treatment and then move on.

Other couples approach ART with a more leisurely pace. These include couples who are younger and those who feel no external pressure, such as an impending insurance change. Because they are not locked into a specific time frame, they can undertake each ART cycle when they feel ready, knowing that they can start—and stop—or take intermissions as needed.

Some couples, especially younger ones, discontinue treatment temporarily and pursue an alternative path to parenthood, knowing they have the option to return to ART later. These couples know that their primary goal is to become parents and that being biological parents is only a secondary goal. Others take a lengthy break from high-tech treatment, not to pursue an alternative family-building method but to reassess their goals and to take an extended vacation from the grueling demands of ART.

The field of high-technological reproduction has grown enormously since the birth of Louise Brown. *In vitro* fertilization, which forms the basis for all the ARTs, has become a widespread and versatile tool: it has virtually redefined reproduction. ART enables couples to procreate without having sex, and bypasses previously insurmountable reproductive problems. Cryopreservation has revolutionized the process of conception by allowing embryos to be frozen, a phenomenon that greatly expands reproductive possibilities. Even physicians specializing in the ARTs cannot keep up with the developments and the vast amount of research that has proliferated as a result. What is clear, however, is that once the ball began rolling it could not be stopped, and although IVF and all its variations have supporters and detractors, the new reproductive technologies are here to stay.

For every couple who faces infertility, there is a difficult and painful journey, sometimes through the rocky terrain of the ARTs. For some couples, that journey leads to the birth of a child or children; for others it leads to a different outcome. As clinicians working in the field, as authors, as parents, and as women who have experienced infertility, we firmly respect every couple's right to say no to ART—whether for personal, financial, religious, ethical, or emotional reasons. Our experience has taught us, however, that couples who try the ARTs have few regrets. Those for whom ART does not result in a successful pregnancy feel the satisfaction of knowing that they have done their best. And for others—those who are fortunate to have successful pregnancies—they have a living, growing reminder of the miracle of modern science and the mystery of creation.

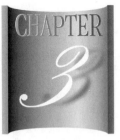

Pregnancy after Assisted Reproductive Technology

While they are undergoing ART, couples fantasize about the joy they will feel when they finally achieve pregnancy. Those who have never experienced pregnancy loss imagine that a positive pregnancy test will usher in nine months of celebration. In fact, many patients cope with the emotional, physical and financial hardships of ART by looking foward to the glorious light they imagine to be at the end of the tunnel.

Unfortunately, pregnancy after infertility is rarely as pleasurable as people anticipate. Even pregnancies that end successfully—and most do—are filled with questions and unsettling feelings. Sadly, some pregnancies do not progress as hoped and end in loss. This chapter will discuss pregnancy after ART, addressing both pregnancy and pregnancy loss.

A Miraculous Conception

Any pregnancy after prolonged infertility—and especially after ART—feels both tenuous and miraculous. After all the months, and probably years of disappointment, it is difficult to believe that a life is finally beginning in what has felt like barren territory. Sometimes women who get news that their test was positive have been known to call the clinic back in disbelief, asking someone to double check the lab results, certain there was an error. Once their pregnancy is verified most women feel as if a miracle has occurred, fearful they will awake and learn it was only a dream. Although, medically speaking, a pregnancy after ART is almost always a normal pregnancy, the mother-to-be never thinks of herself as a normal pregnant woman.

The Physical Experience

Before identifying and discussing some of the ways in which pregnancy after ART can *feel* different from other pregnancies, it is essential that we acknowledge the myriad ways in which pregnancy after ART is not different from spontaneous conception.

All pregnant women undergo a series of physical changes which can produce an array of symptoms—symptoms which may, or may not, be bothersome. These include: breast enlargement and nipple tenderness, nausea and vomiting, frequent urination, fatigue, headaches, mild cramping and increased vaginal discharge. And all expectant mothers are encouraged to find ways of coping with these symptoms, including afternoon naps, frequent small meals, wearing loose, comfortable shirts.

What is different for women pregnant after ART is not the symptoms themselves, but the way in which they may be experienced. While a woman who conceived spontaneously may feel burdened by her nausea and fatigue, women who struggled with prolonged infertility sometimes relish these symptoms, seeing them as clear evidence of a "strong pregnancy." Conversely, while other women will appreciate an easy pregnancy—one that comes with minimal symptoms—women pregnant after ART tend to worry more if they do not feel very pregnant.

Nutrition is important in all pregnancies. Women are encouraged to eat a balanced diet and to avoid alcohol and tobacco. They are also advised to take folic acid supplements—prior to conception if possible—to decrease the risk of neural tube defects such as spina bifida in the baby. What is different for many women pregnant after infertility—and especially, after ART—is not their nutritional requirements, but rather, the emphasis they put upon them. For example, a woman we knew who drank one glass of wine early in her pregnancy was tormented by this transgression for the remainder of her pregnancy. When she "confessed" to her mother what she had done, her mother was baffled, saying, "When I was pregnant with you I drank a glass of wine every night before bed—my doctor told me to."

Unanticipated Questions

To their surprise, many couples find that pregnancy after ART raises questions and prompts feelings that they did not anticipate. They discover that although they were well prepared for ART, they are ill prepared for pregnancy. To some degree this is because they are so surprised—it is hard to believe that something finally worked. However, their lack of preparedness is usually also the by-product of their treatment programs: there are orientations for IVF and GIFT and there is "preconceptual counseling involving nutrition and medication use," but no program (that we are aware of!) prepares people for the emotional experience of pregnancy after ART.

"A Little Bit Pregnant?"

In their 1990 article, "Pregnant Moments: the Process of Conception in Infertile Couples," infertility researchers Sandelowski *et al*, address some of the reasons why pregnancy after infertility is perceived differently than spontaneous pregnancy. They note that unlike spontaneous pregnancy, which is understood to begin at a specific moment in time, pregnancy after ART involves a series of "pregnant moments."[11] Depending upon their perspective, some patients consider themselves pregnant when they learn that they have achieved fertilization. Others regard themselves as pregnant when an embryo has been transferred to the woman's uterus. Most will not "feel pregnant" until there is at least one confirmation of pregnancy through a blood test, and some postpone believing they are pregnant until there is a heartbeat or, possibly, a "good amnio." Sadly, we have known women who have had difficulty believing they were pregnant for several months—even with the convincing "evidence" of a growing abdomen and frequent fetal movement.

The experience of pregnancy after ART contradicts the old dictim, "You *can't* be a little bit pregnant." In fact, pregnancy after ART does seem to begin in steps, promoting the feeling that a woman is "a little bit pregnant" and then "a little more pregnant" and then "even more pregnant" and so forth. As one woman described it, "I had difficulty calling an obstetrician to make an appointment because I wasn't sure how to describe my situation. I could say that I'd had a positive pregnancy test, but I couldn't really say I was 'pregnant'. I thought that sounded like an exaggeration at this point."

How Many Are There?

Most ART procedures involve the transfer of more than one embryo, since this increases the likelihood of pregnancy. As all ART patients are informed, however, the transfer of multiple embryos also increases the likelihood of multiple gestation. While they are undergoing ART, the question of whether they will experience a multiple gestation and what it will mean for them remains distant and somewhat abstract for most couples. Feeling barren, it is difficult for them to imagine that they will have one baby, let alone two or more.

Once pregnancy is confirmed, the question of multiple gestation becomes more real. Some couples hope for twins, feeling that this "instant family" will be a true reward for their suffering and their heroic efforts. Others, especially those who elected to have four—or even more— embryos transferred, reflect back upon their decision and wonder if it was a mistake. "Did we take too much of a chance? Could we now have triplets—or more?"

Although very high levels of pregnancy hormones on early pregnancy tests do suggest that a woman is carrying more than one baby, a multiple pregnancy cannot be confirmed by a blood test. A couple must therefore wait until a six or seven week ultrasound to know how many babies they may be expecting. We say "may be expecting" because the spontaneous loss of one or more babies is a common occurrance in multiple pregnancy, especially in the first trimester.

Some couples react to the news that they may be having more than one baby by saying "Terrific, the more the merrier." Those who paid for their treatment out of pocket—or had limited insurance coverage—feel especially blessed that they are getting "two—or more—for the price of one." Others are more cautious. Having known loss and disappointment, they are reluctant to become excited about being the parents of twins or triplets. They have learned that "bad things happen to good people" and they now remind themselves of all the obstetrical challenges posed by multiple gestation.

Couples are usually upset to learn that they are carrying three or more babies. These couples are confronted with a troubling paradox: their infertility treatment has resulted in a risky form of superfertility. They face the threat of severe prematurity and its associated problems or the disturbing option of multifetal reduction— the process of aborting one or more fetuses in order to decrease the risk to the remaining babies. Those who thought they wanted instant family may look back with guilt and regret, angry at themselves—and possibly at their physician—for forcing nature.

By contrast, couples who learn that they are carrying twins tend to feel a mixture of delight and caution. Most are pleased with the prospect of two babies but are also concerned about prematurity and other complications of a multiple gestation. Some realize that they were naive when they hoped for a twin pregnancy, since a singleton pregnancy usually poses fewer risks.

Physicians do not consider a multiple pregnancy a blessing, especially if there are more than two fetuses. Rather, a multiple pregnancy is a high-risk pregnancy, carrying with it an increased risk of pregnancy loss or prematurity, which in itself increases the likelihood of medical complications. Loss in multiple gestation can happen early in the pregnancy or later (see the section on Loss in Multiple Pregnancy later in this chapter).

Multifetal Reduction

Infertile couples who turn to the ARTs and other new paths to parenthood find themselves in places that they never expected to be. Perhaps no subset of infertile couples experiences this more poignantly and more powerfully than those who consider multifetal reduction. Few, if any, could have imagined that they would find themselves faced with the unimaginably cruel dilemma: the elective abortion of one (or more) fetuses to try to ensure the health and survival of the others.

Multifetal reduction was originally developed to reduce risks to mothers and babies in some instances of multiple gestation. Although it was highly unusual before the use of ovulation inducing medications, women on rare occasion did become pregnant with four or more fetuses. When this occurred, physicians sometimes recommended reduction of one or more of the fetuses, so that the remaining ones would have a better chance for survival. Multifetal reduction was also used sometimes when prenatal testing revealed that one fetus in a multiple pregnancy had congenital defects.

The use of ART—in conjunction with ovulation inducing drugs—in which three, four, or even more embryos/oocytes are commonly transferred, has dramatically increased the number of multiple pregnancies. This has led to increased use of multifetal reduction. Because it is often difficult for a woman to carry three or more babies safely to term, multifetal reduction is now used to reduce a pregnancy to one or two babies. This procedure, performed primarily to obviate health risks to either the mother or the babies, carries with it a high emotional price: the abortion of one or more cherished babies, and the worry that the process could cause injury to the other(s).

Couples who decide to undergo multifetal reduction are overwhelmed with questions, doubts, and fears of regret. Regardless of how many babies the woman is carrying, parents wonder if they are making or have made a mistake. Even when it seems clear that multifetal reduction offers the best hope for a good outcome, the decision to undergo the procedure is a very difficult one. The baby being aborted is neither unloved nor unwanted. Rather, it is the beginning of a long-sought and greatly cherished child.

Although it happens infrequently, there is a possibility that a multifetal reduction will accidentally terminate the entire pregnancy. Aware of this risk, many couples find it difficult to come to a decision. Some are terrified that they will decide on multifetal reduction, lose the entire pregnancy, and then be tormented by regret.

The decision to undergo this procedure is especially perplexing for those who are carrying triplets. Triplet pregnancies represent that gray area in which it is not clear that a reduction will improve the outcome of the pregnancy. Many women do carry triplets successfully, and reductions do not always ensure the health and survival of the remaining babies. Yet women who carry triplet pregnancies are in a higher risk category for prematurity than those who carry twins. Premature birth can result in neonatal death or in potentially serious physical, psychological, or neurological problems for the offspring. Consequently, couples expecting triplets find themselves more perplexed than those carrying larger multiple pregnancies: will multifetal reduction help or hurt their efforts to build a family? In fact many—perhaps most—couples expecting triplets do not elect to reduce the pregnancy. Rather, they live for many months with both fear and excitement about the outcome.

Couples carrying more than three babies frequently decide to undergo multifetal reduction. When they do, they often have a sense of loss following the procedure, perhaps intensified by feelings of guilt. Many couples blame themselves for pushing nature beyond its limits, wondering if they are now getting the punishment they deserve. They may feel guilty in the company of other infertile couples who, longing for a pregnancy themselves, are astonished that anyone could electively abort a baby that was so difficult to attain.

Couples who endure a multifetal reduction may feel anger towards their physician and clinic staff whom they perceive as having inadequately prepared them for the possibility of conceiving triplets or quadruplets. Those whose physicians encouraged them to transfer four or more embryos sometimes feel betrayed, fearing that their doctors cared more about their clinic's success rates than they did about the couple and their offspring. Sometimes couples may even wonder if they were told the truth about the number of embryos/ oocytes that were transferred. They may imagine that the clinic, in an effort to have a high pregnancy rate, transferred "extra" embryos (or eggs).

The experience of infertility can profoundly change people's attitudes and beliefs about life and death. Thus the decision to undergo multifetal reduction is difficult for most couples—even for those who have always supported a woman's right to choose. Having battled infertility, and having endured invasive high tech treatment, it is difficult to imagine giving up any potential children. One woman writes about her experience:

> "If I had been pregnant with four or more, there would have been no questions about reducing the pregnancy. But triplets was such a gray area. In my three IVF cycles, I had never taken a casual view of embryonic life. I had always frozen the extra fertilized eggs for potential (and once, actual) use later, because I could not bear simply to throw them out. And now I was dealing not with a two day old, microscopic embryo in a petri dish, but an eight-week old fetus already implanted and growing in my womb."

When and Where to Seek Obstetrical Care?

When they begin ART treatment couples are instructed to find an obstetrician. This is a "tall order" for many infertility patients, who cannot imagine ever qualifying for obstetrical care and who feel awkward calling an obstetrician's office. Although some do have familiar and trusted physicians whom they look forward to seeing for pre-natal care, many ART patients find themselves pregnant with no clear plan as to who will take care of them during pregnancy.

The transfer of care from an infertility clinic to an obstetrical practice can be confusing. First, there is the question of when to make this transfer. Most ART programs do not have a specific schedule, but rather, they recommend transfer at a point at which the pregnancy is determined to be well established. For some patients this point is around seven weeks. However, others, including those who have had frequent spotting, questionable lab results or who are pregnant with multiples, are often not referred on until later in the first trimester.

The second question that arises for couples pregnant after ART is whether to seek a high risk obstetrician. Those carrying multiples, as well as those with other known obstetrical risks, such as diabetes or a history of premature labor, are generally advised to see a high risk physician, assuming one is available and accessible in their area. Others, who have no known obstetrical risks, but who feel that any pregnancy after ART is "high risk," will also elect to see high risk obstetricians. These patients do so hoping that a high risk obstetrician will take their concerns seriously and will offer them tests and office visits that will help keep their anxiety in check.

Prenatal Testing: If and When to Have It?

The question of whether to undergo prenatal testing—and if so, which tests to have and when to have them—is one confronted by most pregnant women over thirty-five and their partners. However, the implications of prenatal testing—and specifically, of amniocentesis—are more complicated for couples pregnant after long term infertility and ART.

Although prenatal testing has been widely accepted as an opportunity to improve a couple's chances for a healthy baby, in her 1988 book, *The Tentative Pregnancy*[12], feminist Barbara Katz Rothman examines the dark side of prenatal testing, outlining all of the ways in which prenatal testing complicated the experience of expectant parents. Specifically, Rothman focuses on what it means for a pregnancy to feel tentative, especially given the fact that some of the results of prenatal testing are ambiguous.

The "tentative pregnancy" is all too familiar to infertile couples, who experience all of their pregnancies as tentative, regardless of whether they are considering prenatal testing. In their 1991 article, "Amniocentesis in the Context of Infertility,"[13] researchers Sandelowski, Harris and Holditch-Davis examine the ways in which a history of prolonged infertility impacts upon prenatal decision making and they look at ways in which prenatal testing resonates with the experience of infertility. Specifically, they focus on the technological aspects of amniocentesis, contrasting it to alpha-feto-protein (AFP) testing which is a blood test and so does not carry with it associations to reproductive technology. They note that infertile couples appear to accept AFP more readily, seeing it as "a simple thing." By contrast, amniocentesis is not simple—neither the procedure itself, nor the results, can be assumed to be simple.

Sandelowski *et. al.* point out that for infertile couples, amniocentesis is a paradoxical experience: it confirms the existence of a baby to disbelieving couples, but it also interrupts pregnancy in a way that is disconcerting for those who struggled so long and hard to achieve it. Specifically, they are troubled by the sudden intrusion of technology, coming at a time when most are happily moving away from the frequent contact with technology.

For couples pregnant after ART, deciding on prenatal testing may also force them to re-visit questions regarding assisted conception. "Did we make something happen that was not meant to be, and if so, do we have a right to terminate it?" To the extent that they have lingering fears that the use of technology may have somehow contributed to a birth defect, some couples anticipate relief following prenatal testing, hoping it will assure them of the health of the baby.

It is important that infertile couples work with a physician—and, possibly with a mental health counselor—who can help them address their feelings about prenatal testing. Physicians who make recommendations for testing solely based on age—or even on genetic history—will fail to grasp the complexity for many ART couples of making this decision. Those who feel pushed into the process may feel that they have lost their right to decline the procedure. In addition, when they undergo it, patients may suffer undue anxiety during and after the procedure.

Sadly, we have known a few couples who struggled long and hard to achieve pregnancy, only to learn from an amnio that they were expecting a child with a genetic problem. These couples have described to us the anguish they felt when they elected to abort a most wanted pregnancy. Ironically, infertility may have played a significant role in these tragedies— it took each of these women so long to conceive that she was forty years old when she finally became pregnant. This irony is not lost to these grieving parents, who have had to face the sad truth that they wanted the pregnancy, but not the baby it was bringing them.

How and When Do We Tell Family and Friends the News?

While they are undergoing ART, couples make determinations about privacy. Most decide to tell their families and close friends that they are undergoing treatment, but many do not reveal the specifics of that treatment. Even those who do tell others that they are undergoing IVF or GIFT may be deliberately vague about the timing of the procedure, hoping to preserve some privacy following a positive or negative pregnancy test.

Once pregnancy has been confirmed, couples face new decisions about privacy. Some feel that they should have the same rights as their fertile friends, many of whom do not announce a pregnancy until late in the first trimester. Others feel obliged to be more open, feeling appreciative of the support and encouragement they received along the way. They may feel it is unfair to others to withhold this information.

Questions of what to tell—and to whom—are heightened for couples who learn they are carrying multiples. Those who are considering multifetal reduction may well wish to maintain privacy while they are making a decision and many elect to keep this private even after undergoing the procedure. However, even those who are carrying one baby and whose pregnancies are proceeding uneventfully face privacy questions. Although some are proud and delighted that they achieved their pregnancy through ART, others feel uncomfortable telling people about their treatment and prefer to keep the means of conception private.

Couples are not always in agreement about when to tell people that they are "expecting." Just as they moved at different paces through their treatment efforts, so may they find themselves moving at different paces through pregnancy. Often the father-to-be feels eager and ready to tell others before his wife does. For him the positive tests are confirming and affirming, while his partner may be worrying that every cramp or twinge she feels is a sign of impending loss. Since both partners are feeling vulnerable during this time, it is crucial that they make mutual decisions about "telling." This is especially important because they must be prepared for comments and questions from others which may be difficult. These include both overly celebratory "Welcome to the fertile world" messages, as well as intrusive questions about "the problem" and about ART.

Unanticipated Feelings

Couples pregnant after ART treatment almost never feel the way they expected they would. A history of infertility tends to rob them of a "normal experience." Because their pregnancy feels so precious and so tentative, it is difficult to relax and enjoy it. No matter what their obstetrician tells them, women pregnant after ART treatment know they are not normal pregnant women.

Early Attachment

Because they fear that their pregnancy will end in loss, ART couples are often afraid to become "too attached to it." Some vow that they will not think in terms of a baby, but rather, a growing embryo or a fetus. Others attempt to "swear off" bonding entirely, saying that there will be plenty of time after birth for them to develop closeness with their child.

Early blood tests to confirm pregnancy and early ultrasounds, which confirm the reality of a growing baby, promote the feelings of attachment that many ART couples work so hard to avoid. Long before they can feel any fetal movement, couples see their baby moving on an ultrasound screen (and sometimes learn its gender). This early "preview" of their future baby makes the growing life more real and more familiar. Hence, many find that efforts to remain detached are thwarted—there is a real baby "in there" and it is very difficult not to fall in love with it. The result

92

is what some have described as a "collision of emotions"—their minds tell them to protect themselves by maintaining distance, but their hearts move them in a very different direction.

The Loss of the "We-ness" of Pregnancy

In recent years many couples have begun to announce pregnancy with the words, "We're pregnant." This expression seems to be an outgrowth of both the Women's and the Men's movements. Couples who use it are attempting to convey their belief that women and men share roles equally and parenthood is not simply "women's work."

Although the sentiments behind "we're pregnant" are appealing, the words sound absurd to those who have always known that only women can be pregnant. Some are critical of the expression, seeing it as trendy. However, for couples pregnant after ART, the words "we're pregnant" are by no means hollow—they are directly relevant to the couple's experience.

IVF pregnancies, in which conception occurs outside a woman's body, begin with "we-ness." Couples speak proudly and lovingly about "the kids down at the lab," delighted to know they have achieved fertilization and hopeful that at least one of "the kids" will develop into a real baby. Having worked hard in sharing the burdens and challenges of ART, couples are all too pleased to be able to share the joy of newly confirmed pregnancy.

"We-ness" diminishes early in pregnancy after ART. Although *they* are pregnant only *she* is experiencing changes in her body. Although *they* are waiting eagerly for news following each blood test or ultrasound, only *she* is eagerly awaiting fatigue and nausea and only *she* is watching for spots of blood when she goes to the toilet (women have a hard time believing that they can bleed and still have a healthy pregnancy).

Couples pregnant after ART inevitably go through a period of re-defining the "we-ness" of their pregnancy. Most find that although it is in many ways a shared experience, it does ultimately reside in her body and this reality mandates that they will have very different experiences. She is likely to bond earlier, to feel more emotionally involved, to feel more vulnerable and more responsible. He is likely to feel a bit left out, a bit helpless and somewhat less clear of his role in their unfolding experience.

In their 1994 article, researcher Holditch-Davis discusses some of the ways in which infertile couples actually share pregnancy symptoms. Their most interesting observation involves what they identify as "pregnancy attunement," the term they use to describe the ways in which an expectant father's experience resonates with that of his pregnant wife. For example, the following symptoms tended to be experienced by both husbands and wives: backache, hunger, swollen hands, frequent urination, insomnia, fatigue, relaxation, irritability and anxiety. The authors speculate that the shared experience of infertility may set the stage for this attunement. Ironically, they observe that it may be a way for some couples who felt emotionally estranged during their infertility to regain a sense of intimacy and connection.[14]

Isolation

Infertile couples—and especially, the women—long to join the fertile world. Feeling very much like they have been standing on the side lines of life, they look forward to being part of the mainstream. They anticipate that pregnancy will establish this—that when they are pregnant they will cease to feel different. To their surprise and disappointment, pregnancy after ART accomplishes this slowly, if at all.

Instead of feeling "just like everyone else," women pregnant after ART report feeling isolated and alone. They say that others seem to expect them to be relaxed and jubilant, failing to understand the stress associated with pregnancy after ART. They also report feeling that they are being held to a different standard regarding the discomforts of pregnancy: others are allowed to complain, but they are expected to take their symptoms in stride, ever grateful to be pregnant. Finally, they speak of feeling isolated from other women, fitting into neither the fertile nor the infertile world. As one woman commented, "My fertile friends acted like I was simply one of them and my infertile friends said they were happy for me, but tried to avoid me."

Women pregnant after ART sometimes express anger and resentment towards other pregnant women. They envy their innocence—the fact that they can smile and say, "We're expecting," while the ART couple feels like *they* are expecting only loss and disappointment. They envy, also, the fact that others, who didn't have to work as hard as they did to become pregnant, seem to be able to enjoy the pregnancy all the more. This experience contradicts a central belief that many of us have about life—working hard for something should cause you to enjoy it all the more. While ART couples *appreciate* their pregnancies, they find it hard to *enjoy* them.

Loss

As we will discuss in the second section of this chapter, some ART pregnancies do end in loss. However, it is important to acknowledge that even those pregnancies that proceed successfully involve losses. These losses are more difficult to identify and, certainly, to speak about.

One substantial loss is that of time. While they are in the throes of infertility treatment, couples are acutely aware of this loss—they know that time is passing and they worry about this. However, many do not feel the full impact of this prolonged period of "life on hold" until they are pregnant and confronted with the fact that grandparents are older, possibly ill, cousins are older, children of friends are nearly grown.

Another often entirely unexpected loss—is that of infertility treatment. Although this "loss" is one that they had eagerly awaited, some ART patients are surprised to discover that they miss their caregivers, people whom they had come to know and care about. And even the experience of being an infertility patient—so difficult and daunting in many ways—has become a familiar one. Pregnancy, although thrilling, is a strange and foreboding new land.

Although loss is a part of pregnancy after ART, it is but a small part. For the most part, couples who achieve pregnancy feel enormously blessed and take great delight in this blessing.

No Longer "On Hold"

One of the unique experiences of pregnancy after ART involves the movement of time. Having lived their lives for so long in measurements of 28 days, parents-to-be find themselves adjusting to new rhythms and new experiences with the passage of time.

"Pregnant Time" has a very different pace from "Infertility Time" and ART "Pregnant Time" differs from other "Pregnant Time." ART couples, who became acclimated to rapid jolts in pacing—with time sometimes moving in slow motion and other times at a breakneck speed—now find themselves experiencing a very gradual increase in the pace of time. Pregnancies which seemed to literally crawl by in their early hours and days, now begin to move along somewhat more steadily, with someone going from being "five weeks, three days and two hours pregnant" to being "at the end of my eighth week" to a more comfortable, "three months along". In fact, there comes a point in many ART pregnancies when time may even begin to move "too fast." Having waited so long to be pregnant—and certainly, to look pregnant—some women are not eager to have it end.

The unfolding process of pregnancy is not the only reason that couples notice differences in the passage of time when they are pregnant after ART. Past time and future time each look different through the lens of pregnancy. Couples look back on the years spent in pursuit of parenthood and wonder where they went—the years spent in 28 day increments now seem a blur. Future time, by contrast, begins to come into focus, with couples feeling that they will finally be able to resume a normal relationship with time. Gone are the deadlines—"I *must* be pregnant by next Christmas/ Mother's Day/my birthday/my original due date" etc. Couples look forward to finally being able to celebrate holidays and family occasions without feeling the "what if I'm still not pregnant" dread.

Ambivalence

Ambivalence is part of every pregnancy and certainly it is part of parenthood. However, it is difficult for many ART couples to accept and acknowledge their ambivalence because they have worked so hard to become pregnant. There is nothing "accidental" about their pregnancies, and unlike spontaneous conception, which can be considered something that "just happened", ART pregnancy is planned, timed, and clearly, unequivocally sought.

Sadly, many individuals and couples pregnant after ART struggle quietly with their ambivalence. Women comment that they feel different from their fertile friends who can moan and groan about their nausea and fatigue. By contrast, they feel that they should be so grateful to be pregnant that nothing should bother them. For example, one woman whose first pregnancy had been spontaneous and uneventful and whose second pregnancy was achieved after an arduous struggle, observed, "This time it is completely different. Last time I complained to my husband constantly about each ache and pain and twinge of nausea. Now I say nothing. Even if I feel miserable I smile and tell him that I am feeling great."

Planning for the Arrival

When they are in their third trimester, most couples pregnant after ART do feel some degree of confidence that a baby is on the way. Nonetheless, many find that even then, they are different from their fertile friends.

Preparing a Home, a Car, a Job for the Arrival of a Baby

Although some couples who are expecting a baby after long term infertility take great delight in shopping for baby furniture and a car seat, many find this experience unsettling. Still scarred by disappointment and loss, they are reluctant to assume a safe arrival. However, there are practical steps to be taken and many find a way to take them. ART couples have been known to buy car seats and leave them in their boxes until the baby arrives. Others tell of selecting baby furniture, but asking the stores to postpone delivery until a future date.

Some say that they prefer to leave the baby's room in its current state— as a study, guest room or computer room—until after arrival. They note that a newborn can sleep in a basket next to their bed and that there will be several weeks in which they can paint, carpet and furnish a nursery. Similarly, some postpone arranging a leave of absence from work (or resigning, if that is their intent) until the baby's arrival. Although some employers will understand this, others may react with frustration and annoyance, baffled by an obviously pregnant woman's apparent reluctance to make plans for her maternity leave.

A Baby Shower

While they are in the midst of treatment, most infertile women do all that they can to avoid baby showers. They find these to be the most torturous of occasions. Some resolve never to have showers if they become pregnant (or adopt) but others feel differently—"I suffered through other people's showers and now it is finally my turn."

Some women pregnant after ART ask their friends and family to postpone a shower until after the baby is born. Others decide that they want the celebration, as well as the practical gifts it will bring, and opt to have a shower in the final weeks of their pregnancies. Finally, there are those who are not given a choice—their friends surprise them with a shower. Sadly, this can be a very difficult surprise for those who fear that joy and celebration will jinx them.

Having a baby shower also brings up feelings about one's relationship to women still struggling with infertility. It can feel like an ultimate betrayal to have a shower, knowing that an invitation to it would most likely bring pain to an infertile friend (but not wanting to leave her out). It can also feel like a "sell out"—a woman who once complained bitterly about baby showers may feel that she is being a bit of a hypocrite to have one. On the other hand, denying herself that pleasure serves as yet another reminder of the way that infertility lives on in her life.

Childbirth Class

Although there are some childbirth educators who offer special classes or individual sessions for couples pregnant after long term infertility, most expectant ART parents prepare for childbirth alongside fertile couples. This can be another unsettling experience, since many discover that their concerns are very different from those of fertile couples. Some envy and resent the innocence of couples who raise questions in childbirth class about anesthesia, stretch marks, weight loss after birth and other topics that seem so insignificant to them. They report feeling very much alone with their concerns, which involve the health and safety of the baby. At the same time, however, many say that they are tickled to be in a room of expectant couples—at long last members of a club that eluded them for so long.

Pregnancy after Gamete Donation

Pregnancies achieved through donated gametes prompt many of the same feelings as other ART pregnancies, but they also bring with them additional challenges. These challenges will be discussed in the Chapters 5 and 6 (Donor Insemination and Ovum Donation), but are also noted briefly here.

Privacy

As we will discuss at length in the last chapter, pregnancies achieved with donated eggs or sperm raise issues of privacy and secrecy. While we feel strongly that the children born of these pregnancies should be told the truth about their origins, we recognize and respect the fact that many couples will have a need for privacy during the pregnancy and, perhaps, for months and years following delivery. It is therefore important to acknowledge that maintaining privacy may be quite difficult for many people during pregnancy: they may find themselves ill-prepared for how public an event a pregnancy can be.

Although our society has many unspoken rules about privacy, pregnancy is often a time when social boundaries slip aside or dissolve.

Strangers have little hesitation about talking with pregnant women about their condition and frequently ask remarkably personal questions. While some pregnant women are all too happy to talk about when their baby is due, about the fact that they are expecting twins and about their aches and pains, others need to maintain privacy. Among them are women who conceived through gamete donation and who feel that casual conversations may lead to ones more deeply personal.

We have found that some women pregnant with donated gametes struggle to maintain privacy not so much because they fear the questions that others will ask, but rather, because they fear their own desire to tell the truth. Although they may have very clear reasons for maintaining privacy about their conception, it can begin to feel like a secret during pregnancy and that secret can be tormenting. Some women find themselves tempted to be more open but conclude that they cannot be. To avoid the pain of this conflict, they may pull back and say very little about their pregnancies.

Privacy issues arise also when women pregnant with donated gametes seek obstetrical care. Although many are clear that they want their physicians to know the truth about their conceptions, they worry about confidentiality. Will office and hospital staff know about the origins of their pregnancies and if so, will that make the experiences of pregnancy, labor and delivery more difficult?

Privacy issues arise most poignantly in multiple gestation after gamete donation. Because multiple pregnancies—and certainly, multiple births—attract so much attention, those wishing to maintain privacy can feel substantially challenged. Questions begin with "Do twins run in your family?" extend to, "Did you take fertility drugs?" and then take off from there. It can become immensely confusing for women pregnant who are carrying multiples after gamete donation to figure out how to respond to the seemingly endless questions.

Fears and Expectations

Although no pregnant woman can truly know the baby she is expecting, many women have vivid fantasies about their future child. Sadly, women pregnant after anonymous gamete donation are often robbed of the delightful fantasies that entertain and enchant their fertile pregnant peers. Instead of imagining a child who will feel familiar to themselves and their extended families, some find themselves fearing a "stranger." One woman said that this was so frightening to her that she found herself coping by imagining only separate body parts. Rather than thinking about a growing—and possibly, strange—human being, she comforted herself by thinking, "Oh, that's an arm" or "that must be a leg."

Women pregnant with gametes from known donors face different challenges than those whose donated gametes came from anonymous sources: they have far fewer fears of "the stranger." Instead, these moms-to-be find themselves with the psychological task of making the baby their own. This challenge is especially poignant for women whose sisters donated eggs to them. Although they have the confidence of knowing that their child will be a full—and familiar—family member, they still feel challenged in terms of authenticity. Some wonder if other family members will question who the "real" mother is or if they, themselves, will feel a resurfacing of this unsettling question.

Fears that there will be something wrong with the baby abound in pregnancy but can be especially powerful after ART procedures and gamete donation. Some women cannot help but ask themselves if they may have "pushed nature too far" and find it difficult to avoid feelings that they may be punished. Although ultrasounds and other prenatal tests offer them some reassurance, fears of the potential consequences of their non-traditional conception do not vanish.

All couples who achieve pregnancy after ART are thrilled when they are finally in the delivery room welcoming their long-awaited child. However, for those who conceive with donated gametes, this arrival brings with it a special relief—and poignancy. For most it is a huge relief to have a real baby that they can nurture and love to be spared the fears and uncertainties of pregnancy. For many, the arrival marks the beginning of feeling that they are truly entitled to this baby: he/she is their child and they are, at very long last, a family.

Pregnancy Loss after ART

We have no voices to remember. We have no occasions or activities to remember. We have no recollections of smiles or kisses to comfort us. We have only pictures of our two dead babies. We have birth and death certificates of our daughters who were born only to die. Why did this happen to us? We laid down our lives for this pregnancy. We did everything that was humanly possible to be parents. Now we are parents but we have no children.

—A couple whose twin daughters (stillborn at twenty-two weeks gestation) were conceived with GIFT after five years of trying.

If life were fair, all infertile couples who achieved pregnancy would go on to have healthy babies. Far too often, however, long-sought, hard-earned pregnancies end in loss. In some instances, such as advanced maternal age, the same problem that caused infertility in the first place is now implicated in pregnancy loss. However, most of the time, these losses are random examples of bad luck—one in five pregnancies ends in miscarriage and a history of infertility offers no exemption from this experience. In fact, among older women, the chance of miscarriage rises, approaching 50% by the time a woman is in her early 40's.

We now turn our attention to the experiences of couples who endure pregnancy loss—miscarriage, ectopic pregnancy, stillbirth, and loss in multiple gestation—all after turning to the new reproductive technologies. We will also discuss multi-fetal reduction, an ironic form of pregnancy loss that is primarily an outgrowth of the new reproductive technologies.

Early Pregnancy Loss

For several weeks I replayed the scene of the ultrasonographer telling me the bad news. I can picture the screen and the room and the sounds, and most of all, her words. I know that just before she told me, after performing both a vaginal and an abdominal ultrasound, she turned for a moment and faced the sink, while carefully rinsing off the probe—turning her back to me. I remember how her back stiffened, and she raised her shoulders and sighed. I knew, at that instant, that it was over—that she was building the resolve to tell me. She was trying to find a way to say that all that we had sought for so long and attained—was lost.

Miscarriage is almost always a painful and difficult experience, even for those who conceive easily. Women, in particular, feel grief, fear, guilt, and

confusion. When loss occurs following treatment with the assisted reproductive technologies, these feelings may be greatly intensified. Couples
who conceived with ART experience a special kind of anguish as they ask,
"Why did this happen?" "Did we do the wrong thing by forcing nature?"
"Did I somehow cause this loss?" "Could something have been done to
prevent it?" "Was it really meant to be?"

Medical Facts

In order to understand the anguish that couples feel as they ask and
attempt to answer these questions, it is important to begin with some medical facts. Although there is no single and definitive explanation for early
pregnancy loss, miscarriage is not the mystery that it once was. Physicians
have identified a number of factors that can cause or contribute to miscarriage. We begin with a brief discussion of these factors because we have
found that medical information helps couples to grapple with what is often
the most puzzling and troubling question: "Why did this happen?"

Miscarriage, also known as spontaneous abortion, is usually defined as
the loss of a pregnancy in its first twenty weeks. The vast majority of these
losses occur within the first twelve weeks, making miscarriage after the
first trimester much less common. In fact, most miscarriages actually occur
within the first six to eight weeks of pregnancy. However, since some
women miscarry before they even know that they are pregnant and others
experience the physical signs of miscarriage several weeks after the baby
actually dies, the prevalence of very early miscarriage is underreported.
Miscarriage can be caused by chromosomal problems in the embryo or by
problems in the maternal environment. The current understanding is that
most early pregnancy losses are caused by problems inherent in the baby;
estimates are that 60% of miscarriages in the first half of the first trimester
and 15 to 20% of miscarriages in the second half of the first trimester are
caused by chromosomal abnormalities. These defects in the fetus prevent
it from growing beyond a certain point.

Problems in the maternal environment, although more varied, are a less
common cause of early pregnancy loss. For example, there can be uterine
factors such as Asherman's syndrome, a scarring of the uterus that can
occur after a dilatation and curettage (D & C) or abortion or following
an infection. Asherman's syndrome can cause miscarriage by preventing
an embryo from implanting properly.

Another maternal cause of early pregnancy loss is a progesterone
deficiency. However, since most women who become pregnant through

the ARTs have their progesterone levels monitored regularly, it is unlikely that a woman will lose an ART pregnancy due to progesterone deficiency. Women whose progesterone levels are low are given supplemental progesterone preventatively, and many programs prescribe it for all their ART patients.

Placental problems are occasional causes of early pregnancy loss, but more often they cause later losses. *Placenta previa* is a condition in which the placenta attaches to part or all of the cervix. *Abruptio placentae* is a condition in which the placenta separates from the uterine wall. Losses also occur when the placenta does not function properly and denies the fetus essential nutrients. Similarly, early loss can be caused by infections or by systemic disease such as diabetes, thyroid disease and autoimmune conditions in the mother. However, systemic diseases are more often the causes of late losses.

Another potential cause of miscarriage is embryo toxic factor. Physicians are investigating the possibility that some women produce a toxin that destroys their embryos. Some promising results have been reported when women with embryo toxic factor are treated, in subsequent pregnancies, with very high dosages of progesterone. The theory is that the high dosages will overcome the potency of the embryo toxin and permit the fetus to survive.[15]

Finally, there is a new form of early pregnancy loss that is a direct outgrowth of the ARTs: biochemical pregnancy. In a biochemical pregnancy, the first pregnancy test (two weeks after ovulation) indicates a low, though positive, beta subunit number, yet subsequent tests reveal that the pregnancy has not progressed.

Some physicians do not consider a biochemical pregnancy to be a "real" pregnancy. These doctors say that a woman is pregnant (sometimes referred to as clinically pregnant) only after her pregnancy hormone levels have risen twice and a gestational sac in her uterus, with a heartbeat, has been confirmed by ultrasound. Hence, from a medical standpoint, a biochemical pregnancy is not always considered a pregnancy loss. However, from the couples' perspective a very real loss has occurred, for in their hearts they were expecting, if only for a few days.

Feelings

As couples struggle with trying to understand what caused their pregnancy loss, they are plagued by many feelings. The following are among the most common:

Grief

When infertile couples learn that their hard earned pregnancy has ended in loss, most feel profound grief. Even those who tried to shield themselves from disappointment by postponing any sense of celebration feel crushed. In retrospect, they realize that once they learned the pregnancy test was positive, even if the initial signs looked grim, they began to feel attached to the growing life inside them. Now, the baby, on whom they had begun to focus their hopes and dreams is gone.

The grief that couples experience is often intensified by the fact that others rarely acknowledge the significance of their loss, especially when it occurs very early in the pregnancy. Instead, friends and family tend to focus on the "good news" aspect: now the couple knows they can achieve pregnancy. Physicians also try to comfort them by explaining that the pregnancy indeed confirmed that they are excellent high-tech candidates.

It is especially painful when couples who cannot afford the costs of another ART cycle are told, "At least you can get pregnant." Such predictions only serve to heighten their sense of loss.

Although there is some truth to the "good news" aspect of a pregnancy loss, couples who miscarry hardly feel like celebrating. Rather, they need to grieve and to know that their grief is acknowledged and respected. When others focus on their potential for success in future attempts, they feel that their sorrow has been "disenfranchised."

By making a pregnancy visible early on, ultrasound monitoring can foster early attachment. Hence, this technology may contribute to the sorrow couples feel when the pregnancy is lost. They focus on the photographs that they receive from the ultrasound technician and experience them as concrete proof that a baby is beginning to grow. When a pregnancy is lost, these photos sometimes become unexpected treasures— concrete testimony to a life that began and ended before it's time.

Fear

Many people react to the miscarriage of an ART pregnancy with fear. Even those who can afford, both financially and emotionally, to try again will do so with keen awareness that treatment may not work. They may fear that this was their only chance at pregnancy and dread returning to a treatment process that they fear will only result in failure.

A fear that arises with a vengeance is that of another pregnancy loss. Even when there is no medical reason to see this loss as anything other than a random event, some couples worry that it is likely to happen again.

Infertile couples know about the phenomena of repeated pregnancy loss and many fear that this problem will turn out to be the next hurdle in their difficult path to parenthood.

Isolation

Because many couples do not plan to tell friends and family about their pregnancy until it is well established, those who miscarry often feel alone. When they tell people after the fact that they were pregnant, others seldom grasp the full impact of the loss.

Friends and family tend to react with confusion. Since little is written in the popular press about pregnancy loss with the ARTs, there are many people who assume that all women who conceive with IVF or GIFT have a successful pregnancy. Assuming that the loss was a highly unusual event, they expect that the couple can try again and count on a successful pregnancy. Women's magazines and other popular journals contribute to this perception by featuring articles about "miracle babies." Hence, families and friends are often unprepared to offer support and compassion to the couple experiencing pregnancy loss.

Guilt and Self-Blame

Among the questions that plague couples who miscarry an ART pregnancy are the following: "Did I do something to cause this loss?" and "Was there something that could have been done to prevent it?" The struggle to answer these questions often prompts intense feelings of guilt and self-blame, especially in women.

It can be difficult to convince a woman that the miscarriage was not her fault. Although infertility is a shared problem, pregnancy can feel like a solo experience. Women focus on the fact that the fetus was in their body when it died and conclude that there must have been something they did to make this happen. Some are merciless in their self-scrutiny.

Men as well may struggle with feelings of doubt and regret. They look at the outcome of their experience—and especially at their wife's suffering—and wonder if they made a mistake by "forcing nature." Is this loss a punishment, they wonder, for their decision to try the ARTs? Some are haunted by past words of well-wishers who said, "If you're meant to become pregnant, you will." Memories of such pronouncements are especially painful for those whose religious teachings oppose IVF: they worry that God is now punishing them for going against their faith.

Some of the guilt that people feel following a miscarriage seems to be their attempt to gain control over a situation that is beyond their control.

Many scrutinize their past behavior, trying to find explanations. Women who went through IVF are especially vigilant in this process, focusing on everything that they did—or did not do—during the cycle. They revisit their activities—what they ate and drank, how far they walked, how often they showered, the number of times they carried groceries—in search of the cause of their pregnancy loss. Since the medical process is managed precisely and carefully, it is easy for women to assume that whatever went wrong must have been their fault.

Women scrutinize their thinking as well as their deeds. They may torment themselves with thoughts such as, "If I was really a good person, this would not have happened." Some worry that they were not appreciative enough of their pregnancy, that they may have jinxed themselves by feeling ambivalent or by worrying that they were carrying multiple fetuses. Some condemn themselves for the envy and jealousy that they felt of pregnant friends and relatives in the past. Still others reexamine the degree of optimism or pessimism that they brought to the process: "I didn't think positively enough," or "If we hadn't gotten our hopes up ... ," or "Maybe the stress I felt and the constant worrying I did made me lose the baby."

Women who lose an ART pregnancy may examine even their past for "clues" about why it happened. Those who chose to terminate an unwanted pregnancy years earlier are prone to look back on this event and feel that they are now receiving their just punishment. Those who delayed parenting in order to pursue other life goals may feel that had they tried earlier, they would have been spared the trials of infertility and pregnancy loss.

Some women feel that they have a fundamental character defect. They may have no idea what it is but simply believe that if they were a "better person," the miscarriage would not have happened. A woman whose low self-esteem predated her infertility is especially vulnerable to believing she is simply not a good enough person to be a mother.

Some IVF programs inadvertently promote guilt in their patients. Those that recommend a lengthy bed rest following embryo transfer may prompt women to feel that any movement, however slight, could harm their fetus. Moreover, the bed-rest prescription implies that the well-being of the pregnancy is within the patient's control and that she has an obligation to curtail her activities if she wants the embryos to implant and to stay implanted.

Anger

Although some of the anger that couples feel after a pregnancy loss is directed inward, in the form of guilt and self-blame, other angry feelings are directed outward—at physicians and nurses. Couples sometimes wonder if there was something that their physicians could have done to prevent miscarriage. For example, should they have been given more progesterone to support the pregnancy? Others are less specific in their questions but have a sense that if the physician had paid closer attention to their pregnancy, the outcome might have been different.

Sometimes infertile couples who miscarry ask yet another question: Why us? Having endured the unfairness of infertility and the physical, emotional, and financial trials of the ARTs, they feel unjustly teased as well as cheated when the pregnancy ends in miscarriage. Some feel that they were never properly warned about the percentage of ART pregnancies that end in miscarriage.

Couples with strong religious beliefs may express anger toward God and their religion. Some conclude that their faith has betrayed them. Once again, they raise the questions that reverberated throughout their infertility treatment: Why is this happening to us? What did we ever do to deserve this? Why are our best efforts to "be fruitful and multiply" being stymied?

God, religion, and spirituality are forces that help many people get through their infertility, but some reach a point when they feel they have been tested unfairly. Pregnancy loss after ART often represents that point at which the "test has gone too far." Angry and confused, people sometimes turn away from their religion, feeling that their faith—once a source of great comfort—has abandoned them.

The Burden of Technological Monitoring

Many couples who experience a pregnancy loss following ART describe their experience as technologically confusing. Not only was their conception the result of advanced technological interventions, but the course of their pregnancy was immediately monitored and predicted by laboratory tests and by ultrasound. Having mastered the language of high-tech treatment, from embryo transfer to estradiol levels, newly pregnant patients now face new terminology that they feel obliged to learn and understand: HCG levels, progesterone levels, and ultrasound measurements. Although many couples find this monitoring helpful and are appreciative of the up-to-date information that it provides, there are those who find the technology confusing and intrusive.

Couples using ART are often troubled to discover that early pregnancy testing can raise more questions than it answers. Unlike their fertile friends, who do a home pregnancy test and learn that they are pregnant or not pregnant, infertile couples undergo an early blood test that frequently results in confusing information. Dramatic examples of this are biochemical pregnancies, when couples are told that the pregnancy test is positive but the pregnancy hormone levels are low. If this happens, even the most knowledgeable and sophisticated patients are unsure how to react.

Since most clinics measure more than one hormone level—typically estradiol and progesterone levels, in addition to beta sub units (HCG)—couples may be confused to learn that one or more assays may be high (signaling a probable "good" pregnancy), yet others may be low (signaling caution). Another possibility is that the hormone levels will be "somewhat" low and rise "somewhat" slowly. When this occurs, weeks may pass before it is clear whether the pregnancy will be ongoing or is doomed to end in loss.

We have found that couples are confused when they learn that the numbers are equivocal: they begin to feel that there are degrees of pregnancy. Of course this is entirely inconsistent with what they have always been told—that they can't be a little bit pregnant. For some, much of the confusion subsides over the next few weeks, as blood tests first confirm the pregnancy is probably viable and ultrasounds identify the number of gestational sacs (there may be more than one) and their location (a uterine pregnancy needs to be ruled in and an ectopic ruled out). Further confirmation can come at approximately seven weeks (five weeks after retrieval) when ultrasound can identify whether there is a fetal heartbeat.

Miscarriage can still occur after a fetal heartbeat has been confirmed on ultrasound. Although some couples have a warning—they are told that the heartbeat is weak—most do not. In fact, they are often told that it is uncommon for women to miscarry after a fetal heartbeat has been confirmed. Although research bears this out in women under the age of 35 (there is a 2.1% miscarriage rate), women between 35 and 40 have a 16.1% miscarriage rate following confirmation of a fetal heartbeat and this number climbs to 20% in women over 40 who go on to miscarry.[16] Hence it is not an uncommon event in some populations and when it occurs, it is devastating. Not only is there loss, but there is also a sense of being cheated by technology: the monitoring that the couple counted on for accurate information has instead promoted false hope.

Miscarriage after a fetal heartbeat is detected, can be puzzling to physicians, as well as to their patients. Some point to advanced maternal age and the greater likelihood of chromosomal abnormalities in older women. Others suspect that the fertility medications may possibly cause changes in the uterine lining that make it difficult for the embryo to implant properly, and may contribute to miscarriages throughout the first trimester.

Whatever the cause, miscarriage after several weeks of close monitoring is a devastating experience. Although most couples feel that the monitoring is still more of a help than a hindrance, we have also known couples who feel that the high-tech monitoring made their experience more difficult. They say that they would have preferred to go through the physical and emotional pain of a miscarriage at ten or eleven weeks (physicians remind them, however, that the pregnancy could have been ectopic and this needs to be identified early) rather than to suffer the agony of "roller coaster monitoring." Some feel that the frequent tests robbed them of any opportunity to enjoy being pregnant and contributed to their sense that they had forced nature. One woman described her experience as "like the Chinese water torture—a cruel, slow process."

Grieving an Early Pregnancy Loss

Grieving an early miscarriage is a complex process that can continue for a prolonged period of time. The depth and extent of the grief that people feel surprises them, as well as those around them. For those couples who cannot afford more treatment or who do not want to put themselves through more (possible) torment, the experience of grieving is likely to be prolonged.

Following an early loss, most people feel very sad for several weeks. It is important during that time for couples to mark their loss and commemorate the life that ended before it began. In that way they can move on a little more easily and begin to heal from the pregnancy loss. Some plant a tree, others bury some baby clothes, some make a special spot in a family album for an ultrasound photo, or embroider something that represents their unborn child. In so ritualizing the loss, they recognize and acknowledge that although their baby had no name, no face, no clear identity, his/her beginning was—and will remain—a significant event in their lives.

As time passes, as a woman's menses return, and if the couple is able to renew efforts to have a baby, many find that their intense sadness abates. Unfortunately a subgroup of couples re-encounter this grief if their next attempts at conception again end in a pregnancy loss. This second encounter with grief following early loss, can be more powerful and more disturbing because it informs people that miscarriage is not a loss from which they can easily move on.

Since many infertility patients do not become pregnant easily or promptly following miscarriage, their grief can intensify during the early months of treatment efforts. Many focus on their original due date, "feeling desperate to be pregnant" before the dredded date arrives. Those who are not pregnant on their due date can feel as if they are re-living the original loss, a loss that has unexpectedly grown in magnitude with the passage of time.

Second Trimester Pregnancy Loss

During my eighteenth week, I went in for a routine exam. Everyone told me how well I was doing and they signed me up for childbirth class. The doctor told me that I could expect to feel life in another two or three weeks. Then she said, "And now for the fun part—let's hear the heart beat.

Silence. There was only silence. They tried several times, several ways. Finally, they did an ultrasound. I didn't want to look. I knew. Then the doctor said she was sorry—that it looked like the baby had died three or four weeks earlier. I can't believe that all the while that I was busy rejoicing—busy buying maternity clothes and signing up for childbirth class— my baby was dead.

Unlike their fertile friends, who typically breathe a sigh of relief when they complete their first trimester, infertile couples, being so accustomed to loss, may never feel entirely out of the danger zone. Nonetheless, the likelihood of pregnancy loss greatly diminishes in the second trimester, and many infertile couples feel somewhat more relaxed as they enter it. This increased comfort, together with the increased attachment that they feel toward their unborn child (despite the fact that many try hard to avoid attaching), makes later miscarriage all the more startling and difficult when it occurs.

Second trimester losses are accompanied by an intensification of the questions and feelings we have already discussed. In addition, most couples experience an overwhelming sense of shock; even those who had remained cautious and anxious are stunned when a pregnancy is lost in the second trimester. As with early miscarriage, we have found that some understanding of the medical causes helps couples to cope with their loss.

Medical Facts

Late miscarriages, like early ones, can be caused by either maternal or fetal factors. The most common cause of late miscarriages is a maternal factor involving premature dilation of the cervix, sometimes as early as eighteen or nineteen weeks (sadly this problem is referred to as "incompetent cervix", a term that is a insulting as the term "habitual aborter," the accusatory description of a woman who suffers a series of miscarriages.) If the problem is detected early enough a cerclage (suture) can be placed around the cervix to keep it closed. However, if significant cervical dilation is present, little can be done to prevent pregnancy loss. For those women who dilate prematurely, in future pregnancies a cerclage can be put in place at 12-14 weeks of pregnancy. When a cerclage is done as a preventative measure, the success rate is 80-90%. Sadly, many women suffer a late pregnancy loss before the need for this prophylactic treatment is identified.

Fibroid tumors and uterine abnormalities are other maternally-related causes of late miscarriage. A small percentage of women with fibroids will have a tumor that grows so large and so rapidly that it causes the uterus to contract prematurely. A small fibroid located near the uterine cavity can also be detrimental. However, since many infertile women who have fibroids undergo myomectomy (the surgical removal of a fibroid tumor) prior to ART treatment, it would be unlikely that a miscarriage after ART would occur for that reason. And since most infertile women undergo hysteroscopy—an internal viewing of the uterus—it is likely that uterine abnormalities will be detected prior to ART treatment.

Immunological problems, related to the father or to the mother, are another possible parental factor in late miscarriage. These causes are currently being investigated, and we will review them later in this chapter when we discuss repeated miscarriage.

Chromosomal abnormalities are the most common fetal cause of late miscarriage and are thought to account for ten percent of these losses, for although most chromosomally abnormal fetuses do not survive beyond twelve weeks, some do. The fetus can appear to be developing normally but, as with many early miscarriages, there is something inherently wrong with it that causes it to abort. When this happens several weeks into the pregnancy, after a heartbeat has been detected, and after fetal growth has been followed on the ultrasound screen, it is a bewildering—and devastating—experience.

Finally, many second trimester losses are of unknown etiology. In this situation, when no explanation can be found for the loss, women are plagued with doubt and self-blame, often convinced that they "did something to the baby."

Feelings

In addition to all of the feelings engendered by early pregnancy loss—grief, fear, isolation, guilt, anger—late miscarriage prompts feelings of injustice. Infertile couples know that life is not fair, but losing a pregnancy after they had finally begun to believe it was real feels immeasurably cruel. Couples wonder why so much emphasis is placed on getting through the first trimester if a pregnancy remains vulnerable in the weeks that follow.

Couples who go through infertility are vulnerable to feeling defective; their bodies do not work right. A pregnancy after long-term infertility, even if it ends in early miscarriage, may help repair some of these feelings. Couples are comforted to know that conception can occur. They may begin to feel more "normal." However, when a long-sought pregnancy is established, progresses, and then ends in unexpected loss, the experience is jolting, causing them to feel even more out of control. One woman who experienced two second trimester miscarriages following GIFT cycles, said:

> I found that my relationship with other women changed
> when I found that I was infertile, and then it changed again
> when I miscarried. I feel like an infertile woman with a very
> dark rain cloud over my head. It is as though my burden of
> infertility was lifted and then returned, with even more
> weight and force. I feel that I am now a walking symbol
> of the precariousness of good luck.

Some women who have late miscarriages after ART despair that even the most sophisticated technological assistance cannot repair something fundamentally wrong with their bodies. As we noted earlier, the close monitoring that most receive can contribute to the anguish they feel. They saw an actual fetus on the ultrasound screen and now they wonder what they may have done to cause things to go wrong.

The "character defects" that we decribed in relation to early miscarriage also plague women who suffer late miscarriages, especially after the ARTs. When others pronounce, "Maybe it wasn't meant to be," they think, "Maybe

God knew that I would be an unfit mother [or father] and this was God's way of telling me." Some extend their self-blame to their decision to use IVF or GIFT, wondering if they were punished because they tried to tamper with nature.

Grieving a Late Pregnancy Loss

Because of the attachment that occurs as a pregnancy unfolds, a couple's grief after a late loss is intense. Although their grief is more understood and acknowledged by others than are early losses, it is also fraught with anguish. Unlike the grief following early loss, which may not be as startling, later loss comes as a shock and is more devastating, more all encompassing, at the beginning.

In the days following a late miscarriage, most couples are acutely grief stricken. Like others who suffer the sudden loss of a loved one, they are forced to figure out what to do and when and how to do it. Because they are in somewhat of a gray zone, where a funeral and burial are possible, but not assumed, they must make very difficult decisions—decisions which are entirely unfamiliar, but which will have life long implications for them.

Knowing the gender of the baby makes it easier for some couples to grieve their loss. They can select a name and to some extent the baby takes on an identity. The loss, then, becomes more identifiable, more evident. Although they find that others are sometimes uncomfortable, grieving parents can refer to the baby they lost by name and in some instances, can show a photo or speak of the funeral and burial.

Grief following late loss extends for several months. If another period of infertility follows the loss, grief may actually intensify over time. As with early loss, both the due date and the anniversary of the loss become critical points in time in which much of the acute grief is re-visited.

In the weeks and months following both early and late miscarriage, couples often find that they must educate others regarding their loss. Saddened by the tendency that people have to withdraw, to minimize the loss, to focus on the positive—"at least you *know* you can get pregnant"— grieving couples must find ways to let others know that they have experienced a *big* loss that will not vanish. Failure to acknowledge its magnitude only serves to make them feel diminished and even dismissed. When their efforts work—when others are able to empathize—grieving becomes somewhat easier because it is shared.

Repeated Miscarriage

Although many infertile couples fear that a single miscarriage following the ARTs means that there will be others, most are spared this devastating experience (after one miscarriage, the chance of a second remains at 20% for women under the age of 35). But some couples become pregnant after long-term infertility only to face the frustration and devastation of repeated pregnancy loss. For some, the losses are interspersed with long periods of infertility.

Medical Facts

Women who have repeated miscarriages were once called "habitual aborters," an unfortunate term that implied (albeit unintentionally) that the women were responsible for their miscarriages. Psychologists practicing a generation ago frequently offered psychodynamic explanations for the losses. For example, Helene Deutsch, a well known and well respected psychoanalyst, offered two interpretations of multiple miscarriage in her 1945 work, *The Psychology of Women II*. She believed that some women miscarried because they feared motherhood. Other women were said to become habitual aborters because they were so traumatized by their first pregnancy loss that they developed an unconscious compulsion to repeat the trauma.[17] Thus, in the absence of medical knowledge, an elaborate psychological theory was constructed that unfortunately served to exacerbate guilt rather than shed light on the phenonmena.

Although we now have several medical explanations for repeated miscarriage, there is still much mystery surrounding this experience, and many women continue to blame themselves whether or not a medical explanation has been offered. They may wonder if this new problem is definitive proof that they were not meant to be mothers after all.

The possible causes of repeated miscarriage are varied, and as time goes on, more explanations are being found. Current investigation of multiple miscarriage is focusing on embryo toxic factor and potential immunological factors, both alloimmune and autoimmune. The former, according to some physicians, may be the cause of multiple miscarriage because the woman does not develop a necessary "blocking factor" which would prevent her body from rejecting the baby it perceives as a foreign object. Women with alloimmune factors it is thought, fail to develop this blocking factor, thereby allowing their immune system to destroy the baby. Experimental treatments in which the woman is injected with her

114

husband's white blood cells are being used in a few treatment centers. The theory behind this treatment is that the presence of the husband's white blood cells will help a woman to develop the absent blocking factor.

Another possible immunological cause of repeated miscarriage, and one that is more widely accepted, is an autoimmune problem known as the antiphospholipid antibody (or anticardiolipin antibody) syndrome. The presence of these antibodies increases the likelihood that a woman's blood will clot. If these clots occur in placental vessels, blood flow to the baby will be compromised. To treat immunological problems physicians are experimenting with a protocol that involves taking one baby aspirin daily. An alternative treatment is to use a baby aspirin in combination with a steroid, usually prednisone, and heparin, a blood thinner. These treatments aid circulation, thereby enabling the fetus to receive its needed nutrition from the placenta.

It is unusual for a couple to move from long-term inability to conceive to repeated pregnancy loss. Nevertheless, there are couples who manage to cross one new frontier—conception—only to find themselves on another—repeated pregnancy loss. The treatment for this second new frontier is even newer and more experimental than the ARTs. It takes remarkable perseverance, stamina, and hope for a couple to enter into the experimental treatment of multiple miscarriage when they must endure so much to first achieve pregnancy.

Feelings

In addition to their grief, couples who have the misfortune of experiencing both infertility and repeated pregnancy loss have many feelings, including bewilderment, anger, and frustration. Some re-visit questions about "forcing nature" and conclude that the multiple losses are the ultimate evidence that this was "not meant to be." Others approach their experience more scientifically, concluding that their infertility and their losses must all be part of the same problem. For them, the losses then become an extension of the ongoing battle, rather than a signal that they should accept defeat.

Above and beyond all else, victims of repeated miscarriage after infertility feel isolated. Where once they felt companionship in the world of infertility, they now feel different from their fellow infertility patients. Pregnancy, which was once the "promised land," is now a frightening and forboding territory that they have come to fear. Most try to grapple with the paradox of their situation: can they continue to seek the experience which has come to represent such pain and disappointment?

Grieving Repeated Pregnancy Losses

Couples who suffer repeated pregnancy losses after ART find that their grief expands exponentially. Most look back upon their first loss and remember it as a relatively benign (though of course it was not) event. By contrast, each subsequent loss feels increasingly malignant, as pregnancy becomes a terribly stressful, confusing and ultimately distressing experience.

The grief process in repeated pregnancy loss is especially complicated because it is often on-going. If one loss follows another—or if they are interspersed with periods of infertility—there is no time for recovery. Unlike couples who suffer one loss—be it early or late—and who take active steps to honor and commemorate that loss, victims of repeated pregnancy loss after infertility may cope by allowing the losses to almost blend together.

It is as though it would take too much energy to fully grieve each and every loss, leaving little reserve for continued efforts.

Ectopic Pregnancy

Ectopic pregnancy, pregnancy that occurs somewhere other than the uterus—most often in the fallopian tube—is a rare, though traumatic experience, occurring up to 5% of the time after an ART procedure. Not only does it mean the loss of a pregnancy, but it is also physically painful, often prolonged in its resolution, and it forces a couple to delay renewed efforts at conception. Having one ectopic pregnancy puts a woman at increased risk of another, though the risk is still very slim that it will happen again. However, women who have gone through such an ordeal are often terrified that it will be repeated. Some medical facts can help people get a better handle on the experience.

Medical Facts

Ectopic pregnancy is rare in the general population; only an estimated one percent of pregnancies are ectopic. Of these, the vast majority (probably 90 to 95%) occur in the fallopian tubes. The remaining ten percent can occur in the cervix or the abdominal cavity, or an embryo can attach to an ovary. An ectopic pregnancy constitutes a medical emergency. If it is caught early, before rupturing, it may be treated by medical or surgical intervention. Once it ruptures, emergency surgery is required to remove the fallopian tube.

The fact that ectopic pregnancy occurs more often in an ART pregnancy is surprising to many people. Because *in vitro* fertilization bypasses the fallopian tubes, many assume the embryo cannot possibly lodge there. However, if an embryo is placed in a portion of the uterus near where it meets the fallopian tube, it can migrate up into it and become trapped inside the tube, especially if the tube is damaged or malformed.

Although some women who experience ectopic pregnancies following ART treatment have known tubal blockages, which are the most likely cause of their ectopic pregnancies, others are thought to have clear tubes. This group includes women who turned to the ARTs because of unexplained infertility or because of a male factor and still ended up with an ectopic pregnancy. When this happens, they are understandably confused. Most are quite startled to learn that ART treatment, in and of itself, put them at slightly increased risk for an ectopic pregnancy.

Reproductive endocrinologists have several explanations for why ectopic pregnancy is more common in infertile women, especially those using the ARTs. One is that many women who turn to ART treatment do so because they have tubal disease, which might make the embryo more susceptible to migrating there. Another possible explanation is that fertility medications alter the hormonal environment of the fallopian tubes, making it more likely that an embryo will implant there following a GIFT procedure. In addition, since there is often more than one embryo transferred in IVF, or several eggs transferred in GIFT, the odds increase for an embryo to lodge in the fallopian tubes.

Because ectopic pregnancy is rare, fertile women who conceive without difficulty are seldom alerted to the possibility. Some may suddenly find themselves in excruciating pain before they even know they are pregnant. Others may suspect pregnancy but have no idea that an embryo can implant outside the uterus. Both groups, as well as those who may be somewhat more prepared for the possibility of an ectopic pregnancy, are often startled to find themselves en route to or coming out of emergency surgery. Pregnancy has suddenly turned into a life-threatening condition.

The Difficulty of Diagnosis

Because IVF and other high-tech patients are carefully monitored via ultrasonography, ectopic pregnancies that are the result of the ARTS are generally diagnosed early. This is almost always an advantage, since early diagnosis can save the tube as well as spare the patient some of the physical and emotional trauma. However, there are some instances in which it is difficult to diagnose an ectopic pregnancy, even with close monitoring:

- Blood HCG levels that remain low or rise irregularly can indicate an ectopic pregnancy, as well as an impending miscarriage. However, blood levels may be ambiguous. When this happens, the patient is usually monitored more closely, but even then, several days may elapse before it is clear whether the pregnancy is ectopic.
- Pregnancies in the proximal portion of the tube (the part closest to the uterus) cause early tubal rupture. This area, the isthmus, is more muscular and does not distend as well as the midportion of the tube, thus making it more vulnerable to rupture. Even close monitoring may not identify the pregnancy as ectopic in time to avoid rupture.
- There may be more than one implantation site in the tube or a simultaneous intrauterine and ectopic pregnancy in which the ectopic pregnancy was not found because the uterine pregnancy was obvious. In this, case hormone levels would probably be rising appropriately, obscuring the problem.
- Physicians and patients usually base their calculations about what the hormone levels should be on the timing of the GIFT or IVF procedure. However, physicians know that sometimes delayed implantation occurs, and they may assume the laboratory numbers are slightly off but that the pregnancy is probably fine.
- Since gastrointestinal and ovarian symptoms are common after ovulation induction and can mimic ectopic pregnancy, it is difficult for physicians to make a differential diagnosis based on a woman's physical discomfort alone.
- Although bleeding may occur with an ectopic pregnancy, it is not uncommon for women to bleed early in normal pregnancy. Some mistake this bleeding for either their menses or, if they know they are pregnant, for breakthrough bleeding, perhaps indicating an impending miscarriage. This may delay the diagnosis of an ectopic pregnancy.
- Some patients who develop acute pain are rushed to an emergency room and seen by a physician (probably not an obstetrician) who completely misses the diagnosis. Although ectopic pregnancy is a common

cause of acute abdominal pain in women of childbearing years and should be suspected in infertility patients (whether or not they are known to be pregnant), some physicians do miss the diagnosis.

The intense pain of a ruptured ectopic pregnancy and its rapid onset are some other reasons why it is such an upsetting experience. Women report finding themselves in sudden and debilitating pain. The degree of this pain, together with the fact that its origins may have been misdiagnosed or dismissed, intensifies the crisis.

Women who have had ectopic pregnancies and later return to treatment have remarked that they will never forget the pain. Some say that it makes them feel ambivalent about becoming pregnant again; they long for a baby but are terrified that the pregnancy will be another ectopic one. They may postpone treatment until they feel more equipped to deal with this possibility.

Treatment

Ectopic pregnancy can be treated surgically or medically or by both methods. No matter which method is used, however, the treatment can add to the trauma of the experience. Women and their husbands are often startled by the urgency with which surgery is presented to them, especially when it may follow hours, or even days in which the seriousness of their condition was not recognized. Many are confused and angry when they feel that doctors suddenly turn from minimizing their problem to indicating that they are in a life-threatening condition.

Medically, an ectopic pregnancy is treated with chemotherapy, commonly methotrexate. This news can be shocking to a couple who associate chemotherapy solely with cancer. However, chemotherapy is an effective nonsurgical, and hence less invasive, treatment for ectopic pregnancy (it is used to shrink—and eventually eliminate—an embryo that has implanted in a tube). Unfortunately, recovery can be especially protracted, and patients sometimes require several weeks of monitoring. It is also not uncommon for pregnancy hormone levels to decline slowly or incompletely and for patients to require a redosing of medications. This prolonged treatment and surveillance can be very stressful for a woman who wants to end a traumatic ordeal.

Surgical treatment of ectopic pregnancy is also traumatic, especially for those who have only recently gone through oocyte retrieval in an IVF procedure or a laparoscopy for a GIFT procedure. Even women whose ectopic pregnancies were diagnosed early, making their surgery less emergent, are distressed to find themselves back in the operating room.

Prognosis

The degree of risk of a subsequent ectopic pregnancy depends on the original diagnosis and on how the first ectopic was treated. Physicians estimate that up to ten percent of women who have had one ectopic pregnancy will have another. However, women who lost a tube when the ectopic pregnancy ruptured and have a healthy remaining tube may be at less risk for a second ectopic than those who have two partially damaged tubes remaining. Some women in this latter group may wonder why their doctors bothered to save either tube, since the surgery may have left them at increased risk for another ectopic pregnancy.

Feelings

Women undergoing the ARTS are usually aware of the possibility of an ectopic pregnancy. Those who spend any time around an infertility clinic may hear from other patients about their experiences with ectopic pregnancies, especially when those pregnancies may have caused or contributed to further tubal disease. However, those who do not have tubal disease may not realize that the treatments they are undergoing put them at an increased risk. When these women are confronted with an ectopic pregnancy, they may be confused, especially after under- going IVF. It is difficult to understand how embryos that were placed carefully in the uterus could end up in the tubes.

When ART leads to an ectopic pregnancy, patients can feel doubly punished: not only have they lost a much wanted pregnancy but they now know they have a problem that seriously limits their treatment options. Some, who hoped they could return to the less costly and invasive intrauterine inseminations, or possibly become pregnant on their own, may now learn that this is no longer an option. And even IVF—with it's ability to by-pass their tubes—offers them limited protection from an ectopic pregnancy. Sadly, some who tried ART—at least in part to avoid looking back with regret—now wonder whether they have actually caused additional fertility problems.

Whatever the cause of an ectopic pregnancy, couples are devastated by the experience, especially after treatment with the ARTs. They have gone from one medical ordeal to another, usually in the space of a few weeks. It seems doubly unfair that they went through so much to create embryos, only to have them implant in the wrong place.

Grieving an Ectopic Pregnancy

Grief following an ectopic pregnancy takes many forms, depending in part upon whether there was a known tubal problem prior to ART treatment and upon whether the ectopic pregnancy was removed surgically or through chemotherapy—or both.

We have found that most people are so startled after an ectopic pregnancy that their grief begins as a period of emotional turmoil. "How did this happen?" (especially if there was no history of tubal disease and if IVF or GIFT were being used to address another infertility problem). "What can we *possibly* do now?" (especially if there was a known tubal problem and IVF was being used to by-pass it.) "How could I have put myself/put my wife in a life threatening position?" These —and countless other—questions plague those who are trying to find a way to move beyond an ectopic pregnancy.

Because there is so much upheaval following an ectopic pregnancy, the loss of the baby may be temporarily obscured. Couples are focusing on the recovery from surgery or on the ordeal of methotrexate. For many, it is months before they feel confident of a full physical recovery and even then, there are difficult decisions to be made about returning to treatment. Hence, it may take several months for the actual loss of the baby to hit. When it does, people often feel a powerful sense of sadness. Many perceive the baby they lost as a potentially strong young being who simply had the misfortune to end up in the wrong place.

Loss in Multiple Pregnancy

Since any woman who has more than one embryo or more than one egg transferred is at risk for multiple gestation, she is usually followed closely by blood tests and ultrasounds to determine how the pregnancy is progressing and the number of embryos that have implanted. The purpose of the ultrasounds is not only to determine how many sacs are in her uterus but also to rule out that any embryos have implanted outside her uterus. Loss in multiple pregnancy can occur in various ways.

Early Loss in Multiple Pregnancy

A pregnancy in which embryos are discovered both inside and outside the uterus (usually in the fallopian tube) is termed heteroectopic. If found early, it is often possible to save the uterine pregnancy since the ectopic pregnancy can be surgically removed without disturbing the intrauterine pregnancy. If the ectopic pregnancy ruptures (usually not the case in ART pregnancies due to close monitoring), the tube is removed and the patient is followed.

Another kind of early pregnancy loss occurs when early ultrasounds reveal two or more gestational sacs but later ultrasounds fail to detect heartbeats in all of them. Frequently the sac that does not have a developing fetus in it vanishes on its own. Little is usually made of these experiences, and couples sometimes express relief when they occur, especially if the "lost" embryo was a third (or fourth) one. But it is common for couples also to feel a great deal of sadness. Viewing on ultrasound an embryo (or two) without a heartbeat and at the same time seeing at least one embryo that does have a heartbeat can be both an upsetting and a joyous experience. Parents-to-be are thrilled to view an on-going pregnancy on ultrasound but saddened by the loss of a twin or a triplet.

Some parents comment that it is not until much later, perhaps after the birth of the surviving babies, that they experience a sense of loss. Some say that years later they will occasionally look at their twins and wonder what the third would have been like had the embryo survived. If they have a single child, they may be even more likely to wonder about the twin.

In other instances, two or more sacs are identified, all with heartbeats, but on a subsequent ultrasound, one or more heartbeats are undetectable. This loss, which occurs in non ART pregnancies as well, but may not be identified because there is rarely the frequent early monitoring, is known as the vanishing twin. It is very upsetting for the expectant parents, especially if the doctor has not prepared them for this possibility. However, even those who know that losing a twin is always a possibility still experience varying degrees of sadness and loss, coupled with a fear that they will also lose the healthy fetus.

Although the loss of a multiple gestation is frequently discovered by ultrasound, there are times when an actual miscarriage occurs without warning, accompanied by bleeding and cramping. When this happens, couples become terrified, assuming that they are losing the entire pregnancy. This is sometimes the case; however, many women do go on to successfully carry and give birth to the one or more remaining fetusses.

Late Loss in Multiple Pregnancy

Some losses in multiple pregnancies come in the second and even third trimesters, when the parents are attached to each of the fetuses and to the idea of parenting twins or triplets. Although the vast majority of twins (and triplets to a lesser extent) survive past viability, prenatal testing and monitoring sometimes reveals that a fetus has died in utero, or that it will not survive long past birth because of congenital problems. In these instances, a couple is told that the pregnancy must be carried as long as possible for the sake of the other(s). Women then find that their joy has turned to anguish as they must carry a dead or dying fetus for several weeks.

When a couple experiences a later loss in a multiple pregnancy, family, friends, and even physicians frequently fail to understand the depth of their loss. Instead of acknowledging how painful it is to lose a child who is so wanted, they focus on the well-being of the surviving twin(s). The expectation is that the couple will feel so grateful to have an ongoing pregnancy that they will be able to easily recover from the death of their other baby.

The Center for Loss in Multiple Birth (CLIMB) is a support network for parents throughout the United States and Canada who have experienced the loss of one or more fetuses in a pregnancy. In its newsletter, CLIMB members chronicle the pain they have experienced on losing one or more multiples. Their writings emphasize that the survival of one or more babies may mitigate their pain but it does not erase it. Rather, their enduring feelings of loss make the survival of another child bittersweet. One CLIMB member stated, "Two out of three or one out of two is NOT good when it's your baby who has died." Following is a brief excerpt from an essay by Sandy Lee, a CLIMB member, that appeared in the newsletter:

> We had visions of watching Erin smile while riding her tricycle down the street. We had visions of her going to the prom (after carefully checking out her date!). We had visions of watching Erin and Kristen growing up together. So it's with unfulfilled hopes and dreams for this little girl and "our twins" that we grieve....Taking Kristen out in her stroller, we think about the twin stroller we almost bought. When the three of us drive off for a ride in the car, we often feel as though we're leaving someone behind.[18]

Jean Kollantai, president and founder of CLIMB, notes that CLIMB members often go through a great deal medically and emotionally with their surviving child(ren), who frequently require lengthy stays in the neonatal intensive care unit for medical problems that may result from prematurity. These problems vary in nature and severity, but often involve respiratory difficulties. Parents may find themselves taking their children home sequentially, hence coping with the challenges of having one—or more—newborns at home and one—or more—newborns in the hospital. Kollantai adds that this experience, difficult for all parents, is made much more painful by the previous infertility, since people have already endured so much loss and disappointment before even becoming pregnant. She notes, also, that many new parents of multiples have lost one or more babies along the way. Sadly, some of the babies who survive are medically fragile or handicapped, adding to the tremendous parenting challenge and providing another ongoing reminder of loss. Kollantai observes that these parents face a complex grieving process that includes mourning the loss of their special status as parents of twins or multiples.

Loss of an Entire Multiple Pregnancy

Couples are not always prepared for the difficulties that women can encounter carrying a multiple pregnancy. Even some mothers who are in the care of highly skilled obstetricians are grief stricken to find that they cannot carry their babies long enough. All too often, multiples are born so early that none survives. When this happens, the loss is shattering. Often it follows a long, difficult period of bed rest, as well as the use of medication to postpone labor.

The CLIMB newsletter is filled with testimonies to the attachment that parents feel for their lost babies. The essays that describe the collision of joy and sorrow experienced by those who have lost one or more babies and have given birth to a twin are deeply moving. The accounts that tell of the death of both twins or of all triplets speak to the overwhelming grief of couples whose children are with them for too brief a time. Most of these couples lose their babies in the late second or early third trimester of pregnancy. One woman found these words to describe her loss:

When we found out that I was carrying twins, it felt like our wish for "instant family" had come true. I had had a very hard time with the fertility drugs. even to the point of being hospitalized for hyperstimulation, and so we felt especially grateful to be able to put the "getting pregnant" part behind us. Little did we know the difficulties and the pain that would follow.

Our daughters were born at 24 weeks and each lived for just over an hour. During that small window of time, we tried to give them the love of a lifetime. When they died, it felt like our whole family had died. All our dreams. All our hopes. All our expectations. All our children gone before their time.

Kollantai has observed that parents who lose both or all of their babies often feel angry at the technology that was successful in helping them conceive their babies but was unsuccessful in saving them. Parents also feel guilty for having wanted children so much that they resorted to using high tech treatments, which put them at greater risk for a multiple gestation, which in turn put them at greater risk for pregnancy loss. Although the trauma of this experience makes it easy for them to conclude that they were "not meant to have children," most go on to try again. Kollantai offers the following explanation for this phenomenon: "Seeing their own offspring for the first time, even though tiny and dying, is the experience of a lifetime and propels many into further efforts to conceive."

Grieving a Partial Loss in Multiple Gestation

Couples who suffer the death of one or more of their babies in a multiple pregnancy usually find that others do not understand or appreciate their loss. Instead, people tend to say, "You're lucky to have ended up with a healthy baby" or, worse, "Imagine how difficult it would have been if there had been two (or three)!" Couples need to remind themselves that these comments, although intensely painful, are usually not ill intended; others want to help them to feel better and believe that these remarks are supportive. Moreover, some family members and friends may be unaware of what it means to lose a fetus in multiple pregnancy.

To the extent that they feel able, parents can share their grief. As long as they are grieving the loss of the baby who dies, they may need to explain to others that the survival of one fetus does not erase the loss of another. They may wish to explain that if a triplet dies in utero and two survive, the two are surviving triplets, not twins. Similarly, the single baby that survives when a twin dies in utero may actually remain a twin in his or her parents' eyes.

Parents need to seek support from others who do understand and to take all the time and the opportunities they need to grieve for their baby— for "our twins" or "our triplets." This is seldom easy, both because parents are busy caring for their surviving baby and because their family and friends are likely to take a "let's move on" approach. However, we have found that parents who are able to grieve enjoy their newborn and find meaningful ways to remember that child who did not survive. Sometimes it helps is to set aside some time or times during the day to feel sad. It can be planned, for example, when the baby sleeps or when someone else is caring for him or her.

Since most of the people in the couple's lives will want to celebrate the arrival of the child who survived, rather than grieve the child who did not, caregivers can play an especially important role in helping couples. Those who participated in their medical care knew, first hand, that other babies were expected and they should acknowledge this. Rather than avoiding the subject for fear of opening a wound, caregivers should be open and direct, aware that the parents will appreciate someone's thoughtful acknowledgment of their lost child.

Grieving the Loss of an Entire Pregnancy

Couples who lose an entire multiple pregnancy, especially when the loss occurs late in the pregnancy, often feel as though they have lost their family. They realize that the instant family they may have joked about was a reality to them. They had come to expect and anticipate the juggling that comes with twins or triplets and instead feel a huge void in their lives.

When the couple feels ready to attempt another pregnancy, it is important that their goal not be another multiple gestation. Although the arrival of two or three healthy babies would have been a joyous event, they have learned the difficulty of carrying a multiple pregnancy. More important, they need to be prepared for a singleton pregnancy (or no pregnancy, since the odds per cycle are always against success, even when the couple has been pregnant previously).

It is not uncommon for couples who have lost all their babies in a multiple gestation to consider themselves parents and to refer to themselves in this way. Since much of the world will not know or understand this, grieving parents are vulnerable to feelings of isolation and even rejection. Sadly, some find that when others cannot understand the magnitude of their grief, they withdraw and seem to avoid the couple—or the subject.

Stillbirth

Stillbirth after infertility is the unthinkable. How can a pregnancy, hard earned and now well established, end in fetal death? Sometimes there are medical explanations; rarely are there ways of understanding this trauma emotionally. Stillbirth after infertility is the ultimate proof to infertile couples that life can be unfair.

Medical Facts

A pregnancy loss after twenty weeks gestation is frequently referred to as a stillbirth. However, in this section we use the term stillbirth to refer to those instances in which the death of the infant occurs after the point of viability—in the third trimester.

Stillbirth, or intrauterine fetal demise, is relatively rare in a singleton pregnancy, occurring in fewer than one in 100 deliveries.[19] Nonetheless, there are infertile women who have ongoing healthy pregnancies following IVF or GIFT, only to have them end tragically. One medical explanation for stillbirth is that there was some malfunction in the umbilical cord, resulting in a loss of oxygen to the fetus. This may occur late in pregnancy or, perhaps even more tragically, at delivery. If the unbilical cord is compressed during the delivery, or if it becomes wrapped around the baby's neck, it can cut off the oxygen supply and result in the death of the infant.

Placental problems can also lead to intrauterine death. If the placenta is implanted too low in the uterus (placenta previa), it can separate prematurely and cause the mother to hemorrhage. Alternatively, if the baby is postmature, the placenta may begin to malfunction, thereby depriving the baby of oxygen.

Other possible causes of stillbirth include conditions in the mother such as toxemia, diabetes or high blood pressure. Each can compromise the flow of nutrients to the baby. Or, if the mother's water breaks prematurely, the baby may contract a life threatening infection.

Sadly, no explanation can be found for many stillbirths. Grieving parents are then left with the additional burden of unanswered questions, questions which are likely to haunt them if and when they attempt another pregnancy.

Feelings

When a pregnancy goes to completion and then is lost, there are many *what ifs*. Grieving parents look back and wonder what they or their care-takers could have done differently. Could another obstetrician have provided better care? Should they have called the doctor or gone to the hospital earlier? Was there anything damaging about either their attitude toward the pregnancy or their activities? These unanswerable questions and self-blame are very painful, especially in the months following the loss.

As much as people will look back and scrutinize their own actions and judgment, they will also feel anger toward their physician, nurses, and other caregivers. They may wonder if something could have been done to pre-vent this devastating loss. It is also common to feel angry at God. In this age of scientific advances and medical miracles, it is difficult to compre-hend how this tragic event could have happened at all, especially to them, when they had already been through so much.

Grieving following Stillbirth

The grieving process following a stillbirth after infertility is inevitably lengthy. Even those couples who have been remarkably resilient through-out the infertility process, can feel crippled by a stillbirth. Many find it difficult to return to work, to resume social ties, to re-enter the world. In the months following their loss they are reluctant to put themselves in situations which might confront them with babies or pregnant women. Their loss has been too devastating and has left them feeling profoundly empty and vulnerable.

Sadly, friends and family, at a loss for words of comfort, may withdraw from the couple who is griefstricken after a stillbirth. Unable to find words that honor the lost child, or to acknowledge their profound sorrow, it may seem easier to avoid the grieving couple altogether. Unfortunately this abandonment usually intensifies their feelings. By contrast, couples who receive understanding and acknowledgement of their loss, seem to have an easier time healing.

A woman whose son was born at twenty-nine weeks and lived only a short time spoke to us about how much it meant to her when others came to his funeral. She saw their attendance as acknowledgement that her son was a person, whose life, though brief, had meaning. There was nothing that others could do to replace her loss, but their presence at the funeral served to ease her sorrow.

The Role of Caregivers Following Pregnancy Loss

Caregivers—especially those in ART treatment centers—play important roles at the time of pregnancy loss and in the minutes, hours, days, weeks and months following a loss or losses.

The first role that caregivers play is to be available to couples as they are experiencing loss or threatened loss. This is usually a time of great confusion, with people needing information as well as considerable support. It is crucial that caregivers remember how exquisitely sensitive patients will be to each question, comment, suggestion. Not only will they search words and glances for clues about their prognosis, but they will also take recommendations extremely seriously. Caregivers must tread cautiously because their actions and reactions can have so much impact.

Another reason why it is crucial that caregivers within an ART treatment make themselves available to couples has to do with issues of success and failure. Couples who have experienced pregnancy loss report feeling like failures and some say that their caregivers contributed to this sense of failure by avoiding them. Although what they may actually be observing is a caregiver's personal sense of sadness at the loss, some feel that they are being abandoned in favor of more successful patients.

Caregivers wear several hats during and following pregnancy loss. In addition to offering support and education, they also bear witness to lives lost before they begin. This is a significant role because, as witnesses, they are in a position to acknowledge the meaning of a short life, something extremely important to grieving parents. This bearing witness takes many forms. Sometimes it means writing a condolence note after an early loss. Other times it means helping a couple to hold a stillborn baby at a time when they might otherwise try to avoid it. It also means taking pictures of stillborn babies—pictures which will be treasured in years to come. And sometimes it means assisting with funeral or burial plans.

Another role of caregivers involves offering guidance. Whether it be a couple who has had a stillbirth and does not understand the importance of seeing their baby or a couple who has just learned that their cherished pregnancy is ectopic and must be terminated through surgery or chemotherapy, caregivers are dealing with people who are in crisis. A significant component of this crisis is the lack of information that people have—they find themselves in an experience that is entirely unfamiliar to them and they need guidance traversing it.

In addition to the general roles of caregivers after all pregnancy loss, there are specific issues that arise depending upon the nature of the loss. To the extent that the loss also involves a physical crisis, as it does in ectopic pregnancy, caregivers must arrange for appropriate nursing and medical care. All too often couples in the throws of a pregnancy loss find themselves in the most uninviting settings—a busy emergency room, an obstetrician's waiting room or a maternity floor.

It is important that caregivers remind themselves that they have two patients, not one. Although the pregnant woman is the one experiencing the physical crisis, her partner also undergoes loss. Sometimes partners are left feeling like outsiders. Their loss is not always acknowledged, nor are their fears for the safety and well-being of their wives.

Caregivers must remind themselves that their role with grieving parents does not end when people leave the hospital or physician's office. The days and weeks following a loss are a time in which people feel very vulnerable and during which caregivers can plan a crucial role in healing. It is during this time that caregivers can help people to grieve their loss and to begin to move on. They play an important role in helping people determine when they are ready to return to treatment, as well as to help some decide that it is best for them to pursue other options. They also help people maintain a sense of connection to their treatment program, something which is critical during a period of grieving. Without this connection, couples are likely to feel more alone and possibly, they may even rush back to treatment prematurely to regain or secure this connection.

Caregivers also help grieving couples navigate the difficult landscape of dates following a loss. Not only will people have anniversary reactions a year following a loss, but they will also have feelings about an approaching due date or the anniversary of the time they conceived. It is important that caregivers serve as guides, acknowleding the importance of each of these markers and normalizing people's feelings and reactions to them.

Loss in multiple pregnancy requires special attention from caregivers. When a couple loses part of a pregnancy, caregivers must acknowledge this loss, but also help couples prepare for a different pregnancy than they were expecting. This may be especially difficult when a couple has lost a triplet, since it is tempting to focus on the "good news"—it will be an easier pregnancy for them to carry safely to term. Nonetheless a real loss has occurred and must be acknowledged. Caregivers must often take the lead in this acknowledgement since ART couples are not clear that they are justified in their sadness.

When a couple has lost an entire multiple pregnancy their grief is for the loss of their babies as well as for the loss of the specialness of multiples. Caregivers need acknowledge this because this can be another form of "dis-enfranchised grief"—people do not believe they have a right to feel sad that they are not going to experience the attention and recognition that comes when you are the parent of twins or triplets. It is crucial that caregivers help them with this grief so that it does not interfere with future treatment efforts.

The pregnancy losses we have described testify to the depth and breadth of life's unfairness. It is difficult to comprehend how a couple can go through so much to establish a pregnancy and then endure the excruciating pain of losing it. Yet we have witnessed—over and over again—remarkable resilience. Even after devastating—seemingly crippling losses—most couples find ways to move forward, carrying painful, though precious memories.

Pregnancy after ART is complicated and it can be filled with an array of challenges. Although we have gone to great lengths to identify many of these challenges, it is crucial that couples maintain the following perspective: the majority of clinical pregnancies after ART result in the births of healthy infants. These children, so long in coming, are welcomed into hearts and homes truly ready to celebrate their arrival.

CHAPTER
4

*C*hanging Directions

When is enough, enough? This is the question that tortures and confounds today's infertile couples. Many wonder how they will ever decide when it is time to stop the quest for a bio-genetic child when there are always new and ever-expanding reproductive options. For unlike those who struggled with infertility in earlier times, when there were fewer treatments available, couples today are hardpressed to say, "We've tried everything. Now we know that we've done our best"

As we have seen throughout the first third of this book, couples who become involved in the ARTs find themselves in a place that they never anticipated. Having first approached parenthood with the assumption—in most instances—that children would come easily, many were surprised and confused when "doing what comes naturally" did not work. With fear, caution and sadness, they eventually made their way out of the bedroom and into a doctor's office. Later, many moved on to more high tech, state-of-the-art, treatments—treatments which were impersonal, intrusive, costly, time consuming and sometimes, physically painful. With fortitude and hope, couples using ART committed themselves to doing whatever it took to have a child.

For many couples, the journey through ART treatment, though difficult and unexpected, proves rewarding. Some try one IVF or GIFT cycle and go home with a baby (or babies) nine months later. Others travel a bumpier road—through failed cycles and pregnancy losses—but eventually accomplish their goal. For each of these couples, the ARTs are miraculous.

But what of the other couples? What happens to those who also travel through the treacherous terrain of high tech treatment, but who do not end up with a successful pregnancy? How and when do they say, "We have come to the end of this road and we are ready now to travel down a different pathway."? Living in a time of rapid and promising medical advances, how do these couples arrive at a point where they can move on without regret?

Guidance from the Mind

Prior to the development of IVF, many infertile couples were given a definitive infertility diagnosis: there was virtually no chance they would conceive or carry a pregnancy on their own and their options for building a family were limited to donor insemination or adoption. High technology treatment, designed to overcome even the most severe and intractable problems, has left many previously "hopeless" couples in a gray area of uncertainty.

Physicians, whose knowledge of human reproduction allows them to make predictions about outcome, recognize their own predictive limitations. This awareness, together with rapidly improving and expanding treatment possibilities, makes many physicians reluctant to ever say "never." Hence the decision to end treatment usually rests with the couple who must become well versed about their medical situation. Though, as we shall see shortly, objective information is not the only consideration.

Among the key determinants in any couple's decision to remain in treatment or to leave it are their treatment opportunities. Depending on their geographical location, financial or insurance situation, diagnosis, prognosis, treatment history, and age, they will have more or fewer treatment options available to them.

Treatment History

The length of time that a couple has been infertile and the success or failure of past treatment efforts influence their feelings about when to end treatment, regardless of their diagnosis. Most couples can put their lives on hold and subject their relationship to the stress of infertility for only so long. Most women are willing to undergo physically invasive and painful procedures only for a limited time. This length of time varies considerably among couples but eventually most find that they are running out of energy. Their exhaustion is the result of their experiences and is not necessarily reflective of prognosis or duration of infertility. Some couples stay in treatment upwards of ten years; others stop after two or three.

Sometimes couples may want to stop treatment but are reluctant to do so because their physician assures them they still have a good chance of conceiving. This reassurance is confusing. On the one hand, it is wonderful news. After all, their physician is the "expert". On the other hand, they feel exhausted and depleted by their past treatments. Although their physician's optimism is encouraging, they wonder how they can reconcile two conflicting perspectives: pregnancy is possible, but their energy to pursue it is diminishing.

Couples who have had a pregnancy as a result of ART treatment and have subsequently suffered one or more miscarriages are especially uncertain about whether to stop treatment. They often feel saddened and defeated by their experiences and long to avoid further suffering, but at the same time, their pregnancy offered hope. They may have been told that the pregnancy loss was a random event and that they should feel encouraged by the knowledge that they can become pregnant. Those who have suffered two or more pregnancy losses are in a more difficult situation. They do not know if they can become pregnant or, if they do, whether they can carry a baby.

Couples coming to the end of treatment may attempt to set a deadline on their efforts to have a baby: if they are not pregnant by the new year, by next Mother's Day, or some other defined date they will move on to an alternative. Others set a limit on the number of IVF attempts they are willing to do, or on how many more months (or years) they will continue treatment, promising themselves that they will move on once they reach that designated point. A deadline can help couples regain a sense of control, especially if they recognize that they can always alter it if their medical situation or their feelings change.

Age

Because the woman's age plays a significant role in fertility, many couples focus on age when they try to determine whether enough is enough. Women in their twenties or very early thirties and their husbands sometimes fear that their treatment could go on forever. With all the dramatic advances in reproductive medicine and years of potential fertility ahead of them, there may always be something new to try. Some feel torn between their desire to stop treatment and move on and their awareness that they have not tried everything. From a medical perspective they are not pressured by time. One way that some younger couples solve this dilemma is to decide to abandon efforts temporarily, taking an alternative path to parenthood, but planning to return to treatment in the future. Others abandon the effort totally, never intending to turn back.

Women in their late thirties or early forties and their partners usually have a different outlook. They may be exhausted by their treatment efforts but know that this is their last opportunity to bear a child together. Faced with declining fertility, they feel that they had better push themselves now.

Often women identify a maximum age for having children although they may revise that number from time to time. For example, a woman may have assumed that she would have had her first child by age thirty. When she married at twenty-nine, she moved her anticipated childbearing age upward, perhaps to thirty-three or thirty-four. Upon encountering infertility, it may have moved still upward. But not all women who specify a maximum age are comfortable revising it, believing that it is unwise for them to have a child past a certain age. When they reach their targeted age, they conclude that it is time to move on.

The situation for older women is confounded by the fact that their chance for a successful outcome, whatever their diagnosis, is limited. They wonder if it makes sense to take powerful medications or to undergo invasive, uncomfortable procedures when their odds are so poor. They are also aware that age brings with it an increased chance of miscarriage—sometimes estimated to be as high as 40 to 50% in women over forty.

When a woman is in her mid-thirties and has been attempting pregnancy for an extended time, the decision to end treatment can be even more perplexing. Unlike younger women, who can pursue other options and return to treatment a few years hence, women in their mid-thirties know that stopping treatment now probably means ending it forever. If they decide at some point in the future to try again, it will be with diminished expectations of success.

Although most couples focus on the age of the woman in deciding how long to pursue treatment (and her age is reproductively much more significant than her partner's) some couples pay attention to the age of the man as well, for social rather than medical reasons. For example, if the husband is significantly older than his wife, they may decide that in fairness to the child—and to each other—he should not be past a certain age when his wife conceives a child.

More so than in the past, there are couples in which the woman is older than her partner, and her husband's relative youth can influence treatment efforts. Some couples try longer for a pregnancy than they might if he were the same age as (or older than) his wife, feeling secure that the child will have the benefits of a young father. One forty-one-year-old woman whose husband was thirty-one commented that she had never felt odd about being an older wife until she began dealing with infertility. Although her husband reassured her many times that he did not marry her in order to have children, nevertheless, she felt she was letting him down and feared he might leave her for a younger woman.

An increasing number of older women are considering ovum donation. While it is crucial that no one pursue this parenting alternative in order to please a younger spouse, there are women in their early forties who decide to shift from attempting conception with their own eggs to attempting pregnancy with donor eggs (see Chapter 6).

Availability and Accessibility of Treatment

In 1995 there were 281 ART clinics in the United States reporting to SART (the Society for Advanced Reproductive Technologies). SART requires all clinics performing over 100 ART cycles in a calender year to report their statistics to them. Couples who live near these clinics (most of which are located in major metropolitan areas) can seek or continue treatment without having to travel long distances or relocate temporarily. By contrast, couples who live far from treatment centers face significant decisions about travel each time they try another cycle or a new treatment. The toll that travel takes on their energy, their relationship, and certainly their careers, is a major factor in the decision of many to end treatment.

Just as they looked at financial considerations prior to trying treatment, couples re-visit them when deciding whether to continue efforts or move on. Those who have no insurance coverage and who want to preserve a "nest-egg" for adoption, may draw a financial line beyond which they will not go. Ironically, those who have insurance coverage for ART and who are daunted by the high costs of adoption may stay in treatment for a prolonged period of time.

Access to treatment may also be restricted by the policies of a particular program. Some IVF programs limit treatment to women under a certain age or to couples with certain types of infertility problems. Some programs refuse treatment to unmarried couples, lesbian couples, or single women, although such policies can probably be challenged as discriminatory.

Diagnosis and Prognosis

Couples focus on their diagnosis, and even more so, on their prognosis, when they face the question of when enough is enough. Physicians can be helpful to couples attempting to assess their chances for future success. Reviewing their diagnosis, the results of previous treatment, the treatment approaches that have already been tried, and their age can offer a couple a clearer sense of whether additional treatment is likely to prove worthwhile.

The physician's task involves challenges more difficult than trying to make a rational assessment of a couple's prognosis. Experience has taught every physician that infertility brings surprises and that sometimes the most hopeless situations bring unexpected success, while the ones that appear most promising may end in disappointment. Experience has also taught physicians that some couples are looking for guidance and permission to leave treatment, while others want their doctor to offer them yet another treatment opportunity. These factors and others cause many physicians to avoid the difficult topic of advising regarding discontinuing treatment.

Physicians who are able to discuss ending treatment often find that their patients appreciate the guidance. Some cautiously introduce the topic by asking a couple whether they have considered adoption or other alternatives to biological parenting, trying to determine from their response, whether they welcome the opportunity to discuss options. Couples may feel relieved by their physician's cautious approach and view his or her questions as evidence of caring about them. Moreover, these couples may long for some confirmation of their own growing sense that it is time to move on.

Sometimes couples feel that their physician is giving up on them when he or she mentions alternatives. Initially, this discussion can be upsetting, especially for those who feel a strong connection to their physician and suspect that they are being abandoned. Nevertheless, many couples come to appreciate their doctor's willingness to talk about adoption and realize, in retrospect, that his/her broaching the subject, although jolting, introduced them to the possibility of ending treatment. Moreover, their physician's mention of alternatives serves as an endorsement of these other options.

138

Guidance from the Heart

Most couples say that deciding to end treatment would be easier if a physician were to tell them that pregnancy was a hopeless goal. Such news, though devastating, would be clear and would offer them the opportunity for closure. But few couples are given such a definitive prognosis; most are forced to make a decision for themselves. They do so each in their own style and at their own pace. What is enough for one couple is too much for another and not enough for yet a third. Each couple must look deep into their hearts to determine what they need to do—or not do—to minimize future regrets. For although they may never have the bio-genetic child for whom they had hoped, in the end they will more easily reach resolution if they feel at peace with the amount of effort they committed to the process. The following considerations are subjective ones that are important for couples to think about in making their decision.

Feelings about Genetic Continuity

For some couples the decision about when to end treatment revolves around the feelings that one or both of them have about genetics. As we have seen—and will continue to see throughout this book—people have different feelings about genetic continuity and about the significance of parenting a child with whom they have a shared genetic connection. For some, genetic continuity forms the cornerstone of the parenting experience: without it, there is no compelling reason to raise children.

Since people have varying and often even conflicting perspectives regarding the significance of genes, each must examine his or her own feelings about this complex subject. Those with a powerful longing to pass on their genes will probably have difficulty ending their quest for a bio-genetic child. It may feel easier for them to remain in treatment—even with only bleak hope for success—than it is to try to let go of their longing. Those who seek a genetic connection, but are unable to carry the pregnancy might seek gestational care. Those who feel that a genetic connection is neither necessary for nor central to a satisfying parenting experience, move more easily to alternative paths to parenthood.

Partners may not be in agreement about the significance of genetic ties. Some focus on personal genetic continuity while others are moved by the desire to have a child that blends their genes with those of their partner. If the goal is personal genetic continuity more so than blending, an option that offers half a genetic connection may provide a resolution (especially if the person who cares most about personal genetic continuity is the fertile partner). However, in other instances, a couple may realize that pursuing an option that offers half a genetic connection is unwise for them. Included in this group are those in which the infertile partner has very strong longings for genetic continuity (and might envy or resent his/her partner having that opportunity), as well as those in which the fertile partner cares little about personal genetic continuity. In addition, because none of these second choices comes with a guarantee of success, some couples will decide against opting for an alternative that may bring further disappointment and loss.

Couples who decide to try adoption or a third party parenting option, whether it be donor insemination, ovum donation, surrogacy or gestation care, all face the possibility that they may confront the question of when is enough, enough, yet again.

The Nature of the Gamble

ART treatments demand enormous commitments of time, energy, and money. For some couples, the decision about when to end treatment revolves around their feelings about what it means to have committed such substantial resources to this effort. Some feel that having done so much, they cannot quit. Attempting pregnancy can begin to feel more like gambling than like medicine. One woman who was struggling with whether to try IVF for the fourth time stated, "Having a chance sounded good at first, but now it is beginning to feel like winning the lottery. It's beginning to sound like stuck."

Couples who find they cannot quit may be stuck for two reasons. Some feel that quitting would mean that all their efforts had been in vain. Only by remaining in treatment—and achieving success—will they feel their efforts were worthwhile. Others who feel that ending treatment is quitting prematurely view ART as much more of a gamble and feel that their odds of success increase the longer they remain in treatment. (In fact, IVF statistics indicate that the chances of pregnancy are equal for at least four cycles provided a couple produces viable embryos). Such couples wonder how they can end treatment when the next cycle might be the one that works.

There are also couples who, despite the disappointments they have endured, persist in believing that they will eventually be rewarded. They view their bad luck as time limited; if they continue a little while longer things will work out. These couples manage to keep a positive outlook throughout treatment, refusing to believe that life—or their faith—will let them down.

By contrast, still other couples look back on the time, effort, and money that they have committed to treatment and see it as evidence that enough is enough. These couples feel that they do have a great deal to show for their efforts; the thickness of their medical file is proof enough that they have done all they can. They perceive continued treatment efforts as a waste of valuable resources better spent on adoption or on another alternative path. Such couples know that one more cycle—or two or three—holds no guarantee that they will "hit the jackpot". In addition, their infertility experience has taught them that life is not always fair and that often those who have suffered the most are called upon to suffer again.

Avoidance of Grief

There are some couples who appear to be cycling indefinitely. Consciously they believe that persistence will eventually bring success. Unconsciously, however, they are avoiding grief and they stay in treatment because they are afraid to face feeling so vulnerable, knowing that a long mourning process awaits them. Patients who avoid their grief may be afraid that they will not be able to cope with life should they face the reality of being unable to bear children. Paradoxically, they remain stuck in the very treatments that perpetuate their sorrow and self-blame. They do so because each new cycle offers them some small kernel of renewed hope, and as long as they possess that kernel, they are able to avoid their loss.

Difficulty Saying Goodbye

Closely related to the difficulty that some couples have in facing the loss of their dream is the surprising sadness and fear that they often feel about saying good-bye to treatment efforts. We refer to the separations that occur when couples leave a treatment facility. They must say good-bye to the physicians and nurses to whom they feel attached and to their role as ART patients.

Although couples (and in particular women) know they will not miss unpleasant procedures and treatments, most realize they will miss their physicians and nurses. Having at times felt angry and disappointed with their caregivers, these couples may be puzzled to realize that they also feel attachment to them. Many are further perplexed when they recognize that they will miss being ART patients; it was not an identity that they sought for themselves, but most have mastered it.

Many couples do not say good-bye formally. Instead, they never make another appointment and try to walk away without looking back. They may be afraid that their caregivers will be disappointed with them or that the caregivers themselves will feel like failures. Sometimes they are correct.

Caregivers are not always able to help patients with the grief that accompanies saying good-bye. Some providers may feel their own sense of failure and disappointment; these are the patients for whom the miracle treatments have not worked. It can be tempting for physicians to suggest yet one more cycle, rather than acknowledge the sadness that comes at the end of an unsuccessful pursuit. Yet long-term infertility patients also feel relief when they decide to end treatment and we have found that patients consistently appreciate a physician's restraint and support at this time.

Caregivers who understand the sense of failure and disappointment that many couples feel upon ending treatment can help reduce such feelings by expressing positive sentiments about adoption or other alternatives, including the decision to remain child free. They can thus convey to their patients a clear sense that their decision marks a successful resolution to infertility.

Feelings about Alternatives

In the course of infertility treatment, many people identify a "light at the end of the tunnel." Recognizing that they may not succeed in having their first choice—a bio-genetic child—they look to alternatives. Most find that although they may not initially embrace the idea, they can imagine another pathway to parenthood—or a satisfying child-free life.

Individuals and couples have different feelings about the light at the end of the tunnel. These feelings are determined by their experience with a given option (i.e. a man or woman whose best friend was adopted may have very positive associations to this option,) as well as by their feelings about the significance of pregnancy and genetic continuity. What is most important in deciding to move on is that a couple be able to reach agreement about this second choice. For some couples, this is relatively easy; for others, it seems nearly impossible.

Some couples are unable to identify an alternative second choice, but most can engage in this emotionally charged and complex decision making process and eventually arrive at a decision. Many are relieved to discover that they were never as far apart as they had initially feared: each needed to be able to make the decision at his or her own pace. Additionally, couples tend to balance each other: one member may be able to move forward with more determination because the other is cautiously holding back. Similarly, the partner who expresses reluctance about moving on may be doing so because he or she has confidence that they will still continue to move forward as a couple. Sometimes they switch positions at a later date. It is common for couples considering adoption, for example, to take turns advocating for this parenting option. When one feels enthusiastic about it, the other may think of several reasons why it is an untenable option. Later, each may change his or her viewpoint. In short, delicate balancing often occurs as couples prepare to move beyond ART treatment, and this balancing can be a necessary part of deciding that enough is enough.

In examining their second choices, some couples focus their attention on their feelings about the pregnancy experience, while others look more carefully at genetics or at the social aspects of parenting. Couples who feel strongly about experiencing a pregnancy together, even if it will not result in their full genetic child, may look more carefully at donor insemination or ovum donation—options that offer a shared pregnancy. Those for whom a genetic connection is most important but who cannot carry a child together may consider gestational care. The majority of couples, however, even among ART veterans, probably look first to adoption, finding it the most familiar, successful, and predictable alternative path to parenthood.

Couples who, after considering parenting alternatives, conclude that genetics and gestation are prerequisites to parenthood often decide not to pursue alternatives, determining that being child free will be more satisfying for them. Many begin by identifying other ways they can have children in their lives. Some have nieces or nephews with whom they hope to spend more time; others think about becoming a big brother or big sister to a child in need. Although most could not have imagined that they could go from being childless to embracing being child free, they emerge from a period of exploration and mourning with a renewed sense of optimism and energy.

Sadly, there are some couples who are unable to reach a decision about a second choice. They find themselves at an impasse, with a strong desire to move on but without a place to go. These couples are in crisis. Counseling can be useful in helping them sort through their feelings, attitudes, beliefs, and prejudices about the alternatives that are available to them, and one spouse may eventually come to feel more comfortable with his or her partner's preference.

Couples who cannot come to any agreement have a bleak future. Their inability to identify an alternative they can both embrace increases their sense of isolation from each other, as well as from both the fertile and infertile worlds. Sometimes these couples fear for their marriage, and some infertile couples' marriages do end in divorce (as do the marriages of many fertile couples). Nevertheless, many clinicians agree that couples who struggle through the pain of infertility often find that the struggle has brought them closer to each other. Many feel comforted by this evidence of their resiliency as individuals and as a couple.

Couples select their alternatives based not only on feelings about genetics and gestation but also on the availability and accessibility of other options and on the degree to which their outcome is predictable. Some couples might find the idea of a particular alternative appealing but will not pursue it because geography, cost, or some other factor makes it virtually inaccessible. Conversely, they may decide against an option, even if it is readily available to them, because they believe that it is unlikely to result in a successful outcome. Having been on the roller coaster ride of infertility for too long, such couples are reluctant to enter into another process that may result in disappointment.

Adoption.

When they are in the midst of infertility treatment, many couples receive unsolicited, and often unwelcome, advice about considering adoption. In addition to ignoring what the decision to adopt means for couples from an emotional standpoint, these well-meaning but uninformed individuals may believe that it is easy and inexpensive to adopt. State run agencies may have lower fees than do private adoption, but they often have excessively long waiting lists—upwards of five years in many cases. Even those couples who have "waited" through several years of heartbreak often cannot imagine waiting that long to build their family. The adoption of a healthy infant is an expensive process, as much as twenty thousand dollars. Independent adoptions (in which couples attempt to locate birthparents themselves), may involve a series of disappointments before couples achieve their goal of parenthood.

Finances aside, adoption can still be a difficult process. International adoption often means traveling to another country and may also require staying there for a prolonged period of time. And foreign governments are known to change their adoption policies frequently. Domestic adoption too is a process filled with uncertainty; while changes of heart after placement are rare, it is not uncommon for birth- mothers to change their minds at the time of birth, leaving adopting couples with yet another loss.

Another reason why adoption can be difficult is that couples are not always eligible for the adoption program of their choice. Some agencies, as well as some foreign countries, have age or religious restrictions or requirements for length of marriage. Others take extensive medical and psychiatric histories and may exclude certain couples because of past problems. However, there are no universal requirements for adoption and most couples intent on adopting can identify a viable route to it. We will not explore adoption further in this book, but those who wish to have more information may wish to read *Adopting after Infertility* by Patricia Irwin Johnston (Perspectives Press 1992).

Donor Insemination.

Donor insemination (DI) is available and accessible to virtually all couples with male factor infertility. The process is neither costly nor especially time-consuming to pursue. In fact, some couples with male factor infertility who might otherwise lean toward adoption decide on donor insemination at least in part because of financial factors. Another important consideration for these couples is that donor insemination is an alternative offering a high probability of success, especially for couples with no identified female problem. Although it can take several months to achieve a pregnancy, most fertile women conceive via DI in less than a year. Despite its convenience, however, there are many reasons why couples who are candidates for DI elect not to pursue it. (We will explore DI in detail in Chapter 5.)

Ovum Donation.

Ovum donation is available and accessible to some couples in whom the woman has ovarian failure or the inability to conceive is thought to be a function of aging eggs. In couples with few other identified problems, ovum donor pregnancy rates are surprisingly high. Those who have a known donor, as well as those who have access to an anonymous donor program and live near a medical center that offers this treatment, may decide to try this option. Others will be deterred from pursuing it for financial, geographical, or emotional reasons. (Ovum donation is explored in detail in Chapter 6.)

Surrogacy.

Surrogacy is available to couples with documented female infertility when the male partner is fertile. It generally has a predictable outcome: the vast majority of surrogates who have proven fertility become pregnant in a reasonable period of time (under six months) and go on to have successful pregnancies. And only in the rarest of circumstances do surrogates refuse to relinquish the child they bore. However, surrogacy is not accessible to many couples because it tends to be a very expensive option, with fees often ranging above $30,000. In addition, most couples do not live near a professional surrogacy program, and many are reluctant to travel or to become involved in a long-distance arrangement. Some couples get involved in "do it yourself" surrogacy arrangements, but those, although much less expensive, may be riskier. Historically surrogacy has been surrounded by controversy. Of all the parenting options, it is the most objectionable to the greatest number of people. Couples pursuing surrogacy must be prepared to face criticism for their decision. (Surrogacy is explored in detail in Chapter 7.)

Gestational Care.

Gestational care is an option for couples who can produce healthy embryos (through IVF) but cannot carry a pregnancy. This too is a costly option and one that does not come with a high probability of success (although the younger the genetic mother, the more likely the carrier is to become pregnant). In addition, gestational care is not easily accessible to many couples since it relies on highly specialized legal and psychological services, as well as on a skilled medical team. (Gestational care is explored in detail in Chapter 8.)

Embryo Adoption.

Embryo adoption is an option for couples who are unable to provide gametes, but who wish to share a pregnancy together. Among such couples are those who feel that the gestational connection to a child is important and significant as well as those who may regard pre-pregnancy adoption as a safer option than adoptions in which placement is made after birth. Because embryo adoption is not readily available, may be costly and offers limited chance of success (no greater than 20% per cycle), few couples are currently pursuing this option. (Embryo adoption is explored in detail in Chapter 9.)

146

Child-free Living.

Child-free living is available to all couples. Like adoption, it is not discussed in this book because it does not involve medical intervention. However, from an emotional perspective, it can be a satisfying resolution to infertility and thus deserves careful consideration. Though childfree living means not parenting one's own children, most childfree couples find many ways to involve themeselves in the process of nurturing and mentoring young people. We encourage readers who are interested in considering this lifestyle alternative to read *Sweet Grapes : How to Stop Being Infertile and Start Living Again* by Jean & Michael Carter (Perspectives Press, revised, 1989), a well-written and uplifting book by an infertile, child free couple, about the process of resolving their infertility through child free living.

In examining options, infertile couples are often influenced by other infertile couples whom they come to know in the course of their treatment. Relationships that begin spontaneously in a physician's waiting room or are outgrowths of RESOLVE and other support group experiences are often instrumental in helping couples begin to take steps to end treatment. Many couples gain the confidence to pursue a particular option when they hear about the experiences of their friends. There is no better "advertisement" for adoption, for example, than a couple who is bubbling over with enthusiasm over their newly adopted infant.

Couples moving on must think about how they will—or will not—tell others about their decisions. Those who are adopting will face a variety of reactions from others, and those who feel tentative about the decision are likely to be especially sensitive to others' questions or criticisms. Positive reactions from family and friends will help reinforce the rightness of their choice, but the inevitable insensitive comments are likely to bring renewed questions and doubts. Those who are moving on to collaborative reproduction may have more difficulty telling others that they have decided to end treatment leading to a biogenetic child. These couples may be attempting to reconcile their need for privacy with their desire to be truthful.

All couples who are embarking upon a new plan should take some time to renew their relationship and to look back with some perspective on where they have been and where they are going. Although there may be pressures to move on without delay, those who are able to take even a short break from treatment will benefit from the time off. For many couples, one of the hardest parts of moving on is facing the fact that their second choice may also pose some uncertainty and that sometime in the future they may have to identify and pursue yet a third choice.

Grief, Resolution, and Celebration

As we have acknowledged, couples sometimes extend their treatment experience in an effort to avoid grief about their inability to have a bio-genetic child. Although this effort may temporarily spare them some pain, the truth is that most people feel worse about themselves if they prolong treatment in order to avoid their grief.

The grief that comes at the end of infertility treatment takes different forms for different people, depending on their past history and current life circumstances and their feelings about pregnancy, genetic continuity and genetic blending. Individuals who have had earlier losses in their families often find that leaving treatment prompts them to revisit those losses. For example, a man who had looked forward to naming a son after his deceased father may feel that the loss of his expected son adds to the depth of his earlier loss.

Individuals whose lives are otherwise rich and full may find that their grief paves the way for relief; it frees them up to enjoy and celebrate other aspects of their lives. By contrast, those who are experiencing frustrations and disappointments at work, or with family and friends, may find their grief more burdensome because the rest of their life feels empty and unfulfilling. In these situations some soul-searching, counseling, or reaching out to others may help them identify new goals and in turn feel a renewed purpose in life. This sense of optimism will help them find a second choice.

Personality styles also influence the ways in which individuals grieve at the close of treatment. Some tend to be passive, accepting their sorrow as something that will end when it will end. Others take a more active approach, creating rituals and ceremonies that help them move on. They may plant trees in memory of their unborn children, write poems, or even invite friends to participate in this important, though painful, passage. For example, one woman invited several of her close friends to a "healing circle" in which drums, song and personal statements were combined into a very personal ceremony of loss and renewal.

For some couples, a religious ceremony plays a critical role in helping them mourn and move on. One couple modeled their ceremony upon a

Passover seder, finding the images of a journey, of plagues, of destruction and rebuilding, and of fertility all very relevant to their personal journey.

When couples decide that they have truly had enough of treatment and that they have successfully identified a second choice, they commonly combine grief with celebration. Although this sounds contradictory, joy and sorrow can be two sides of the same coin. As sad as couples feel upon ending treatment, because it signals the end of shared biogenetic parenthood, they also feel a sense of relief that the medical ordeal is over. One woman describes this merging of grief with relief.

> Our grieving took the form of celebration. Alex and I went out to dinner, had a bottle of wine, went home and threw out the remaining vial of Pergonal and all the ovulation predictor kits. Then we made love. For the first time in nearly four years, our love-making felt like a sign of our success as a couple, rather than our failure. We still felt profoundly sad that we would not "make a baby" together, but there, in bed together, that sorrow was not with us. We were too busy enjoying the love and tenderness that remained strong between us.

Donor Insemination

Donor insemination—the process by which a woman is artificially inseminated with the sperm of a man other than a husband/partner—is not a new reproductive technology. Dating back approximately one hundred years, donor insemination can more aptly be considered a longstanding reproductive option for couples with male infertility. Over the years, however, donor insemination has been mistakenly identified as a *treatment* for male infertility, yet it has never been a treatment in the way that surgical procedures or pharmacological regimens are. The latter are designed to improve the quality and quantity of sperm so that conception can occur; DI is an alternative path to parenthood.

One of the problems with presenting donor insemination (DI) as a treatment, is that the word "treatment" implies "cure," and donor insemination, though a cure for childlessness, is not a cure for male infertility. The question—one which is not often asked—is why donor insemination is presented to infertile couples as a treatment, rather than as an alternative childbearing method? In order to answer this question it helps to reflect back on the history of DI and on the history of male infertility. By looking at these separate but intertwined histories, we can better understand why this case of "mistaken identity," occurred, and how, along with many other factors, it has shaped the history and the practice of donor insemination.

Setting the Stage:
A Climate of Shame and Secrecy

The history of male infertility begins, in the Western World, with the Bible. The Old Testament commands men to produce heirs to inherit their property and carry on their names. Although barren women were pitied and held responsible for their condition, men who did not have offspring were seen as tragic figures and were shamed. They were out of compliance with God's law.

The importance (and necessity) of paternity in biblical times is illustrated by the fact that a man whose marriage was childless after ten years was instructed to find a concubine to bear children for him. Even more extreme measures were mandated posthumously for a man who died without children: his brother was obligated to marry the widow (his sister-in-law) and have children with her. The resulting offspring were considered the dead man's children, bearers of his name and evidence that he did not die without heirs.

The process by which a man impregnates his dead brother's wife is referred to as a Levirate marriage. Although some biblical scholars have pointed to such arrangements as the earliest form of donor insemination, there are obvious differences between the two. Nevertheless, the Biblical Levirate concept of creating a child from another man's sperm and raising the child as the legal offspring of the husband is similar to the modern concept of donor insemination.

Although our biblical ancestors realized that semen is necessary to achieve pregnancy, they did not understand why. Not until thousands of years later, in 1677, did Anton van Leeuwenhoek, inventor of the microscope, discover the presence of sperm. Even after his discovery, however, it took two more centuries before the mechanics of reproduction were understood,

Van Leeuwenhoek subscribed to the preformationist school, believing that a single spermatozoan contains all the elements essential to create an adult human being and that during the embryonic period that individual would emerge. The woman was necessary, he thought, because she provided the gestational environment, but she did not have a role in the conception of the child. Van Leeuwenhoek therefore believed that the man plants the seed of his future child in much the same way that a farmer plants seeds in the ground. If the soil is not fertile, the land will be barren.

152

Thus, it is easy to understand why our ancestors believed that women alone were responsible for infertility. Since sperm could not be seen in an ejaculate—let alone be counted, as they are today—our ancestors must have assumed that if a man ejaculated his seed, he was fertile.

Over the past hundred years, and especially in the last few decades, much has been learned about human reproduction, including that both men and women have an equal stake in the creation of their offspring and that infertility can occur in either partner. Knowledge about the causes of male infertility and the ways to diagnose it has increased several-fold, especially in the last decade. Understanding a problem, however, does not necessarily mean it can be cured. Although physicians are able to identify many reasons for male infertility—for instance, low sperm count, poor motility, too many abnormal sperm, the presence of antibodies—the ability to "fix" these problems has been limited. Although *in vitro* fertilization, and more recently microinsemination techniques, have enabled couples with male infertility (who have the financial means) to become biological parents, the source of the problem in these situations has not been corrected.

Historically, there have been two approaches to treating male infertility. The first has focused on trying to improve sperm quality and quantity either through medicine or surgery. This approach, although effective in some instances, has had limited success. The second approach has been to attempt to by-pass the problem by bringing egg and sperm closer together. Traditionally this was done through artificial insemination, the process of introducing sperm into the female reproductive tract through the use of instruments or other artificial devices.

Artificial insemination (AI) was used with animals long before it was used for human beings. The practice dates to the fourteenth century when Arabs used AI to breed horses. Yet it was not until 1799 that the birth of a human conceived by artificial insemination (with the husband's sperm) was recorded in London. The first such birth in the United States was recorded in 1866, and since then the technique has become increasingly popular among physicians.

Artificial insemination is performed by placing the sperm in the woman's vagina, cervix, or uterus. Placing it in the vagina is effective only when a mechanical problem precludes semen from being deposited there via sexual intercourse. Placing sperm in the cervix (intracervical insemination) brings it closer to its ultimate destination, the fallopian tube, where, hopefully, an egg awaits. Whether conception rates actually improve as a result of intracervical insemination has been a topic frequently debated among reproductive endocrinologists.

Placing sperm—rather than semen (which may cause severe cramping)—directly in the uterus, thereby bringing it even closer to the egg, is a treatment that has been widely available since the early 1980s and is now employed much more frequently than the other two methods. This treatment, known as intrauterine insemination (IUI) has not been especially successful in treating severe male infertility; many such couples undergo years of IUI treatment without having a pregnancy. Some of these couples turn to IVF and ICSI.

As we noted in the first half of this book, the development of *in vitro* fertilization and the further development of microinsemination techniques have revolutionized the field of reproductive medicine. This development was of special significance to the treatment of male infertility, since it presented an opportunity to truly bring sperm and egg together, providing an opportunity for men with severe male factor infertility to become biological fathers. IVF was also a revolutionary diagnostic tool, providing clear evidence of whether fertilization could occur.

When eggs do not fertilize via *in vitro* fertilization, or with microinsemination, or if pregnancy does not occur, some couples then turn to donor insemination. Couples who do not have access to IVF or to ICSI, also frequently turn to donor insemination as a way to form their families.

Although artificial insemination was performed for several decades using the husband's sperm, it was not until the late 1800s that the first case of AI using a donor was documented—by William Pancoast, who claimed to have performed the procedure in secret. Thus began a trend that continued for one hundred years and still continues today for most couples choosing DI: that of secrecy. The theme of secrecy, as we will see throughout this chapter, has governed the theory and practice of DI, from the way donors are selected, to the way in which physicians speak to couples about this option, to the way in which DI parents conduct their relationships with their children. Unfortunately, as we will also see, shame is a byproduct of secrecy. Sadly, shame only serves to increase men's feelings of inadequacy and to decrease their ability to form close relationships.

Because male infertility still bears a shameful stigma and is associated with impotence, or a lack of virility, physicians tend to feel uncomfortable speaking to couples about the emotional aspects of this problem. Accordingly, most do not address the overwhelming sadness that infertile men and their partners feel upon learning their diagnosis. Nor do most physicians recommend counseling for couples who are facing this alternative and dealing with their loss. Thus many couples find themselves DI parents without ever grieving the loss of having a child who is the joint product of their genes—and without having explored the implications of donor insemination on their relationship as a couple and as a family.

Current donor insemination statistics are difficult to gather; physicians' records are confidential, and many couples are beginning to perform their own inseminations without using a physician as an intermediary. An estimate of the number of U.S. births per year resulting from DI is approximately 30,000[20], a number not much smaller than the number of non-relative adoptions in the U.S. each year. Thus donor insemination plays a prominent role among family-building options for couples with male factor infertility.

$\mathscr{D}$*iagnosing Male Infertility*

Teenage boys learn that only one sperm is needed for conception. Yet it is also true that at least 20 million are usually needed to be stored in the woman's reproductive tract to begin their race when the egg is ripe. But it is not only the numbers that matter. The percentage of motile sperm moving at the right speed and in the right direction should be 40 to 50% normal, and the morphology (appearance) should be at least 60% normal.

Medical knowledge about male infertility is constantly shifting. At one time the count was thought to be the most important statistic. In recent years motility has been thought to be more important, and even more recently, greater emphasis is being placed on morphology. There are, in addition, other factors that affect sperm and can cause infertility, such as antibody problems, infections, and varicoceles (varicose veins in the scrotum).

Male infertility appears to exist on a continuum. Although there are some men who have no sperm (they are azoospermic and therefore sterile), most men suffering from infertility do have some sperm (they are oligospermic). The closer the man's numbers are to the ideal parameters, the greater is the likelihood of an eventual pregnancy. As long as some live sperm are present in the ejaculate, a pregnancy via sexual intercourse is always possible, though in many cases it is highly improbable.

Until IVF, couples with male factor infertility who never had a pregnancy had no way of knowing whether the sperm were capable of fertilizing the egg, even if one should reach its destination. The only diagnostic test that gave any indication about whether fertilization was possible was the hamster egg penetration test in which a sperm sample from the husband is obtained, several ripe eggs are extracted from a female hamster (whose eggs are remarkably similar to human ova), and insemination is attempted under laboratory surveillance. Although the test can predict the likelihood of fertilization, it is often inaccurate. Many men who have "failed" this test have subsequently impregnated their wives without any intervention.

In vitro fertilization, though much more expensive, time consuming, and invasive than a hamster egg test, is understandably a far better diagnostic tool. Assuming that several good eggs are retrieved, a couple will learn whether fertilization is possible. Although there is still no way to know with certainty whether fertilization can occur in the fallopian tube if it does not occur in the laboratory, physicians usually assume it probably cannot.

Candidates for Donor Insemination

Couples arrive at DI for very different reasons and with very different medical histories. However, most heterosexual couples who turn to donor insemination do so because of male factor infertility. Exceptions may include men who are carriers of genetic disorders and, in some cases, men with spinal cord injuries.

The largest group of infertile couples who consider donor insemination do not have an identifiable cause for their problem. Their infertility is considered *idiopathic*—the nature of the problem can be identified, but its cause is unknown. They, like most other couples, approached parenthood assuming fertility, unaware that the man had a low sperm count, poor motility, or abnormal morphology. In the course of a workup, the diagnosis was made.

Depending on the severity of their condition, and the degree of hope offered by their physician, most couples go through a great deal of anguish upon learning of their infertility. The unknown cause creates additional frustration, as many men rack their brains attempting to find reasons—

perhaps a forgotten sports injury, for example—for their condition. Many go through years of testing and treatment, often including the ARTs, and especially ICSI (see Chapter 2), before turning to donor insemination.

A second group of candidates for donor insemination include men who have been successfully treated for cancer. Although the number of couples who comprise this group is still small, advances in the treatment of testicular cancer, Hodgkins disease, and other cancers that strike men of reproductive age have led to an ever increasing population of men who survive cancer at the cost of their fertility. Some who have had cancer were instructed to bank sperm prior to undergoing radiation or chemotherapy, in order to preserve fertility. Those who have done so have varying degrees of success with their samples. Sometimes *in vitro* fertilization is used in combination with the frozen sperm of cancer survivors, even in situations with no identified female problem. IVF maximizes their chances of pregnancy and is an efficient way to use frozen sperm. Due to limited samples and the fact that freezing sperm can damage its overall quality, many of these couples will still not achieve pregnancy and may turn to donor insemination.

Cancer survivors often have a multitude of conflicting feelings. They are grateful to be alive, but once their survival is reasonably assured, feelings of loss may re-surface. These feelings intensify for those who must now confront infertility, and very possibly, sterility. Not only does it feel like the ultimate unfairness that they must face yet another crisis—often at a young age—but the inability to reproduce prompts additional feelings about the cancer. Although "cured" or "cancer free" they are left with a feeling that the disease still has a hold on them and on their futures. As one man who had survived cancer fifteen years earlier, when he was an adolescent, commented upon learning he was azoospermic, "I thought I had put cancer behind me, but now it feels like it is back taking control of my life."

A third group of candidates for donor insemination are those who have congenital infertility. Examples of congenital problems are absence of the vas deferens (the tubes that carry the semen from the testicles to where it is ejaculated); Klinefelter's syndrome, in which a man is born with an extra X chromosome in his XY complement, rendering him sterile; or an undescended testicle that was not surgically corrected at a young age. (This is not correctable as an adult.) Some cases of male infertility due to congenital abnormalities can be treated with microinsemination, by extracting sperm (if there are any) from the epididemis, or from testicular tissue (if sperm are found) that has been biopsied and cryopreserved.

Although men with congenital conditions resulting in infertility may have lived most of their lives aware of the congenital problem, as adults who are prepared to become fathers, these men may find that new feelings of sadness and anger arise.

A fourth group of candidates who consider donor insemination are those whose infertility was caused by an illness such as mumps, occurring post-puberty, or trauma to the testicles resulting from injury. Similarly, infections—often, but not always gonorrhea—can cause blockages in the epididymis or in the ejaculatory ducts. Although men in this group may at least know why they are infertile, this knowledge does not necessarily diminish their loss.

A fifth group of men who may turn to donor insemination are those who have had vasectomies. Some believed they would never want children. Others had vasectomies in an earlier marriage after having all the children they thought they wanted. Although vasectomies can be reversed, the success of the surgery is linked to time. Those who had the procedure done many years ago—more than ten—are less likely to have a successful reversal. Unlike those infertile men who feel damaged or defective, men who have had vasectomies tend to be tormented by guilt, self-blame, and regret. They look back upon past decisions—ones often made with great care—and wonder how they could have been so shortsighted.

A sixth group of candidates for donor insemination are men who have suffered spinal cord injury. Although some of these men can impregnate their wives with the help of electroejaculation (a procedure by which the penis is electrically stimulated to ejaculate), others have a very low sperm count making success unlikely. Although ICSI offers renewed hope for many of these men, the procedure, which is very expensive and needs to be performed by skilled embryologists, may not be available or accessable to some of these men. Sadly, many who have already suffered an extraordinary physical trauma and who have now endured the physical and emotional intrusions of electroejaculation, are faced with the likelihood that they will not genetically father a child. Some pursue donor insemination.

A final group of DI candidates—though a small group—have no history of infertility. They do, however, have family histories of genetic disorders that they do not wish to pass on to their offspring. If the gene in question can be detected by amniocentesis, it is unlikely the couple will choose DI, unless their religious beliefs preclude abortion. However, if the gene is not detectable until after birth, many couples elect not to take the risk of passing it on. If the problematic gene is autosomal dominant, as in the case of Huntington's disease, any offspring of the father would have a 50% chance of inheriting the syndrome. If the disorder is one that is auto-somal recessive, such as Tay-Sachs disease or cystic fibrosis and the woman is also a carrier, their offspring have a 25% chance of inheriting the disease. Afraid to attempt pregnancy with such odds, a number of these couples turn to donor insemination. Many approach DI reluctantly, feeling cheated out of a biological child but not suffering from the feelings of shame that burden infertile men.

Treatment for Male Infertility

Although male infertility can almost always be diagnosed by a semen analysis and its causes sometimes identified as well, it is difficult to cure. Medical advances in this area have been few, and prognosis is generally worse than for female problems. Treatment for male factor involving count, motility, or morphology can be attempted through the use of medication for hormonal problems or through surgery for problems such as a varico-cele or a blockage of the epididymis. Nevertheless, both medication and surgery frequently fail to cure the problem by normalizing semen parame-ters. Microinsemination—though a means to a potential biological child—bypasses the problem, rather than curing it.

Artificial insemination procedures attempt to bypass problems of count, motility, or morphology by depositing sperm closer to the egg—closer than when it is ejaculated during sexual intercourse. Because semen carries prostaglandins, chemicals that cause severe cramping, sperm must be washed to rid them of the prostaglandins as well as any bacteria present that would impede fertilization. Sperm washing concentrates the sperm so that only the most motile, normal ones are used for insemination, in hopes of overcoming problems of low volume, poor motility, or abnormal morphology. Sometimes this treatment works, (especially if the infertility is not severe) and the woman becomes pregnant, but it may take several cycles, and the couple is never sure how long to keep trying. It is common to combine IUI with superovulation therapy, in which case not only are the sperm getting a head start, but they also have more possibilities for fertilization.

Although *in vitro* fertilization was designed to overcome female infertility problems that involve blockage of the fallopian tubes, it has proven to be an effective treatment for couples with male infertility as well. IVF is a means of bypassing a low sperm count or poor motility or morphology. When sperm do not have to travel (in IVF they are placed directly in a petri dish with an ovum extracted from the woman), the numbers of normal sperm and the speed and direction in which they move are not as important as when they are required to make a long journey. Thus, a significant portion of male factor couples who attempt IVF are able to achieve fertilization (and hopefully a pregnancy as well).

Until recently, couples who had poor fertilization with IVF, or none at all, usually concluded that they needed to move on to alternative parenting options. However, microinsemination techniques (ICSI) are now available in many ART clinics and are very enticing to some couples who might otherwise pursue donor insemination. ICSI is recommended (and frequently effective) when the numbers of viable sperm as measured by a semen analysis are too low even for IVF or when attempts at IVF do not yield fertilization. ICSI is also recommended in situations when sperm can be extracted from the epididymis or from testicular tissue but none is found in the ejaculate (see Chapter 2, Microinsemination). This technology has improved greatly over the past few years, yielding an on-going pregnancy rate of upwards of 35% in the better programs and a live birth rate of approximately 25%.[21] Hence, ICSI has enabled many couples who never would have been able to conceive together to produce biogenetic offspring. Unfortunately its cost, limited availability, limited success (in any given cycle, the odds are against it working) and unknown long term ramifications, are major deterrants to many couples now dealing with male infertility.

The treatment of male infertility is indeed difficult and often confusing. IVF is an effective tool with or without microinsemination, but it is not without its limitations. Repeated attempts at IVF or microinsemination that result in failed fertilization or poor fertilization rates or poor quality embryos are upsetting and frustrating for a couple. At the same time, however, these couples—certainly those who have access to ICSI— know they have had the benefit of the ultimate diagnostic test and treatment. Unlike those couples who do not try IVF and may go from month to month wondering if fertilization is possible, couples who pursue high tech treatment and then turn to alternatives know that they have made their best effort to have a biogenetic child. Many such couples turn to donor insemination.

$\mathscr{D}$eciding on Donor Insemination

Although many physicians continue to present DI as a "treatment" for male infertility, the medical profession has come a long way in recent years towards acknowledging that donor insemination is not a simple medical procedure, but rather it is an alternative parenting option that has many emotional, social, and ethical ramifications for a family now and in years to come. In response to this growing appreciation of the complexities of DI, the American Society for Reproductive Medicine has recommended that referral for counseling and evaluation may be very useful to some couples before proceeding with this choice. We feel that counseling should be mandatory. Unfortunately many couples face decisions about DI alone, with little guidance. And because male infertility often engenders feelings of embarrassment and shame, it can be difficult for couples to face the emotional and psychological issues that donor insemination raises.

Considering donor insemination is a painful process; it raises intense feelings of loss, confronting couples with their mortality and with their longing for genetic continuity. Couples embarking on this path must think about what it means to be a parent and how parenting a child who is genetically connected to both of them may be different from parenting a child who is genetically connected to only one of them. Furthermore, DI couples must also think about parent/child relationships and how they develop. They must examine how the addition of a third party, known or unknown, will affect their feelings about themselves, the relationship between partners, and most importantly, the parents' relationship with their potential child. The process of expressing and examining these issues can test the strength and resiliency of a couple's relationship.

A 1986 study done in Canada of 120 couples using DI supports the notion that the use of donor insemination generates intense and troublesome feelings both within and between spouses—feelings that need to be resolved for everyone's well-being. The researchers concluded that common reactions for men are loss of self-esteem, emotional withdrawal, and temporary impotence. Anger, guilt, and a wish to make reparations are part of the woman's experience. The researchers emphasize that if these conflicts are not resolved, they can lead to more serious ones.[22]

Loss of Genetic Continuity

An important issue facing couples considering DI is the loss of genetic continuity. Infertility forces people to think about the importance of bloodlines and of producing biogenetic offspring who will inherit their traits. The value that each person assigns to these concepts is an important determinant in how much effort a couple will expend in order to conceive a child together.

Most couples fantasize—even before attempting pregnancy—what their children will be like: how they will look, what talents they will possess, and the kind of personality they will have. Although children almost always turn out to be different from these fantasies, most have some qualities of each parent that are recognizable. Couples who are confronting male infertility and contemplating donor insemination must face their feelings of sadness about not being able to see some of the father's traits reflected in their children. They must recognize that no matter how carefully they select a donor so that he strongly resembles the father in terms of physical, ethnic, and personality characteristics, he will still be a different person. Some couples are so troubled by this reality that they ask to have the husband's semen mixed with the donor's, hoping to hold on to the possibility that he will be the genetic father. This request, although received with compassion, is rejected on medical as well as emotional and ethical grounds.

For years scientists, sociologists, and psychologists have debated the nature/ nurture question. Although no one has come up with the exact equation—how much of who we are is determined by genes and how much by environment— the balance seems to be shifting in the direction of nature. No one disputes that environment is extremely important in helping us to reach our potential, but recent evidence supports the belief that traits once thought to be solely acquired as a result of upbringing are now understood to have strong genetic components. This knowledge may make some couples even more determined to have children who are genetically connected to them.

The complicated and multifaceted nature of genetics leads some people to believe in a *unique gene pool*. Recognizing that there is no one else in the world who is exactly like them, they place a great deal of importance on the unique combination of genes that they received from their parents, who in turn received genes from their parents. Passing on these unique genes may feel like an imperative, and the inability to do so is therefore a greater loss than for those who identify more with the humankind gene pool philosophy.

Couples who feel rooted in their family tree, and for whom bloodlines are important, may view donor insemination as severing their ancestral ties. Thus it is common for infertile men to feel as if they will be greatly disappointing their families should they choose donor insemination. They may worry that if their family knew about DI, the grandchild would not be loved or accepted in the way a biological grandchild would be. There is reason for such concerns. Sadly, (and cruelly) children who were adopted into their families are occasionally left off family trees or out of a grandparents' will.

There are other people, however, for whom genetic continuity is not very important. They believe in a *humankind gene pool*. Recognizing that no one person has a monopoly on any specific gene, they feel strongly that we are random combinations from a humankind gene pool. Hence there is never any certainty that a particular child will possess curly hair or musical aptitude or any other desired (or undesired) trait of their parents. Similarly, the concept of "bloodlines" is virtually irrelevant to such people, since they believe that we are all part of the same genetic pool.

Concerns about Attachment

When a couple is deciding about donor insemination, the husband often wonders whether he could love "another man's child." Some men voice this concern openly; others express it indirectly. Women considering adoption or ovum donation, on the other hand, tend to have fewer worries about becoming attached to a child who does not come from them. Much of their play as young girls involves being in relationships—playing house or playing with dolls. Teenage girls frequently babysit and grow attached to the children for whom they care. They thus tend to enter adulthood with the understanding and faith that emotional bonds develop through nurturance, not through genetic ties. Since most men had different experiences growing up, they may assume that the reason parents love their children is because they come from their genes. Thus, some men initially reject the idea of donor insemination out of fear they will not be able to love a child they did not create.

Men do not necessarily understand their fears, but over time many are able to acknowledge them. Once these fears are on the table, they can be explored. Couples can talk with one another about their fantasies of parenthood and what they hope for their children. Focusing on parenthood in this way can help with resolution.

Couples who are facing the possibility of adoption or donor gametes frequently find themselves considering whether they could love a particular child they know or whom they observe. Couples in this situation may think more about their friends' children and ask themselves whether they would want to have Joey for their child, or Julie, and on down the list. They think about whether they could love the child they see having a temper tantrum in the supermarket or the one whose nose is always running. Women who believe strongly that they could love a child who did not come from them still wonder if they could love any child, especially one who is unappealing on the surface. Men, who have less faith to begin with about their ability to love a child who did not come from them, may find themselves carefully observing children of all ages, in all situations, in an effort to confirm or deny their feelings.

Adulterous Feelings

A final issue that couples must consider before embarking on donor insemination involves their feelings about having another man's semen placed inside the woman. For some couples this process engenders thoughts and feelings about adultery, as the following example illustrates.

A couple who had been treated for male infertility for three years had just finished their second and last IVF cycle in which they did not get fertilization. Their previous treatment had included several IUIs over two years. They made an appointment with the psychologist to discuss donor insemination. The husband stated that he was ready to move on to DI; he had dealt with his sadness over not being able to produce a biological offspring and wanted to be a father more than he wanted to be a biological father. His wife was far more hesitant, telling the psychologist timidly, "I've never told anyone this, but my husband is the only man I have ever had sex with. I'm afraid that having another man's sperm inside me would make me feel like I was sleeping with someone else."

Men similarly may express feelings of hesitancy about DI due to fears that if their wife conceives, they will feel as if she is carrying another man's child. Couples who ultimately choose this alternative means of family building must be able to separate the act of lovemaking from the act of procreation. Long before couples decide on DI or on any other alternative, most have given up the notion that sexuality and family building are connected. Yet donor insemination represents the need for an even greater emotional separation between the two experiences.

Adoption or Donor Insemination?

The first issue a couple with male infertility must consider when they decide to end treatment is whether they wish to pursue an alternative path to parenthood. Some remain child free. They decide that if they are unable to have a child who is genetically connected to both of them, they would rather not parent at all. For these couples, this alternative is more acceptable than the other two paths open to them: adoption or donor insemination.

In considering alternatives, some couples are clear from the outset that donor insemination is unacceptable for religious, moral, social, or psychological reasons. Others are just as clear that if the child cannot be totally biologically theirs, at least he or she can be half biologically theirs. Still others—and this is a large group of couples—approach the end of treatment knowing they want to become parents yet uncertain about which alternative will work better for them.

Biogenetic Inequality

Biological and genetic equality is an important consideration for many couples. Some fear that the inequality of DI may eventually threaten their marriage. They worry that if a crisis developed with their child, the father would distance himself. They wonder whether he would always feel unauthentic or second class. These couples prefer the relational equality that adoption offers: neither parent is genetically or biologically connected to their child. In adoption, both people ultimately suffer the losses of infertility, and both people begin the parenting venture on equal footing.

Couples leaning toward donor insemination generally feel more comfortable knowing half of the genetic origins of their offspring. They believe their child will feel more familiar to them since he or she is likely to resemble the mother—and members of her family—in physical traits or in personality. They believe that the child will feel equally theirs and that the genetic inequality will not matter.

The Experience of Pregnancy and Childbirth

Of all the potential losses involved in the experience of infertility, the pregnancy-childbirth experience is the most difficult one for many women.

Donor insemination, unlike adoption, offers women the experience of gestating and giving birth to a baby. It also offers the couple the opportunity to share a pregnancy. Many women point to this reason as the major force behind their desire to create their family through donor insemination.

Prenatal Care

Couples who decide on donor insemination rather than adoption know that they will have control over their child's prenatal care, an issue about which most adoptive parents worry. Although adoption agencies obtain as much information as they can about a birthmother's pregnancy, they can never be completely sure that the information is accurate. In some cases, they receive very little information, and many parents who build their families through adoption begin parenthood wondering whether anything in the prenatal environment was problematic, potentially causing problems later in life.

Social Acceptability and Support

Some couples feel that adoption is more socially acceptable than donor insemination. The process of adoption is well known, common, and non-secretive, and it offers a large, identifiable peer group with whom couples can relate. Although adopting a child can feel like embarking into unknown territory, adoptive parents are not pioneers. There are many resources open to adoptive couples, including numerous books on the process of adopting and on raising adopted children, support groups for adoptive parents, play groups for adoptive parents and their children, conferences and other continuing educational opportunities, and family service agencies and therapists who specialize in working with adoptive families.

Compared to adoption, resources for DI families are scant. It is also unlikely, unless they decide to be publicly open, that DI couples will find other donor parents willing to share their experiences. Hence a couple may feel that deciding on donor insemination will lead to future isolation.

Privacy and Legitimacy

Some couples choose DI for the privacy it can offer. For them, the adoption of a child becomes a public statement about their infertility, a statement they may not wish to make. Couples who opt for DI may view adoptive couples as conspicuously different from friends and relatives who were privy to the adoption.

Many couples who choose donor insemination over adoption also express fears that if they adopted they might be made to feel different from other parents by virtue of not having given birth to a biological child. Women fear they might be seen as unauthentic—not legitimate mothers— if they adopt. They anticipate that pregnancy and childbirth will make them feel like legitimate parents.

The Likelihood of Success

Some couples choose adoption over donor insemination because it seems more certain. Donor insemination does not always work, especially if there is a female problem in addition to a male factor. Many couples, after years of trials and tribulations in the world of infertility, are hesitant to get back on the emotional roller coaster and are reluctant to continue the uncertainty of time-consuming, invasive treatment. They are ready to put treatment behind them and move on. While adoption is its own roller coaster, it generally affords them the security of knowing they will eventually become parents. (Certain kinds of adoptions, however—independent, private, or legal risk adoptions—provide less security; there is a chance that adoptions can fall through.)

On the other hand, many couples are convinced of the woman's fertility and believe DI to be an easier and quicker route to parenthood. Others who choose donor insemination are not worried about the risks; after years of uncertainty, they feel hardened to disappointment and are not convinced that any route to parenthood is a sure bet. Having been disappointed many times, no matter which alternative they select, they select it with skepticism.

Financial Cost

Some DI couples who might for other reasons prefer adoption choose DI because it is less costly; they cannot afford a private agency adoption and do not wish to wait years for the placement of a child from a public agency. Infant adoption costs at private agencies currently run between $10,000 and $30,000. The price of a vial of sperm is usually between $150 and $300, plus the fee for the insemination. Frequently these costs are covered by medical insurance, but even when they are not, DI is still a much smaller financial investment than is the adoption of a baby.

Choosing DI means trusting that once a pregnancy is achieved, both members of the couple will begin to feel that it is their child. This acceptance does not mean that couples should pretend they conceived in the usual way, at least not to themselves. Rather, they must acknowledge the special means of conception through which they formed their family.

Couples who have allowed themselves to feel the range and depth of emotions that stem from their loss are in a strong position to face the decision-making process inherent in donor insemination. Though the feelings of loss probably never disappear completely, the hope is that the joys of parenting their child will far outweigh the loss of a genetic link to it.

$\mathscr{K}$nown versus Unknown Donors

One of the first decisions DI couples must make is whether to use a known or an unknown donor. Although the population of couples who opt for a known donor is growing in numbers, most couples do not consider asking someone they know. Thus, the vast majority of DI couples use anonymous sperm from a sperm bank to create their families. Perhaps this is due to the fact that secrecy and shame have always been an inherent component of male infertility, and rarely has anyone—including physicians—questioned that aspect of the process. A recent survey compared eighty-two programs that offer gamete donation. Not surprisingly, the author found that although the majority of these programs allowed known ovum donation, the majority did not allow known sperm donation.[23]

When choosing donor insemination—known or anonymous—there are many questions to consider. The first is an underlying ethical one previously discussed in Chapter 1: *Is it morally right to intentionally bring a child into the world with an unknown genetic parent?* Historically this question has been overlooked. Perhaps one reason is that nurture was once thought to play a far greater role than nature in human development. Those who felt that people's genetic makeup was unimportant to their development, did not see a need for an individual to know its genetic parent(s). The rationale seems to be that if nature is not very relevant, except for physical attributes, it should be almost meaningless to an individual that he or she has no access to a genetic parent. If, on the other hand, nature is believed to be a primary force in shaping human beings, then it becomes less clear about whether it is ethical to create a child who has an unknown genetic father. The shifting emphasis of the nature versus nurture debate, once more heavily weighted on the side of nurture, is making all parties to DI rethink what it means to be born with little knowledge about or access to one's genetic parents.

We can speculate that another reason that this ethical consideration has been overlooked has to do with fears of jeopardizing or compromising the role of the social father. If the importance of the genetic father is acknowledged, some might fear that the importance of the social or rearing father would be minimized. The evolution of donor insemination involves a cover-up—i.e. a public pretension that the social and the genetic father are the same person.

Decisions regarding social policy in the use of donor gametes have been discussed by Elias and Annas, a physician-geneticist and attorney-ethicist, respectively. They refer to donor insemination as a contractual agreement between parties and as the accepted paradigm for other methods of non-coital reproduction. They argue that donor insemination places "the private contractual agreement among the participants regarding parental rights and responsibilities above the 'best interest of the child,' and ... raises a series of societal issues that remain unresolved." The authors go on to say:

> Assuming that deciding about parenthood by contract is
> socially accepted as currently practiced, we ignore the rele-
> vance of legitimacy, lineage, and individual identity tied up
> in kinship, and thus bypass fundamental questions about the
> definition of fatherhood and its role in the family and the life
> of the child.[24]

They then argue the other point of view, suggesting that since issues of legitimacy are no longer important social concerns in the United States and hereditary titles are not bestowed by lineage here, questions about genetic parenthood may be irrelevant. It is noteworthy—and testimony to the fact that these ethical issues are extremely complicated—that even these prominent figures seem uncertain about whether the intentional creation of a child with unknown genetic origins should be acceptable.

Known Sperm Donation

The decision to use a known donor is profoundly different than the decision to use an anonymous donor. These differences prompt many couples to view them as two distinct routes to building a family, each of which has profound ramifications on the child and on the family—both nuclear and extended. Although, as we have previously mentioned, the numbers seem to be growing, couples who choose known sperm donation are a minority. (Lesbian couples and single women appear to be choosing known donors more frequently, however, than do heterosexual couples.)

Choosing Known Sperm Donation

Prior to making the decision, couples must give careful thought to the varying psychological, social, and emotional issues that surround each choice. Most likely those who choose known donation arrived at their decision after a lengthy process and have clear reasons for their decision. The following reasons seem to be important to couples who choose known donors.

Avoidance of Genealogical Confusion

We know a great deal about the importance of genetic ties from the field of adoption, as more and more adoptees have been speaking out about the need to know where they came from. The concept of genealogical confusion refers to a sense of not knowing who one is or to whom one belongs. Some adoptees describe feeling unrooted and biologically disconnected. Because of this genetic void, they feel a piece of themselves —of their identity—is missing. This need for information frequently propels adoptees to search for birthparents so that they can fill in the void in hopes of developing a stronger sense of self.

Professionals, in recognizing the role that genetics plays in the unfolding of a person's life, are attempting to provide adoptive couples with as much information as they can gather about their child's birthparents—information about their medical, physical, social, and emotional histories. In many adoptions (a decreasing number), however, information is lacking about the birthfather; he is unknown or unavailable, or the birthmother refuses to identify him. There are those who argue that if it is acceptable to couples to adopt a child under these circumstances, then it must be acceptable to create a child using sperm from an anonymous donor.

The key ethical issue, however, is the idea of intentionally creating a child with unknown parentage. In the case of adoption, children are not created in order to be adopted. For various reasons, the birthparents are unprepared to provide for their children and look to adoption. This unintended situation is different from a deliberate attempt to create a child from donor gametes.

Some couples who choose known donors do so primarily because they believe that it is unfair to create a child who could suffer from genealogical

170

confusion. They feel that it is emotionally healthier for a child to grow up knowing who the genetic parents are so that his or her identity will be more solid. Even if the donor is not someone who is in the child's day-to-day life or is geographically close, the child may still be able to meet him someday.

Genealogical confusion can become social or relational confusion when relatives agree to be donors. When there is an already established familial relationship—for example, the father's brother is the child's uncle—the fact that he is also the genetic father can be confusing to all. Another point of confusion is that if the donor has children, those children are social cousins and genetic half siblings to the donor offspring. Couples must carefully sort through their feelings about belonging and legitimacy, and discuss these issues with their donor before embarking on a course of action that could wreak emotional and social havoc on the family.

Control over the Source of the Gametes

Choosing a known donor provides the couple some control over the gene pool of their offspring. Infertility has taken away their sense of control in regard to reproduction, and using a known donor will help them reclaim some of it. Although no parents ever have control over their child's particular genetic makeup, couples who select a known donor feel more secure that their child will not seem like a stranger.

Many couples hope that a relative, frequently the husband's brother, will be willing to donate. Preserving the family genes is important to them, as is maintaining a sense of control over their source. Genetically speaking, biological siblings are very similar: because they come from the same two gene pools they share fifty percent of each other's genes.

A potential problem with siblings as donors (and to a lesser extent, any other known donor) is that it stirs up issues of competition. Children growing up in the same family develop feelings of competition about all kinds of issues—power, competence, status in the family, etc.—and these feelings do not necessarily cease when siblings reach adulthood. When an infertile man accepts sperm from his fertile brother, emotionally he may feel that he is in a "one down position." Those feelings may rekindle earlier feelings relating to the power dynamic between the two of them. (We encourage readers to review the Ovum Donation Chapter—unlike men, women often turn to their sisters for egg donation and this form of donation has been regarded very positively, by and large).

A case example illustrates this point regarding sibling competition. A male infertility patient who set up an appointment with a clinical social worker to discuss donor insemination mentioned that he had three brothers. His proposal was to ask each of them to donate sperm and have the physician mix them together prior to the insemination. That way no one would know which brother was the genetic father to the child. The social worker saw the proposal as a red flag and sensed that if he could not tolerate knowing which brother was the genetic father of his child, that he was not emotionally prepared to accept his brother's sperm.

Further discussion revealed that the inability to reproduce was a grave loss for this man, and he believed that his parents would be devastated if he were to tell them about his infertility. In using his brother's sperm, he felt satisfied that he would not be letting his parents down—one brother's genes were as good as another's—and therefore he would not feel guilty about keeping it secret from them. As the interview continued, it also became clear that he had strong competitive feelings toward all of his siblings. Although he had hoped to neutralize these feelings by mixing sperm from all three brothers, the husband realized that this action might even magnify his feelings of competition rather than diminish them. He concluded that he would always wonder, perhaps even to the point of obsession, which brother was the *real* father. The couple decided to attempt pregnancy with anonymous donor sperm.

The request to "pool" sperm from more than one brother (or more than one friend) is not unusual. In-depth counseling in such situations usually uncovers (as it did in the above example) strong resistance to the process, which in turn may serve as a mask for feelings of shame, inferiority, and impotence. Understanding the nature of one's resistance, and resolving the painful feelings that accompany it, can help men and their partners make a decision that is best for their family and with which they can feel comfortable throughout their lives.

One known-donor situation that sometimes arises and is both psychologically and ethically troubling to many mental health professionals is cross-generational donation of parent to child, or vice versa. In the case of a son donating to his father (in a second marriage), many feel strongly that because of the nature of the parent-child relationship (most children always feel indebted to their parents to some degree), a child is not truly free to say no to a parent's request in the same way he is free to say no to anyone else. In the case of a father donating to a son, some professionals feel more supportive, because the concept of a parent giving to his child is already built into the parent-child relationship.

Access to Medical Information

Using a known donor allows the family to have current medical information, something which is important to many couples because of the genetic components of illness. Unlike anonymous donation, which provides people with considerable medical *history*, but not with *ongoing* information, known donation offers families access to medical information as it unfolds in the life of the donor and in his family.

Motivations for Becoming a Known Sperm Donor

What motivates a man to donate sperm for a relative or friend? To our knowledge there has been no scientific research done that can answer this question, however, our anecdotal experience can shed some light on it. There seem to be two primary reasons why men become known donors: either they want to help a friend or relative, or they wish to become a father.

In the first instance, the donor is usually approached by his friend, brother, or other relative. Frequently in these situations the donor is someone who already has children. He may be an appealing candidate because he has proven fertility, has his own family and may therefore be less likely to intrude on the recipient family's life, has desirable genes, and most likely has children who also have admirable characteristics.

Such donors tend to regard donating their sperm much as blood donors view giving blood: solely as an altruistic act. Donors reason that since they have extra blood/sperm and someone else can use it, that not doing so would be selfish. Although they are aware that donating sperm means creating a life, as opposed to sustaining a life, which is the purpose of blood donation, the two acts feel very similar. Typically, these men are able to separate genetic ties from family ties, and when it is pointed out that their children will be half siblings to the donor offspring, they usually respond that they do not view it that way.

Men who donate primarily because they wish to be fathers, but not necessarily full-time rearing fathers, make up a substantial group of donors. They tend to be single and do not know whether marriage and family are "in the cards" for them. Some of these men may be gay and being a full-time father may not fit into their lifestyle or be desirable to them. Men who donate because they want to be fathers frequently, though not always, donate to lesbian couples or to single women.

If a man is donating sperm to a heterosexual couple primarily because he is interested in fatherhood and secondarily because he desires to help his friends, the situation may become extremely complicated. Couples choosing a known donor who does not have children of his own need to be very careful about the donor's true motivations. Although any situation involving a known donor necessitates careful deliberation (ideally involving a mental health clinician) and legal consultation as well, situations in which the donor wants a parenting role can be problematic unless all parties are in agreement about one another's roles and relationship to the child.

Psychological and Legal Counseling

Because of the many questions and concerns involved in using known donors, couples and their donors should have comprehensive counseling from a mental health professional specializing in reproductive medicine before embarking on this venture. It is generally wise for the counselor to meet first with the donor, before she or he has any knowledge about or becomes acquainted with the prospective couple. The counselor can then assume an objective stance and help the prospective donor decide if donating is in his best interest. If the counselor has met with the couple prior to meeting with the donor and has come to know them and feels invested in helping them, it becomes more difficult to remain objective.

Couples and their donors need to be in agreement about the basic issues raised by the process. They must agree on who they will tell about the arrangement, how and when they will tell the child, how frequently the donor will see the child, what his role will be with him/her, and how the families will interact, if he is part of a couple. If the donor has children and/or is married, his spouse should also be included in the counseling and feel comfortable with the agreements. Everyone involved must anticipate that their needs will change over time, and that as the child matures s/he will have a voice in how they relate to one another.

Couples who are using a known donor should also seek legal counsel from an attorney who is well versed in reproductive law. The law in this field is continually changing, however, and varies from state to state. All parties should familiarize themselves with the statutes that apply before entering into an agreement. Both the donor and the parents will want to be protected from future suits or legal entanglements, no matter how close or trusting a relationship they feel they have. The donor needs to know that he will not be required to provide any means of care or support for the child, and the parents need to know they will be protected from any claims on their child, legal or otherwise, from the donor. Such legal contracts may or may not be binding, however, and do not assure couples that future lawsuits will not arise. Nevertheless, the act of consulting with an attorney will afford the couple another opportunity to think through many of the crucial issues involved in known sperm donation.

Anonymous Sperm Donation

Couples who form their families via anonymous sperm donation are part of the vast majority of DI couples. Although there is societal pressure —and frequently pressure from physicians as well—to use an anonymous donor, most couples who choose this route do so because they feel that they are making a rational decision, one that is in their family's and their child's best interest.

Choosing Anonymous Donation

Many couples never seriously consider asking a man they know to donate sperm for them. They imagine that all sorts of social and emotional complications would ensue, and view anonymous donation as an "easier" route psychologically. Although there are no studies done to date which compare the two possible DI avenues, it is not necessarily true that one route is easier than another. Nevertheless, couples who choose anonymous donation share several reasons in common.

Belonging and Authenticity

Those who choose anonymous donation most often feel that in a known situation they and/or their child might be confused about his/her identity and to whom s/he belongs. Specifically, they worry that their child might experience "social or relational bewilderment;" that is, the child might be confused about having "two fathers." Many fear that if the donor lived close by and would be part of their lives, then there would be a greater likelihood of social bewilderment. If the donor were a relative, say a brother, the child may be confused about who is the father and who is the uncle.

DI couples—especially husbands—may have concerns that if the genetic father were known, the social father might feel cast aside. It is extremely important that the husband feel that he is the authentic father of his child and that he is entitled to assume that role. Whatever choice— known or anonymous—DI parents make, they must be convinced that their child will belong to them. Couples selecting anonymous donation see this choice as offering them that opportunity. They fear that if the donor were known, particularly if he is someone who interacts frequently with the couple, the husband may not feel like the real father.

Privacy

Couples to whom privacy is very important tend to prefer anonymous sperm donation. This situation allows them to feel more in control of information regarding their child's conception—a right that fertile couples are unquestioningly granted. Donor couples are aware that when other people have information about them, there is no guarantee it will not be shared. Even though they may fully intend to be truthful with their offspring about all aspects of his/her conception, the knowledge that there are others who are stakeholders in how and when this information is shared violates their need for autonomy over this issue. And although they may find the idea of choosing their donor appealing, it is not worth relinquishing their privacy.

Lack of a Known Donor Option

Not all couples who prefer to use a known donor have this choice. They may not have a friend, relative, or aquaintance whom they feel comfortable asking, or they may have asked someone who refused. People who have been turned down by the donor of their choice have two remaining options: to turn to anonymous donation or advertise for a known donor. Advertising for a genetic father for one's child is unusual but does occur. The February 1993 issue of *Boston Magazine* contained an advertisement in the personal section for a sperm donor. The ad, placed by a single woman (it might just as well have been placed by a couple), was lengthy and offered a detailed description of her motivations for having a child, as well as her reasons for wanting to identify the donor. Toward the end of the advertisement she wrote: "Why such an unconventional route? Concern re: child's identity formation. While anonymous donation is ideal for some, I want to spare my children the burden of mystery regarding paternal identity."

Whether it is morally right to bring a child into the world with unknown parentage is a question that each person must ponder. Currently our society sanctions anonymous donation and is more equivocal about known gamete donation. As society evolves, however, public opinion changes, and what is thought by the majority to be in a child's best interest today may be regarded differently tomorrow. Because there is a growing recognition that our genes form a basic blueprint that relates to our human potential, more people than ever before— albeit a still small percentage— are turning to known donors.

The Selection and Practice of Anonymous Sperm Donation

The practice of donor insemination has changed remarkably since AIDS (acquired immunodeficiency syndrome) has become a health crisis (Ironically, Donor Insemination was commonly referred to as AID—Artificial Insemination by Donor—prior to the AIDS crisis, which created a possible confusion in acronym.) Before the AIDS epidemic, most donor insemination was performed using fresh semen from a donor who had been selected by the local physician or infertility clinic. The clinic would arrange for the donor to deliver his sample prior to the woman's appearing for the insemination procedure. Although everything was done anonymously, at least one person on staff knew the donor personally. Couples were frequently told that their donor was handsome, or that he was a medical student, or a wonderful athlete, or they were offered some other piece of information that was positive and enabled the couple to feel a connection to their donor.

In 1986, in light of the increase in numbers of people being infected with the AIDS virus, the American Society for Reproductive Medicine revised its guidelines pertaining to the use of anonymous sperm donation. The guidelines now strongly recommend that all donation be done with frozen sperm that has been quarantined for at least 180 days, at which point the donor must be retested before the sample is used. Although not all physicians made the transition from fresh to frozen semen immediately, most did in subsequent years, recognizing the importance of using frozen sperm as a safeguard against disease. This practice, although necessary to protect the health of everyone involved, has led to a reduction in pregnancy rates, because frozen sperm is not as viable as fresh semen. When donor sperm are used in conjunction with the new reproductive technologies, however, the fact that sperm were frozen does not seem to affect the fertilization rate.

Emotionally, a drawback to using frozen donor sperm is that the process can feel more remote to the recipient couple. The donor becomes truly anonymous; he is not even known to the couple's physician or to the clinic staff. In recent years, however, sperm banks have begun providing extensive information to couples about their donor in an effort to make him seem more familiar. (See later section, Sperm Banks.) This greater degree of anonymity, though, can be a relief to some couples who know they will not worry about whether their donor was the man sitting next to them in the waiting area.

American Society for Reproductive Medicine Guidelines

The American Society for Reproductive Medicine (ASRM), formerly the American Fertility Society, is a very large, international organization of professionals involved in fertility. ASRM is a private, nonprofit which includes the Society of Reproductive Endocrinologists, the Society of Reproductive Surgeons, and the Society for Assisted Reproductive Technology under its umbrella. In 1993 ASRM revised its previous recommendations pertaining to the use of semen donation in *Guidelines for Gamete Donation: 1993*.

According to the guidelines, donors are required to be in good health, free of systemic diseases, and free of genetic abnormalities. A complete family and medical history should be taken in order to rule out the potential for offspring with genetic problems. Donors should not be in a high-risk group for AIDS. In order to screen thoroughly for sexually transmitted diseases, donors should be tested for syphilis and every six months for serum hepatitis B antigen and hepatitis C antibody. Donors should also be tested for cytomegalovirus every six months, and donors who test positive should be used only with positive recipients. Screening for HIV antibodies (human immunodeficiency virus, the virus that causes AIDS) should be performed every six months, and semen obtained at the time should be cryopreserved and used only if retesting after 180 days confirms the antibodies are not present. Donors should be above legal age but below the age of forty.[25]

The guidelines also suggest obtaining several samples before undergoing more extensive testing. The criteria for sperm parameters after two or three days of abstinence are motility greater than 60%, concentration greater than or equal to 50 million motile sperm per milliliter, and at least 60% normal in appearance. These criteria are strict; a man is considered fertile with considerably lower numbers. They are, however, necessary in order to offset the negative effects of freezing. Because the guidelines are so strict, in many clinics only about one in ten men who apply to be a donor is accepted.

Sperm banks are urged by these guidelines to develop ongoing procedures for monitoring the health of donors. The guidelines do not specify the amount of compensation a donor is allowed to receive for his time and expenses, but they state that monetary compensation should not be the prime reason for the donation. (The standard fee paid to donors seems to be between twenty-five and fifty dollars per ejaculate.) The ASRM guidelines also advise limiting the number of pregnancies resulting from a particular donor to ten, which should ensure that the danger of consanguinity from a particular donor—a worry that couples frequently mention—is virtually nonexistent.

The ASRM guidelines suggest ways to match the male partner with the donor, advising that clinics ask couples to list the physical characteristics of a donor that are important to them and make reasonable efforts to comply with their wishes. At this point in time it is our belief that almost all clinics allow couples to select their own donor—a choice we feel is essential in promoting a couple's autonomy and in allowing them to have some control over the process. Since sperm banks are providing psycho-social information about donors as well as medical and demographic information, it is important for couples to think about the personal qualities and attributes they would like their donor to possess, and to give that information equal weight in selecting a donor.

RESOLVE Inc., the national organization providing advocacy, education, counseling, support, and referral to infertile couples, offers a list of questions to their members regarding sperm banks. RESOLVE urges people to learn the answers before proceeding with a particular bank. RESOLVE suggests that couples inquire about whether the banks keep medical histories on donors, whether they keep track of the number of pregnancies per donor, how long they keep records, and whether the same donor's sperm can be available for a second child. RESOLVE lists criteria for selecting donors and provides a list of diseases for which donors should be screened.

Sperm Banks

Couples who elect to use anonymous sperm from a sperm bank make a giant leap of faith. They must be able to trust that their physician is dealing with a reputable and responsible sperm bank that is performing the necessary screening and evaluations on donors. They need to feel confident about the selection process and believe that the donors are physically and emotionally healthy and are free of any identifiable genetic disorders.

The process of banking and freezing sperm is nationally unregulated; no official body regulates and oversees the practices of sperm banks. The American Society of Reproductive Medicine (ASRM) has a listing of approximately 100 banks. However, since there is no requirement that a sperm bank register with ASRM, it is likely that there are many more than 100— estimates are about 200—in operation. Some programs and clinics operate their own banks, and while they might encourage their patients to choose from among their own donors, most also offer the use of other banks as well. Two states, California and New York, require sperm banks to be licensed in order to operate.

The American Association of Tissue Banks is an organization that encourages sperm banks to become members. In addition to providing guidelines for sperm banks to follow, the Association also offers an accreditation process, which includes visits to their laboratory and scrutinization of personnel and of standard operating procedures. Although many banks may comply with their guidelines, only a few have actually gone through the process to become accredited. Couples who go through accredited banks have the satisfaction of knowing that they have met the strictest standards possible.

Sperm banks, like any other industry, vary in size as well as in the services they provide. In recent years, in response to the needs of consumers, sperm banks have greatly increased the range and repertoire of services they offer. Individuals and couples from all over the country are asking for more information about donors— information about their physical, ethnic, medical, and social backgrounds as well as their personalities, temperaments, interests, and philosophies of life. Some banks offer photos of donors; some provide baby pictures; some provide assistance in matching physical appearance to that of the husband; others provide statements or essays from donors to the offspring; still others provide audio cassettes of an interview with the potential donor.

Although we did not attempt to obtain a cross-section, we have chosen to discuss three banks that offer a range of services that are appealing to couples. These banks consider the needs of all parties, especially those of the children being created. (We do not wish to give the impression, however, that these three sperm banks are the only ones that are considering the best interest of the child and of DI families.) Couples should feel free to call any of the more than two hundred banks to obtain information about their policies or programs.

The larger the bank is, the greater its pool of donors and the more choices available to couples. California Cryobank, the largest in the world, maintains a list of over 250 donors, updated monthly. It also offers the largest group of minority donors. Donors accepted into the program are required to complete a twenty-seven page form that asks extensive questions about their personal characteristics, hobbies, interests, and preferences, in addition to genetic and medical information. This information is available to couples for a nominal fee. If they prefer, they can receive free of charge a short form about their donor, which consists of two pages—the first two pages of the long form. This information is also available on the World Wide Web. In addition, California Cryobank offers audiotapes of its donors to interested couples.

This extensive information about the donor is significant to couples. Through various descriptions, writings, and statements, the donor emerges as a real person rather than as a product. Couples can begin to imagine what he is like and may even feel emotionally connected to him. Some couples have commented that having this information about the donor helps them to fill in the void and to feel a positive connection to the donor.

Another service that California Cryobank offers is its Openness Policy. The bank saves donor records indefinitely, recognizing that unborn children cannot make agreements about their future wishes in regard to the donor, and that sperm donors, especially those who are in their late teens and twenties, cannot know how they will feel several years hence about making themselves known to an offspring. Therefore, if at a later date a donor offspring or the parents wish more information about the donor, California Cryobank will obtain it for them. If the offspring wishes to know the identity of the donor in years to come, the bank will act as middleman and ask the donor whether he will agree. If the answer is no, it will not attempt to force a meeting or reveal the identity of the donor.

Another service provided by this sperm bank is stem cell storage. The umbilical cord of newborns contains stem cells that can be frozen and stored as a kind of biological insurance against future serious illness, including certain types of cancer and genetic blood disorders. Stem cells must be obtained immediately after birth, and the procedure, which is painless, takes about ten minutes. California Cryobank is now able to freeze these cells as insurance against future tragic illness.

Xytex, another fairly large commercial sperm bank, requires all donors to write essays, sharing personal information about themselves or their family, including facts about their upbringing, background and personality. Xytex encourages donors to include messages to the unborn offspring about their reasons for becoming a sperm donor, their philosophy of life, and/or their wishes for the offspring. These messages serve the purpose of making the donor become more real to the couple as well as to their child—the donor becomes a person who has a history, a character, and a purpose in life.

Approximately half of Xytex's donors provide head and shoulder photos of themselves; another group of donors provide baby or childhood pictures of themselves. An additional service that Xytex offers is a Patriarch Program; it stores cells from the donor, which become his genetic file. These cells can be used later, if additional information is needed about a donor's genetic history. Information about Xytex is also available on the World Wide Web.

Larger does not necessarily mean better: small banks may also provide specialized services not offered by other banks. The Sperm Bank of California, in Berkeley, is one of three or four banks (at the time of this writing) that offers a pool of identity-release donors who agree in writing to be identified when the offspring is eighteen, should the latter choose to have this information. This fairly small sperm bank, which began in 1982, is a non-profit organization, with approximately forty active donors, one third of them in the identity-release group. An additional thirty-five or so donors are on an inactive list, available to couples who already have one donor child and would like a biological sibling for him or her. The philosophy of the Sperm Bank of California is that the potential child is the key stake-holder in terms of his or her identity—the most affected by the process of donor insemination.

Identity-release donors are carefully screened, according to Barbara Raboy, director of this sperm bank. They must understand thoroughly the implications of their agreement. They are asked about whether they have shared their interest in being a donor with family and friends and what those people's reactions were. They are encouraged to tell their current partner and are urged to think about whether they would tell a future partner and to anticipate how that person might react.

Potential identity-release donors must be comfortable with separating the nurturing aspect of parenthood from the genetic aspect. Raboy explains that she is very "tough" on these candidates, suggesting various future scenarios that could be problematic. In particular, she wants identity-release donors to think about how they would feel should one (or several) of their genetic offspring request a reunion at a later date, particularly if the donor in question has a family of his own. Donors who hesitate or believe that it may be difficult to be sought out in the future are asked to join the anonymous pool. Their hesitation is taken as a no. Donors who do not have a problem with being identified later are also reassured that since their semen must be quarantined for a minimum of six months, they can change their mind during that period.

Although the sperm banks we have referred to differ in size and style and to some extent, philosophy, we feel that what they share is more significant than the differences among them. They—like many other sperm banks—appear to have an increasing appreciation of the psychological and ethical issues involved in donor insemination. Within the past ten years in particular, they have developed policies and programs that work on behalf of the voluntary participants in donor insemination —the parents and the donors. Moreover, sperm banks seem to have increasing respect for the rights of unborn children—especially those who are the involuntary participants in donor insemination.

Donor Counseling

There is clearly a double standard in terms of how male sperm donors have historically been treated and how female donors are being treated in ovum donation programs. In the next chapter we speculate on the reasons for some of these differences. It is worth noting here, however, that none of the three banks we highlighted, as well as others with whom we checked, provide extensive psychological counseling to their anonymous sperm donors. They may perform thorough medical and genetic screening, but apparently there is little or no mention to potential sperm donors of potential long-term psychosocial issues, the exception being that provided to identity release donors associated with the Sperm Bank of California.

It is interesting to note that although sperm banks are recognizing that donor families have long term needs that must be addressed and are adapting their services accordingly, they do not seem to be acknowledging that donating sperm—even anonymously—may have ramifications for a man's future. Thus it is not surprising that counseling about psychosocial issues is not a part of the screening and recruitment process of donors. Perhaps if donors were encouraged to think about sperm as being part of a biological continuum leading to the creation of a person, rather than as a bodily product that is merely going to waste, there might be fewer donors. Annette Baran and Reuben Pannor, in doing research for their book, *Lethal Secrets*, interviewed thirty-seven men who had been semen donors and found that the emotional implications of being a donor may surface much later.[26] The following story illustrates this point.

A psychologist had the opportunity to meet with a thirty-five-year-old physician who had been a sperm donor several times while in medical school. For years after he graduated, he rarely thought about having been a donor. As his donor offspring were about to enter adolescence, however, he found himself wondering whether he might accidently bump into a young man who looked and was built just like him. The donor himself was the spitting image of his father, a fact that countless people had remarked on throughout his life. He had always assumed that if he had sons, they too would carry on this family resemblance. This thought had begun to plague him more frequently, occasionally intruding in his work, and he was contemplating whether to seek counseling. Another reason that this issue probably surfaced was at the time he was engaged, and he and his fiance planned to have children. He wondered about whether he was still fertile and how he would feel if he learned otherwise.

Ken Daniels, a researcher in New Zealand, where the law requires that all donors be registered, takes a strong stand about the necessity of raising psychosocial issues with prospective donors. A potential donor, he says, needs to think about the fact that he will have offspring whom he will not know. Furthermore, if the donor has children of his own, they will have half-siblings whom they do not know. A donor must think about whether he would tell his children about their unknown genetic siblings. Daniels suggests also that a donor consider whether he will tell his spouse (or future spouse) and how his spouse might react to the information. Preselection counseling should also include thinking about whether he wants to know how many (or if any) offspring were created as a result of his sperm donations and how the information would affect him over the years. Donors must be made aware of the changing trends in record keeping and the fact that future anonymity cannot be guaranteed. Donors should also consider whether they believe a child should have access to information about his or her genetic parent, or whether that child should even be told that the father who reared him or her was not the genetic father. Donors should consider whether they are concerned about who gets their sperm. Do they have a personal stake in whom they are helping to bear a child? In essence, potential donors must explore both the short- and the long-term issues of providing sperm anonymously and whether it is in their own psychological best interest. Daniels states emphatically:

> It is the professional's responsibility to ensure that such consideration occurs. Without consideration of these issues, it is not possible to say that the donor has given "informed" consent. Consent will have been given, but it has not been informed, in that the issues associated with and arising from the donation have been considered and understood. To receive appropriate consideration, the psychosocial factors have to be recognized as having a significant and legitimate contribution to make.[27]

Because donating sperm is not the same as donating blood, we hope that sperm banks will begin to offer counseling to potential donors—counseling that addresses the long-term psychosocial issues involved in semen donation. In the interest of helping infertile couples create families, it is important that we not overlook the emotional needs of donors, or they may surface later. Donors need guidance in exploring what it really means for them to donate their gametes, not only at the time of donation but also over the course of a lifetime—and for future generations.

Social Policy Regarding Donor Information and Record Keeping

There is no legislation unifying the practice of anonymous sperm donation, including the screening and selection of donors, so there is no available model of record keeping ensuring that recipient couples have access to important descriptive information about their donor. Thus, the practice of record keeping varies from sperm bank to sperm bank and from physician's office to physician's office. Many couples are so eager to conceive—and to conceive quickly—that their judgement regarding medical, genetic, and social information may be eclipsed. Couples should be encouraged to question both the sperm bank and their physician about their record keeping. The ASRM guidelines state

It is highly desirable to maintain permanent confidential records of donors, including a genetic workup and other nonidentifying information, and to make the anonymous record available on request to the recipient and/or any resulting offspring.[28]

The Purpose of Record Keeping

Attitudes toward all aspects of donor insemination are changing, including the necessity of obtaining and preserving extensive information relative to a donor's social, medical, and genetic history. There are two main reasons why record keeping is important. The first is for the parents, so that they can develop a positive feeling for the donor prior to the insemination and feel that he is familiar to them. A second reason is for the child, so that he or she has access to the donor's medical and social background—information that will undoubtedly be helpful in identity formation. Furthermore the role that heredity plays in the transmission of personality traits as well as medical conditions is increasingly well documented. An understanding of those aspects of an individual can help to illuminate, and in many instances alleviate, similar problems played out in the subsequent generation.

Although many couples initially approach donor insemination with the conviction that it will be secret, many change their minds. Once the opportunity to get the information has been passed up, it may be too late to retrieve it later, should the parents or the child desire the information. Couples choosing donor insemination should obtain as much genetic, medical, and psychosocial information as they can from the sperm bank. Those who think they want to keep DI a secret can preserve the information in a safety deposit box or in some other safe place. They are likely to change their minds and the information will then be very important.

Donors' Willingness to Provide Information

The history and practice of donor insemination in the United States has followed the lines of secrecy and anonymity. Prior to the change in policy from fresh to frozen semen, physicians urged secrecy for the contracting couple and felt a similar urgency to protect donors from ever obtaining any information about offspring created or the parents who were raising the child. Physicians feared they would be unable to attract donors if they could not guarantee that they would be untraceable. They also feared that if donors were asked to fill out lengthy questionnaires describing their physical, social, psychological, and medical background, they would not be willing to do so. Thus, couples who chose anonymous sperm donation in the past received minimal information about important characteristics of their donor.

In November 1984, Australia banned payment for human gametes and mandated counseling as well as obligatory record keeping for gamete donors. More recently, Canada has followed suit. Although this book focuses on the United States, the trends, practices, and laws of other countries do influence thinking and decision making regarding these same policies. There is reason to believe that donors in the United States would also be willing to provide far more information to the sperm banks that contract with them than they have been asked to do previously. A look at some recent studies, one in New Zealand and one in the United States, sheds light on this issue.

Ken Daniels has conducted several studies that offer insight into the characteristics of semen donors as well as their willingness to share extensive information— identifying or nonidentifying—with sperm banks and/or couples who use their gametes. Daniels found that about half of the donors involved in six Australian programs believe that a child has the right to nonidentifying information about their donor. Eleven percent of donors (as opposed to five percent of couples) believed the child who knows she or he is a DI offspring will want to learn the identity of the donor. The study also indicated that at least one-quarter of the donors would still donate even if there was a possibility they could be traced in the future. An additional 30% said they were uncertain.[29]

A study published in the United States in 1991 by Patricia Mahlstedt and Kris Probasco yielded similar findings. The purpose of their research was to determine the extent to which donors were willing to provide extensive social, medical, psychological, and genetic nonidentifying information about themselves on their applications and to learn what their attitudes were in regard to sharing this information with recipient families. The researchers studied seventy-nine donors from two programs—one in Texas and one in Louisiana. All were between the ages of nineteen and thirty-nine, with a median age of twenty-four.

The results of the Mahlstedt and Probasco survey undoubtedly surprised many people, from physicians who perform inseminations to sperm banks that recruit donors. Of those in the sample, 90% returned the new application form that requested extensive information about physical characteristics, personal characteristics, family history, personal health history, and a statement about themselves. Almost all (96%) of the donors responded positively to the question, "How do you feel about descriptive, but nonidentifying information about you being given to the recipient family?" Their answers indicated they felt it was important for donor families to have information about the donor. When donors were asked whether they would donate if anonymity could not be guaranteed, 36% said they would. In response to a slightly different question, 37% said they felt positively toward openness, suggesting that they would be willing to meet the offspring some day; 38% felt uncomfortable with openness; and 14% were uncertain. Although these results seem to indicate that fewer men would be willing to donate if they were not guaranteed anonymity, they do not indicate by any means that the donor pool would be depleted.[30]

There are no laws in the United States requiring sperm banks to obtain and preserve records of donors. Many in the field of reproductive medicine, like the researcher-clinicians in the previous study, would like such a policy. Elias and Annas, the physician and attorney referred to previously, argue that the policy of secrecy was created mainly to protect the sperm donor from claims arising from his resulting offspring rather than from a consideration of the offspring's best interest. They make a case for allowing donor offspring to have access to identifiable information about their donor parent and refer to a study of sperm donors that indicates 60% of them would still donate even if anonymity were not guaranteed. The authors state:

> Since it may turn out to be an extremely important psychological (and possibly medical or genetic) issue to the child seeking information about his genetic heritage, records should be kept of all births in a way that they can be matched with donors.... The donor can effectively waive any right to access to such records, but no one should be able to effectively waive the child's future access to genetic, medical, and perhaps even personal information about the donor. These records could have two "levels": Level 1 would be medical and genetic history, but not identifiable; Level 2 would contain the donor's actual identity. Access to Level 1 information should be guaranteed. Access to Level 2 should be possible but only if the child can demonstrate a "need to know."[31]

Although it seems that the United States is a long way from adopting such a policy, it may be moving in that direction. Couples using anonymous sperm banks must understand that by the time their children reach adulthood, banks that were once anonymous may be mandated to open their records.

Selecting a Donor

The process of attempting pregnancy begins with selecting a donor. DI couples are curious about sperm donors, wondering what kind of men would be willing to donate semen, and why they would do so. Fantasies run the gamut from those who are down and out, seeking financial compensation, to those whose narcissism compels them to disseminate their genes. Actually most sperm donors fit into neither of these categories. Sperm donors are recruited from a number of locations, graduate and undergraduate colleges being the most common. They undergo a highly selective process which eliminates approximately ninety percent of applicants—usually for physical, medical or genetic reasons. Although undoubtedly their reasons for donating vary, Daniels, who conducted a small study on the motivations of sperm donors, found that 91% indicated that the desire to help infertile couples was the main reason or a reason for being a donor; 59% indicated it was the sole reason.[32]

Selecting a donor is one of the most important decisions a DI couple makes. Couples who are able to regard the donor as a person, with unique characteristics and features, generally seem to be more comfortable with donor insemination. But not all clinic staff are equally informed about the psychosocial issues involved in this alternative, and many unwittingly undermine a couple's sense of control and autonomy as they attempt to create their family through DI. Some clinics—we hope not many—believe that the couple should not be involved in the choice of a donor. In these programs, staff (usually nurses) select a donor whom they feel is a good match for a particular couple. How they make this determination is unclear.

Sometimes couples, in their urgency to become pregnant, readily agree to let the clinic pick their donor. Their need to deny the reality of DI may encourage them to see the selection process as part of the medical procedure, thus leaving it in the hands of clinical staff whose judgment, they think, must be more astute than theirs. Others feel at the mercy of their doctor and staff, never questioning policy or procedures for fear the clinic will reject them as patients. Sadly, many of those couples discover that they have questions and feelings *after* they become pregnant. We have known women, pregnant after DI, who sought counseling because their absence of information about the donor made the pregnancy more stressful. One such woman, who had almost no information about the donor, told her therapist that her lack of information about him caused her to focus more on her own ethnicity. During her pregnancy she "talked" to the baby about her family and imagined imparting her traditions and customs to the child. These rituals helped her feel that when she gave birth to her child he would seem familiar.

Although there are undoubtedly a few couples who may appreciate not having to make the selection, most feel strongly, sooner or later, that they need to make it. Having someone who barely knows them make this crucial decision feeds into their sense of helplessness. Most clinics allow couples to choose their donor, and most have access to more than one bank. All sperm banks provide at least minimal information (many provide extensive information) to recipient couples about the donor(s) they have selected. The information is published in a catalog that is updated regularly and includes certain characteristics: height, weight, build, eye color, hair color and texture, ethnic background, blood type, number of years of schooling, including the donor's major field of study, and key hobbies or interests. We encourage couples to work only with banks that provide extensive information about their donors. We have found that the more they know about the donor, the more secure they are with their choice to create their family with donor sperm.

Most couples try to select a donor whose physical characteristics are similar to the husband's. Although it is natural for them to want their child to physically "fit in" with his/her parents, it is crucial that the couple not be trying to replicate the husband. Hopefully having other information about the donor—his personality, character, interests—helps them acknowledge that he is an individual in his own right, distinctively different from the husband. In fact, this information should help them to develop positive feelings about him—feelings that will be especially reassuring during pregnancy, when DI couples commonly have second thoughts about the conception.

Confronting differences before conception helps couples prepare for pregnancy and parenting after donor insemination. Once they have grappled with the fact that their child will probably be unlike his/her father due to genetic influences, they can feel better prepared to establish and enjoy the major role that the father will play in shaping the child's values, attitudes, character and sense of self.

Attempting Pregnancy

A significant percentage of infertile couples have both male and female factors contributing to their infertility. In many cases the woman has already undergone infertility diagnosis and or treatment prior to donor insemination. When DI does not work after several tries, additional treatment may be recommended, which may include the use of ART. Other couples who elect to attempt DI know that they must use it in conjunction with IVF or GIFT, or pregnancy will not be possible.

For some DI couples, pregnancy occurs in the first few months of trying. Most feel fortunate that they are on their way to becoming parents. Sometimes, however, the feelings are more bittersweet, as the wife's fertility stands in marked contrast to the husband's infertility.

When pregnancy does not occur after about three to six months, couples face a dilemma about whether to change donors, extend the female medical workup, or continue trying with the donor they have selected. Changing donors can be psychologically difficult because couples frequently become attached to their donor, even an anonymous donor, feeling a kind of loyalty. Nevertheless, many couples do make a change, hoping that the failure to conceive was due to the wrong mix of sperm and eggs and was not an indication of an undiagnosed female problem. Sometimes clinics advise couples to change donors if they feel that the samples have not been optimal.

Couples using a known donor face a difficult dilemma. If the donor's sperm count was less than ideal to begin with, they must decide how long they are willing to continue with him before moving to a different donor. If the sperm samples are normal, the couple will probably want to continue, assuming that a female problem may be at work. Because many couples carefully choose their known donors, it is not easy emotionally or logistically to make a change.

A brief struggle with conception can become a positive experience for DI couples. Though feeling mostly resolved about their decision, many begin inseminations acutely aware of their ambivalence. When a few months go by without a pregnancy, the majority of these couples become very disappointed, and their ambivalence gives way to a feeling of confidence about their choice of DI—a confidence now tinged with worry.

When several months go by without a pregnancy, the focus shifts to the woman in an attempt to discover what may be wrong, if anything.

191

Sometimes in the process of her work up, the male factor is forgotten as couples once again focus on whether conception is possible, rather than on how they will feel about a donor child. Men (and sometimes their partners), though feeling disappointed, may also feel a bit relieved that infertility is now shared.

It is common for problems that were previously diagnosed as minor in the woman to be regarded as major when conception does not occur after a reasonable time. In other cases, new problems are discovered that may have been overlooked when the emphasis was on the man. Couples in this situation are now faced with a series of decisions about treatment, which may include the use of ART.

When conception does not happen easily, DI couples find themselves back on the emotional roller coaster, experiencing many of the same feelings and fears that they had during their initial infertility experience. Some, especially those who agonized for a long time before deciding on DI, may begin to question whether they made the right decision. Others decide that adoption is a better alternative for them or elect to live without children.

Fear of Error

Because the process of becoming pregnant through DI is, to a great extent, in the hands of others, couples must have faith that nothing out of the ordinary will occur. They must have faith in the sperm bank that screens the donors and freezes the sperm and in the clinic that processes it and performs the insemination. They must believe that their goal of a normal, healthy child is not only possible but probable under these circumstances.

Many couples describe the process of donor insemination as feeling very strange. The starkness of the examining room, in contrast to the warmth of their bedroom, can give rise to images of well-intended but mad scientists and experiments gone awry. It is common for couples to worry about a mix-up, afraid they will get the wrong sperm. So much must happen between the donor selection process and the actual insemination that it is easy to see how those fears arise.

In fact there have been some distressing cases that have hit the media in recent years, involving errors made by a laboratory or by a sperm bank. One such case was that of Julia Skolnick whose husband had vials of sperm frozen prior to his treatment for cancer in 1985. She gave birth in 1986 to a mixed-race daughter and subsequently sued the physician who performed the insemination and the sperm bank that sent her the wrong vial. Such errors are extremely rare, but the fact that they occur at all is worrisome to many couples using donor insemination.

Pregnancy after Donor Insemination

Pregnancy after donor insemination can bring mixed feelings. Couples who had difficulty conceiving with DI may be able to move beyond their fears and concerns with relative ease, feeling grateful for the eventual conception. Those who conceived soon after the inseminations began, however, may feel their ambivalence more keenly, or for a longer period of time. Pregnancy for DI couples can rekindle old worries, in both husband and wife, about genetic inequality, attachment to the child, and social acceptibility if they are planning to be open about donor insemination. If they are planning to keep donor insemination a secret, they may worry that their child will appear marked in some obvious way.

Like all other pregnant couples, expectant DI parents worry whether their child will be healthy and whether their pregnancy will be a good one. Once they feel secure in the pregnancy, they may begin to think more about the donor. They wonder in what ways their child will resemble him. (For a more extensive discussion of pregnancy after gamete donation, see Chapter 3).

Pregnancy Loss

Although more often than not, DI couples end up with healthy children, this is not always the case. Women pregnant after donor insemination experience pregnancy loss at the same rate as everyone else—approximately one in five times. When a couple loses a child after many years of infertility, it is especially sad. In addition to the universal feelings of loss they share with all other infertile couples, there are a few issues unique to DI couples.

The loss of a donor pregnancy, especially for couples who struggled with religious proscriptions before deciding on DI, can bring up feelings (or fears) that they are being punished—that perhaps they made a wrong decision. Such couples may view the loss as a warning from God not to tamper with nature—or, worse, that they are not meant to be parents.

When a couple experiences a pregnancy loss, family and friends frequently address their expressions of sympathy to the woman. After all, she is the one who carried the fetus and suffered the pain of the miscarriage. When sympathy is expressed only to women, it is hurtful to men, and it is especially hurtful to husbands using DI who already feel like outsiders. If the couple has been open with others about DI and sympathy is directed to the wife, the husband may feel that this is confirms his fears that he is an unimportant and unnecessary player. (For a discussion of pregnancy loss after assisted reproduction, see Chapter 3).

When Donor Insemination Is Unsuccessful

Some couples may not conceive, no matter how hard and how long they try. This situation seems especially unfair to those who spent years trying to overcome male infertility and eventually turned to donor insemination after careful counseling and deliberation. Now they must reevaluate their situation and make a third choice: to become parents through adoption or to be child free. Making yet a third choice is emotionally draining. Couples have been disappointed so many times that they may feel unable to choose any option that involves risk. At the same time, those who have not discussed DI with anyone may feel especially isolated. Others will not know they are suffering, and the couple will feel alone, unable to share their grief. (We refer the reader to Chapter 4, Changing Directions.)

Male infertility has been a painful burden throughout history, and remains so; from Biblical days to modern times, men have been shamed for not producing children. Donor insemination, a viable path to parenthood, provides a resolution to childlessness, but it does not offer a cure for the inability to reproduce, and it is not without consequences. Although DI has been available for about one hundred years, and has been used extensively in the last several decades, its social, emotional, and ethical ramifications have not been explored until recently. Couples making this important decision must realize that donor insemination is not a one time event. Rather, it is a life-long process that has profound implications on everyone in the family.

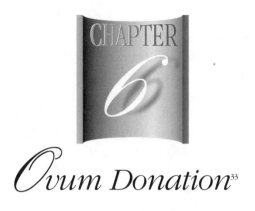

$\mathcal{O}$vum Donation[33]

The practice of using donated gametes to achieve a pregnancy has long offered couples with male infertility the opportunity to experience pregnancy and to have a child that is half genetically theirs. Although it would stand to reason that couples in which the woman is unable to produce healthy eggs (ova) might also seek donated gametes, until recently they have not had this option. Unlike sperm, which can easily be obtained (and frozen), until the development of *in vitro* fertilization eggs could not be removed from a woman's ovaries. [Ova still cannot be frozen successfully, although as this book goes to press we are hearing the first reports of babies (twins) born from cryopreserved eggs. It will probably be several years, however, before this technology is readily available to embryologists in ART clinics.] Once the procedure for maturing and removing eggs from a woman's ovaries was developed, the road was paved for eggs to be transferred from one woman to another. In 1984, just six years after the birth of the first IVF baby, the first pregnancy through ovum donation (also called oocyte donation) was confirmed.[34] With this event the biological clock for women was altered forever.

Although both sperm donation and egg donation have psychological, ethical, and legal issues in common (see Chapter 5, Donor Insemination), there are many differences between them. One important distinction is that ovum donation appears to offer more parity, enabling both parents to have a biological stake in their offspring. The man, through his sperm, and the woman receiving the donated ova through gestation, each make a biological contribution to the creation of their child.

Another distinction is that ovum donation, which necessitates ART, is much more costly and far more medically complicated than donor insemination, which does not even require medical assistance. Although it is not yet a common path to parenthood, ovum donation is becoming one, as more and more IVF centers offer this technology. Because only young donors are involved, the pregnancy and delivery rates for IVF with donated ova are appreciably higher than for standard IVF procedures.

Although IVF makes it medically possible to obtain eggs, there are few donated eggs available. This relative scarcity of ova, the complex reproductive technology required to achieve pregnancy, and the high financial cost deter many couples who might otherwise choose this option.

A further distinction between sperm and ovum donation is that women never see their eggs; they come from deep inside them. Men, on the other hand, have ejaculated sperm since puberty; it is a part of them with which they are familiar. Thus, the concept of removing eggs from a woman's body is foreign—almost mysterious—to most would-be donors and recipients, yet the concept of removing sperm is familiar to all.

Because ovum donation has existed only since 1984, there has been limited psychosocial research on this alternative. Similarly, little has been written about it from an ethical and legal perspective. As a result, all who become involved in ovum donation are pioneers.

Who Uses Donor Ova?

A woman might be a candidate for using donated ova for a range of reasons, some relatively undisputed and some highly controversial. What is important to understand at this point is that as long as a woman has an intact uterus and she is given hormonal supplements in order to make her uterus receptive to the embryo, she should be physically able to carry a pregnancy to term.

A large percentage of women seeking donated ova—those for whom the procedure was developed—are women with premature ovarian failure (POF). They are relatively young women whose ovaries are not producing eggs and who have ceased to menstruate. A woman is generally considered to be suffering from premature ovarian failure if she ceases to ovulate before she is forty years old. Although a forty-one year old woman whose ovulatory function has ceased is young to experience menopause, menopause at age 41 is not considered premature.

Some women have premature ovarian failure after undergoing radiation treatment or chemotherapy for cancer. Others have had their ovaries surgically removed due to severe infection, endometriosis, or tumor. In rare instances, a woman is born with a congenital absence of her ovaries. Other causes are familial (POF tends to run in families). Autoimmune diseases such as thyroiditis and environmental toxins are additional causes of POF. In many instances, however, there is no identifiable cause, and the woman's ovarian failure is considered to be idiopathic. These women have the added emotional burden of not knowing how or why this happened. Whatever the cause—medical, surgical or organic—once the ovaries have stopped working, as measured by follicle stimulating hormone (FSH) levels, there is no treatment available that will "start" them again. It is important to note, however, that there is a spontaneous pregnancy (i.e. cure) rate of 10-15% in young women with POF. The current estimate is that one to three percent of women suffer from POF.

A second category of candidates for receiving donated ova consists of women who are perimenopausal. (Perimenopause refers to the five to ten year period just prior to the onset of menopause.) Although these women continue to ovulate and to have menstrual periods, the quality of their eggs seems to be impaired due to the normal aging process. Many perimenopausal women are identified in the course of an IVF cycle. They may undergo ovarian stimulation, but their cycle may be cancelled due to poor stimulation, or to their poor egg or embryo quality, or to nonfertilization of eggs. Some professionals in the field of reproductive endocrinology are questioning whether these aging women are appropriate candidates for this new technology since their infertility is the result of the normal aging process. Others argue that these women should be offered donated ova because they are still chronologically in their childbearing years.

A third category consists of couples who have completed several IVF cycles without becoming pregnant. Although they have had eggs retrieved and fertilized and have undergone embryo transfers, their pregnancy tests are always negative. In the absence of a definitive cause for these failed attempts, physicians sometimes conclude that the problem is poor egg quality or, in the case of older women, "aging eggs." These women are questionable candidates for donated ova since there is no proof that they will not conceive on a subsequent treatment cycle or on their own.

A fourth category of ovum recipient candidates are women who are known carriers of a genetic defect or disease that has a high likelihood of being passed on to their offspring. If the genetic problem is one that is autosomal dominant, the offspring have a 50% chance of inheriting the problem; if it is autosomal recessive but the father carries the same defective gene, the offspring has a one in four chance of inheriting it. Using donated eggs virtually eliminates the autosomal recessive problem (except in the unlikely event that the donor is a carrier of the same defective gene). In these situations, however, it is much simpler, less risky, and less costly for the couple to use donated sperm rather than donated ova.

The final category of candidates for ovum donation—and many would say that they should not be candidates at all—are postmenopausal women in their late forties, fifties or older who are aware that the technology of ovum donation can push reproduction beyond its normal limits.

$\mathscr{P}$otential Ovum Donors

Donated oocytes are not readily available. Unlike sperm donation, which takes only a few minutes and involves no physical risk whatsoever to the donor, ovum donation is a lengthy process that is physically uncomfortable, inconvenient and involves possible, though rare, medical risks. In addition, there are emotional risks to consider.

Potential donors include infertile women undergoing IVF, fertile women electing to have a tubal ligation, fertile volunteer donors known to their recipients, and fertile women donating anonymously. The last two groups of donors are the most common.

The hormonal stimulation of an IVF patient's ovaries, especially in young women, may produce far more eggs, and result in many more embryos, than can be safely placed into her uterus. Although most couples undergoing IVF are involved in programs in which cryopreservation of embryos for later use is available and the vast majority of couples choose this option, some couples are opposed to freezing their embryos for moral or religious reasons. Couples fearing the long-term side effects of cryopreservation (unproven to date) may also elect not to freeze their embryos. These couples may be asked by their physicians if they are willing to donate their extra eggs to other infertile women.

Couples undergoing IVF are not a common source of donated eggs, because practically all of them agree to freeze extra embryos for their own possible later use. Additionally, many clinicians have ethical concerns about asking an infertile woman to donate oocytes to another infertile woman.

The major concern is psychological—the possibility that the recipient will become pregnant and the patient, who is her donor, will not. Clinicians worry about what it would mean for the donor to live with this knowledge or—should she be involved with a program that withholds this information—left to struggle on her own with unanswered questions. An ethical question is raised by the possibility that if both give birth, the result would be half-siblings with no knowledge of one another.

Some programs offer a sizable reduction in the cost of a cycle to women who undergo *in vitro* fertilization if they agree to donate some of their eggs. Although this reduction enables some couples who might not otherwise be able to afford IVF the opportunity to attempt ART treatment, it does so at a substantial ethical cost: inherent coercion. Recognizing that an infertile woman's despair might cause her to agree to something that could cause her psychological harm, many clinics will not offer reduced fees in exchange for eggs.

Another potential source for donated eggs is women undergoing elective tubal ligations. The incentive for these women to donate is a free or reduced rate for the sterilization procedure or payment for the time and effort involved in harvesting and procuring their eggs. In order to donate oocytes, they must receive hormones to stimulate their follicles and undergo frequent monitoring via blood drawings and ultrasounds in the month prior to their scheduled tubal ligation. After the oocytes are retrieved, the donor's fallopian tubes are tied.

While this may seem to be an ideal pool, women undergoing tubal ligation have not proved to be a predictable source of donated eggs. It is unclear why this source of potential donors remains largely untapped, but it may be that many women have health plans that cover the cost of their sterilization procedure and the offer of a free tubal ligation has no value for them. Referrals from gynecologists who routinely perform this surgery as a source of revenue are rare, possibly because of the financial disincentive. Furthermore, the communication and ongoing coordination necessary to achieve a working partnership with a local gynecologist may be too difficult to maintain in most infertility clinics.

Women undergoing tubal ligation may be reluctant to donate ova even in instances where the financial incentives are attractive. Some have read upsetting articles about fertility medications and do not want to undergo unnecessary health risks. Others are concerned that super-ovulation might accidentally lead to the very situation that they are trying to avoid: an unplanned pregnancy occuring just prior to ligation.

Friends or relatives—known donors—are a popular source of donated oocytes, appealing to couples who wish to both preserve their genetic lineage and to know the source of the gametes. Sisters, in particular, are often a preferred choice, though other relatives have also been known donors. Couples less concerned with maintaining a genetic connection with the wife/mother prefer to ask friends, acquaintances, or co-workers, or to take other steps to locate their donor.

The recruitment of anonymous egg donors from the general population has become a popular means by which oocytes are obtained for donation. Anonymous donors are usually recruited through advertisements in local newspapers, magazines, or university newspapers. As ovum donation is becoming more common, ads like the following are seen with increasing frequency in major cities throughout the United States:

Oocyte Donation

Healthy female volunteers aged 34 and under are needed to serve as anonymous oocyte (egg) donors. Donors will be required to take medication, have blood screening, and undergo a minor surgical procedure. Compensation will be made for time and expenses. If interested please call.....

The Medical Process

Ovum donation is a medically complicated process involving the use of fertility drugs and advanced reproductive technology. The major medical challenge of ovum donation is to synchronize the harvesting of the eggs from the donor with the receptivity of the recipient's endometrium. Synchronization is important because at this point in time the technology to freeze eggs has not been perfected. The first reported birth of twins from cryopreserved ova was reported in October 1997. Unless the endometrial lining is ready to receive the embryos, pregnancy cannot occur. Although eggs cannot yet be cryopreserved, embryos can be frozen, and they are if the best efforts at synchronization fail. However, pregnancy rates using frozen embryos are generally not as high as pregnancy rates using fresh embryos.

The donor, like any other woman undergoing *in vitro* fertilization, is put on a strict regimen of fertility drugs in hopes that she will produce multiple oocytes. These oocytes are surgically removed when they are ripe—just prior to when they would be released by the ovaries if she were ovulating on her own. They are inseminated shortly after retrieval with the recipient's husband's sperm. Two or three days later, a predetermined number of embryos (usually between two and four) are placed into the uterus of the recipient, utilizing the same process as in a normal IVF cycle. GIFT can also be used in the course of ovum donation and may be recommended as a preferred treatment in some instances.

In order to achieve a normal endometrium, the recipient's estrogen and progesterone supplementation are carefully administered and monitored. Recipients usually wear estrogen patches and take progesterone by injection if ovarian function has ceased. If ovarian function persists, recipients are frequently given Lupron to suppress their normal ovulation pattern and a similar regimen of estrogen and progesterone supplementation is then given. Many clinics insist on a trial cycle for recipients prior to stimulating the donor, in order to understand how long it takes for the recipient's body to adjust to the hormones and for her endometrium to be ready. The hormones are timed such that when the donor's eggs have been fertilized with the recipient's husband's sperm and the embryos are ready for implantation, the recipient's uterus will also be ready. If extra embryos exist, they can be cryopreserved and used by the recipient couple in a subsequent transfer cycle.

Medical Screening *of Egg Donors*

Because of the possibility for the transmission of disease from donor to recipient and/or child, donors must be thoroughly screened. They must also fully understand the medical process so that they can give informed consent. And, due to the invasive nature of the procedure, the ethical and emotional issues are even more extensive for ovum donors than they are for sperm donors.

The American Society for Reproductive Medicine (ASRM) guidelines state that anonymous donors should be of legal age but no more than thirty-four years old, since younger donors are much more likely to respond well to follicular stimulation and older donors create an age-related increased risk of chromosomal abnormalities. If the oocyte donor is over 34, this fact should be discussed with the recipient couple as part of an informed consent discussion pertaining to risk, and the recipient should be offered amniocentesis or chorionic villus sampling should a pregnancy result. Although it is preferable that donors have documented fertility, ASRM does not suggest that it be a requirement for donation.[35]

ASRM guidelines specify that all donors, known and anonymous, need to be clear about the procedures involved in ovum donation, because the steps include drug therapy for ovarian hyperstimulation, close monitoring, and an invasive procedure for oocyte recovery (ultrasound-guided transvaginal follicular aspiration), each of which carries potential risks. Although these risks are small, potential donors must be counseled thoroughly regarding these risks, and they must think carefully about their motives and their reasons for wanting to donate.

A major concern for programs utilizing donated gametes is the transmission of the HIV virus. Sperm banks routinely test all donors for the virus, freeze and quarantine all donated sperm for six months, and then retest the donor for HIV. If a sperm donor tests negative for antibodies to the virus, couples can be virtually assured that the semen frozen six months previously is free of infection. Because eggs cannot be frozen, the same precaution against transmittal of HIV cannot be utilized with ovum donors. It is unclear whether HIV can be transmitted through ovum donation, however immunologists tend to agree that follicular fluid is a possible means of transmission. All applicants for ovum donation who have risk factors for HIV infection, such as intravenous drug use or a sexual partner who uses these drugs or who is HIV infected, are to be screened out immediately as potential donors. Then the ASRM guidelines suggest that couples entering an oocyte donor program be given the choice: to assume the low risk of acquiring HIV and use fresh embryos, which yield a better pregnancy rate, or to have the donated oocytes fertilized and the resulting embryos frozen for six months, after which point the donor is retested. If the donor still tests negative, the embryos can be safely transferred into recipient's uterus.

The ASRM guidelines specify that serological testing be routinely performed for syphilis, hepatitis B and C, and HIV I-II and that genetic screening should be performed on a potential donor before allowing her to donote oocytes, ruling out the possibility that she will transmit an identifiable genetic disease. In regard to record keeping, the guidelines state that a permanent record designed to preserve confidentially should be made available on request to the recipient and any resulting offspring. The ASRM guidelines also recommend psychological counseling for all parties involved in the ovum donation process to ensure that they are giving informed consent, are not being coerced to donate, are aware of the potential medical risks, and are aware of the potential psychological risks.

While such is not the case with sperm donation, most programs which offer counseling to ovum donors look to the mental health clinician as a gatekeeper who determines whether a potential donor is psychologically appropriate. The screening may consist of psychological interviews, personality assessments, or other psychological batteries. Most programs reject donors who exhibit psychopathology, as measured by their test results or as determined in a face-to-face interview. Donors who have a history that includes psychological conflict and appear to be consciously or unconsciously donating as a way to make up for an unresolved past event may also be rejected.

In a survey published in 1993, of eighty-two ovum donor programs, 78% stated that they require psychological screening for donors. The survey did not state what percentage of ovum donation programs also offer counseling to recipients.[36] We can speculate from speaking to a number of clinicians working in several programs, however, that most programs that screen donors also require counseling for recipients. The purpose of counseling for recipients is to make sure that they are giving informed consent, are aware of the medical and the psychological risks involved, and understand the ethical and emotional issues involved in creating families through the process of ovum donation.

Ethical Considerations of Ovum Donation

The technologies that make ovum donation possible are continually improving, and more and more couples are taking advantage of this technology. As with all of the other new reproductive options, however, our capacity to reflect on the profound and serious ethical issues they raise is compromised by the rapid proliferation of programs. People are undergoing ovum donation before researchers and ethicists have the opportunity to develop an adequate understanding of the life experiences of families created from this option. It will probably be years before we understand the impact of these technologies on the families participating in them—both donors and recipients.

Many of the ethical issues raised by the technology of ovum donation are shared with sperm donation—for example, questions about the psychological effect on a child of intentionally bringing him or her into the world with unknown parentage, and whether a person has the right to know the truth about his or her genetic heritage. These shared ethical issues pertaining to gamete donation (and other forms of third party parenting) were discussed in Chapter 1. Now we will focus on those issues that have been raised solely as a result of ovum donation.

The Changing Nature of Family

Many social changes in the last half of the twentieth century have challenged the traditional definition of family, including the increasing incidence of divorce (approximately 50% of all married couples), the increasing number of single women choosing to have children, and the increasing number of lesbian couples bearing and raising children together. Couples who divorce are not intentionally creating nontraditional families. Yet many single women and all lesbian couples by definition are intentionally creating families without fathers in the home. More and more frequently they are requesting technological assistance or gamete donation in order to have families, and these requests pose ethical dilemmas for some reproductive health practitioners, centering around the question of whether it is in a child's best interest to be brought into the world under such circumstances. Although research is scant, one recent study indicated that children conceived by donor insemination (all were under eleven years old) and raised by single women or lesbian couples were as well adjusted psychologically as children conceived by DI and raised by heterosexual parents.[37]

Ovum donation further challenges our traditional understanding of family because it allows women to bear children after menopause—at an age when many of their peers are becoming grandparents. The fact that children will be raised by parents who look and probably have life expectancies much more like grandparents is an objection that many clinicians raise on ethical grounds. They feel it is not fair to children to be raised by parents who may not have the stamina for middle-of-the-night feedings, for scout outings, or for the worrisome adolescent years. When single women or lesbian couples opt for ovum donation, especially if they are older, they are creating families that are even more nontraditional.

Other forms of nontraditional families are being formed by individuals who choose to use ovum donation in conjunction with some other alternative path to parenthood such as gestational care or sperm donation. Although these situations are now relatively rare, we are concerned that these deliberately engineered "fourth party arrangements" approach the concept of "designer babies." Evidence of increased acceptance of such uses—or mis-uses—of reproductive technology is now seen in the advertising and marketing tools of some programs that offer both ovum donation and surrogacy.

The Definition of Mother

Prior to the new reproductive technologies, the definition of mother was fairly simple: mothers gave birth to and raised their children. Although adoptions and foster care created a distinction between the roles of birth-mother, legal mother and rearing mother, those were the only variations on the definition of motherhood. The new reproductive technologies, by enabling eggs to be harvested in one woman and implanted in a second woman, allow us to distinguish between the genetic and the gestational mother, as well as the rearing and legal mother.

Traditionally, motherhood and gestation have been linked, so that the notion of genetics seemed incidental. However, over the years we have come to understand the importance of genetics in shaping a person's life. Although it is impossible to separate the exact roles that nature and nurture play in one's life, all agree that each is important in creating the adult. The genetic mother—the ovum donor—is therefore extremely important to the child's identity, regardless of whether she donates anonymously or is known to the parents. Those who question the ethics of intentionally separating the genetic and gestational aspect of motherhood believe that it is not in a child's best interest to be deliberately brought into the world surrounded by this confusion.

Although the new definitions of mother are easily understandable, even to those not involved in reproductive technology, in the legal sense they can be baffling. Many argue that the woman who delivers a child should legally be considered the "real" mother, unless or until she gives up her rights to rear the child. Those who argue this point believe that even in situations in which a gestational carrier is used, she is the "real" mother despite the fact that her gamete was not used in creating the child. Others argue that the genetic mother is the "real" mother, regardless of whether she carries her baby. Our intention is not to argue the legal issues in this chapter but to attempt to elucidate the role that each woman plays in the life of the offspring, and to emphasize that everyone—professional as well as lay—has an opinion, not only about whether it is in a child's best interest to have two (or three) mothers but about who is the "real" mother in the event of a conflict.

The definition of mother becomes even further complicated when we consider that many lesbian couples are choosing to have children make the point that they are both mothers to their offspring. One might argue that only one of them is the natural or real mother, but what about the couple who applied to an IVF program requesting that one woman donate her eggs to her partner, who would then gestate the pregnancy? Even King Solomon would be hard-pressed to argue that one of those women was more the mother than the other.

The Right to Bear a Child

In the May 1997 issue of *Fertility and Sterility*, doctors at the University of Southern California School of Medicine and Loma Linda School of Medicine reported that a 63-year-old woman had given birth.[38] This case, which received considerable media attention, highlighted one of the central ethical questions associated with ovum donation: does an individual or couple have an absolute right to have a child? Given that the technology of oocyte donation can extend a woman's childbearing years indefinitely, many professionals and ethicists debate the question of whether something should be done because it can be done. Perhaps ovum donation, more than with other type of ART, exemplifies the quandry of the desires of prospective parents pitted against the best interests of an unborn child.

Many professionals working in ovum donation programs feel a moral obligation to address the question of what is in the best interests of the potential children they are attempting to create. This question arises in a variety of situations, but the most common is maternal age. Those who set policy must struggle with whether they will set an age limit beyond which they will not allow couples to cycle. Most programs do have age limits, arrived at after careful deliberation. For example, a program in the greater Boston area set the age limit for receiving donated ova at forty-five after checking actuarial tables. Although no child is ever born with a guarantee that the mother will live to see him or her enter adulthood, the practitioners that established the program wanted to feel reasonably secure that children born as a result of their ovum donation program were likely to be raised by their mothers. Recognizing that the role of the father is equally important, however, practitioners at that same clinic also take his age into consideration. If he is under forty-five and the combined average age of the couple is equal to or less than that the couple will be considered for the ovum donation program.

Other programs believe that it is not their place to decide how old (or young) someone must be when she becomes a parent. Those programs have a higher age limit for ovum recipients or none at all. In a survey of 82 IVF programs offering ovum donation, 22 reported they had no upper age limits. Of the remaining 60 that did have upper limits, the average was 55 years—an age that to most seems more suitable to grandparenting![39]

According to their report in *Fertility and Sterility*, the physicians who helped achieve pregnancy in the 63-year-old woman were unaware of her true age. They state that upon entering the program, she lied to them, claiming to be ten years younger than she really was, having falsified medical records so that they were consistent with her stated age. The reporting physicians say that they learned during her pregnancy that she was actually 63 and not 53. Although these physicians may have been duped, there are many other physicians who claim openly that they have helped women in their late fifties and early sixties achieve pregnancy through ovum donation.

Risks to Donors

Infertile women considering high-tech treatment must determine whether they are willing to take the risks—some known and some as yet unknown—inherent in the process. Most couples struggle to a greater or lesser extent with whether the gains outweigh the risks. However, when healthy young fertile women are recruited to be egg donors, especially if they have not completed their families, a question is raised about whether it is ethical to subject them to the possible risks of treatment, including the risk of becoming infertile.

As we reported in Chapter 2, two studies completed a few years ago have indicated a possible relationship between the use of fertility-enhancing medications and ovarian cancer, while many other studies have come to different conclusions. Ovum donation requires these medications, and until we know definitively that they are safe, an ethical question is raised about whether healthy, fertile donors who do not receive reproductive benefits should be taking these drugs.

All who agree to donate assume risks. These risks must be clearly explained by a physician and understood by the donor in order for her to be capable of informed consent. Donors must understand what the ovarian stimulation protocol involves and the potential risks of the medication, as well as the risks associated with egg retrieval. Although most programs will not accept women under 21, many clinicians question whether a woman in her 20s—especially if she has not had children—can possibly give informed consent.

There are psychological risks to potential donors as well. Donors must give serious thought to what it will mean to them over the long term to give their genetic material to someone else, and whether they could suffer long-term emotional consequences as a result of this decision. They must be able to separate the genetic from the gestational and the rearing aspects of motherhood. Those who have not completed their families must try to imagine how they would feel about having genetic children in the world should they become infertile themselves. Some must consider the meaning of anonymity. All donors must do some serious self exploration—often with the guidance of a mental health clinician—to be certain that they are undertaking donation for reasons that are right for them now and in the future. Since many donors are only in their twenties and may have great difficulty anticipating how they will feel much later in life, the mental health counselor will probably need to be very active, asking difficult, thought-provoking questions.

Another concern is whether the donor has health insurance that will cover any medical complications that might arise. Although complications are rare, hyperstimulation can occur, and serious hyperstimulation may require hospitalization. If the donor does not have health insurance, provision must be made for unanticipated medical costs.

Risks to Recipients

Pregnancy, labor, and delivery take a toll on even the healthiest and youngest of bodies and carry the risk of medical complications. As women grow older, these risks are compounded. Once, all pregnant women over

40 were considered to be at high risk. Now, many physicians believe that for women over 40 (or even over 50) who are in good health, pregnancy is unlikely to present serious risks.

Still, when oocyte donation is used for an older woman, she must be adequately counseled regarding the risks of pregnancy with advanced maternal age. Included should be discussion of risks associated with multiple gestation, the incidence of premature delivery, and other neonatal problems.

Financial Compensation of Donors

Egg donation is medically risky, physically invasive, painful, and time-consuming. As a result, payment for anonymous egg donation is considerably higher than the average $30 for sperm donation. In 1993, Braverman's survey reported that payments ranged from a low of $750 to a high of $3,500, the average compensation being $1,548.[40] Some programs have attempted to break down the time commitment a donor must make into a set number of hours, in order to illustrate the point that, hour by hour, donors are being paid only a small amount of money. Whatever the compensation offered, however, there are those who argue that it is tantalizingly high, inducing women to donate their eggs for the wrong reasons; while others feel just as strongly that it is insultingly low, tantamount to exploitation.

Some ethicists view donating gametes in the same way they view donating blood: ovum donors should be encouraged to provide their gametes to infertile couples as a public service, without payment, even for time and inconvenience. Others believe that donors should be reimbursed for actual expenses, such as lost wages, but no payment should be made for time and certainly not for the actual oocytes retrieved. Still others feel that additional payment for pain, risk, and inconvenience is warranted, considering that an egg donor undergoes hormonal stimulation by injection, blood and ultrasound monitoring, and a surgical procedure. Again, the primary ethical concern regarding compensating egg donors is that the money will serve as a coercive inducement to donate, potentially obscuring any social or emotional reasons indicating that donation is not in a particular woman's best psychological interest.

In pondering the issues of ovum donation, ethicists address the potential for commercialization and competition in the marketplace—that these important life-producing cells will be viewed more as commodities seriously affected by the laws of supply and demand. Although many find this argument a gross exaggeration of the realities of infertility treatment, it is also true that more and more couples are choosing ovum donation. It is not out of the question that the increasing demand for donor oocytes, in combination with a limited supply, will cause programs to raise the level of compensation they offer donors, not to mention what they charge recipients.

Two other forms of compensation previously discussed do not involve the direct exchange of money: the offering of free tubal ligations to fertile women and the offer of substantial reductions in the cost of their IVF cycle to infertile women. Both forms of compensation raise the question of whether subtle coercion is involved. If the offer were eliminated, some couples could never afford to try IVF. On the other hand, donating oocytes is an act that an infertile woman cannot take lightly.

Insurance Payment

The health insurance industry has been going through enormous changes. A trend manifested in the managed health care industry limits treatment and pays less and less for "unnecessary" treatment. In 1997, only ten U.S. states have mandates to offer or cover infertility treatment In Canada, only one province (Ontario) mandates coverage for IVF and then only for women with blocked or absent fallopian tubes. The extent to which infertility services will be covered in the future remains unclear.

Serious questions exist regarding insurance coverage for ovum donation. Does society have a moral obligation to pay for this procedure, and, if so, under what circumstances? On the one hand there are young women who lose ovarian function naturally or following cancer treatment and who seek ovum donation as their only opportunity for pregnancy. Many would argue that their treatment should be covered by medical insurance. On the other hand there are women of normal peri-or post-menopausal age, who turn to ovum donation in an effort to tamper with the laws of nature. Few believe that the costs of their ovum donation attempts should be borne by their insurance carriers.

Additional questions arise regarding the health care coverage of donors. Should their health insurance cover complications that might develop as a result of their voluntary donation? What if the donor experiences emotional complications during or following this procedure? These questions illustrate but a few of the dilemmas surrounding ovum donation.

Known Ovum Donation

Donor egg programs offer the opportunity for both partners to have a biological stake in the creation of their child—one through the genetic connection, the other through a gestational one. When a known donor is involved, the couple has control over the source of the gametes and they have a medical history as well. Additionally, if a relative is the donor, the couple is able to preserve genetic continuity.

Choosing Known Ovum Donation

One of the key differences in the practice of sperm and egg donation is that known donors are frequently used for ovum donation, but rarely used for sperm donation. In fact, according to Braverman's survey of 82 ovum donation programs, the majority of infertility programs offering donor gametes offer known egg donation, while the majority of programs do not offer known sperm donation.[41] One possible explanation for this discrepancy involves gender differences. Professionals involved in donor insemination (see Chapter 5) have traditionally sought to protect men from the shame associated with male infertility. Physicians, promoting secrecy, have encouraged couples to use anonymous donors. Although occasional couples have objected to anonymity and have intentionally sought a known donor, most couples using sperm donation accept anonymity as integral to the process. Although infertility is painful to women, it is not usually associated with as much shame as is male infertility.

In addition to gender differences, there are other important reasons why many couples prefer known over anonymous ovum donation. These reasons are egg scarcity, control, and medical history.

Egg Scarcity

As discussed earlier, eggs are difficult to obtain because donors are required to go through assisted reproductive technology, whereas sperm donors can produce a sample in just a few minutes through masturbation. The former procedure is invasive, potentially risky, and physically uncomfortable; the latter, though awkward, is easy and under different circumstances, even pleasurable. Hence anonymous ovum donors are much more scarce than are sperm donors.

Another difficulty in obtaining eggs is that, unlike sperm, eggs cannot be frozen and stored for later use, making logistical arrangements a tedious part of the process. As we explained earlier in this chapter, an egg donor's cycle must be coordinated with the recipient's, which involves careful monitoring. Thus two people—each on her own biological calendar— are involved in the ovum donation process, whereas with sperm donation medical monitoring is only necessary for the woman, and her cycle does not have to be coordinated with anyone else's. Since semen can be thawed in minutes, the only necessary logistical arrangement for sperm donation is that it be shipped to the clinic on time. In other words, because anony- mous sperm donation can be done so easily through the use of frozen sperm, this makes it a practical as well as attractive option. Since anony- mous ovum donation is no easier to accomplish than known ovum donation, expediency does not make it more attractive.

Because the process of retrieving eggs is difficult, and because they cannot be frozen once they are retrieved, most programs do not have a large pool of donors available to donate. There are a few clinics who claim to have a catalog of carefully screened donors, but most clinics have long waiting lists of recipients and few donors. The scarcity of anonymous donors is one of the main reasons that many recipient couples turn to known ovum donation.

Control

Recipients of known ovum donation often feel that they are more involved in the process, and are taking an active role in building their family. After years of feeling helpless and out of control as a result of infertility, choosing a known donor gives the couple a sense of control over the source of their gametes and allows them to feel more in control of their lives than they have in a long time. They are usually familiar with the donor's personality, temperament, and physical attributes and presumably have positive feelings toward her.

Medical History

Medical science continues to uncover more and more data indicating that heredity plays a large role in a person's health history. Although few medical problems appear to result from an unalterable genetic blueprint, individuals are born with hereditary predispositions toward certain diseases or physical problems. Although many conditions are passed on through recessive traits and cannot be anticipated, known donors provide recipient couples with baseline information—nearly as much as they would get if the recipient's gametes were used—about a potential child's likelihood (or not) of developing certain medical conditions.

Known donors are also preferred by many couples because it gives the child the option of knowing his or her genetic parent. Although the extent and nature of their relationship must be negotiated, couples choosing known ovum donation often feel relatively confident that their child will have a more secure identity if s/he knows the donor.

Selecting a Known Ovum Donor

Couples hoping to work with a known ovum donor usually begin with the question: "Who can we ask?" For some, the answer to this is clear: the woman has a relative or friend—preferably under age 35 and with children—whom she feels comfortable asking or who may already have offered. For others, the decision of who to ask is much less straightforward.

Relatives

Many couples turn to a close relative for donated ova. Women with sisters often feel they are ideal donors because of their similar genetic makeup, assuring the continuity of the bloodline which is important to many recipient couples. Since most ovum recipients are infertile due to aging, chances are that only a younger sister—probably significantly younger—will be fertile. Some recipients have more than one sister and must decide whom to approach. Their decision may be influenced by many factors, including proven fertility, completion of her own family, physical proximity, overall health, and the relationship that exists between them.

Ovum recipient couples unable to use a sister may approach another relative, perhaps a cousin or a niece. Depending on the nature of the relationship, however, it can be difficult for recipients to ask such an enormous favor of someone who is not a close relative.

Although women with adult daughters may view them as ideal donors, and the daughters may be willing to donate, many professionals, in particular, mental health clinicians, scorn this controversial practice. They see it as inherently coercive, given the nature of the parent-child relationship in which children may always feel in some way indebted to their parents. They believe that adult children are not psychologically free to say no to a parent in the same way they are free to refuse others. In fact, when an informal poll was taken of approximately 80 mental health professionals attending the American Society for Reproductive Medicine's Psychological

213

Special Interest Group post-graduate course in 1994, only two professionals indicated that they would support this form of inter-generational ovum donation.

The reverse situation—a mother donating to her daughter—brings less opposition. Clinicians observe that since it is the nature of the mother-child relationship for mothers to be caretakers of their children, that this caretaking might theoretically extend—in certain circumstances—to the donation of eggs. However, situations in which a mother is fertile enough to donate to a daughter who is old enough to have a child are extraordinarily rare.

Nonrelatives

Couples may seek a friend or acquaintance if a relative is not available or if they prefer a nonrelative. The latter brings with her the advantages of known genes but not the social and emotional entanglements that could occur in the family if their child say, has an aunt who is her genetic mother and cousins who are her half siblings.

A nonrelative who bears a physical resemblance to the recipients may also be desirable. The recipients may feel the child will fit into the family better and will be less likely to be the brunt of questions such as, "Whom does he look like?" Couples who prefer a nonrelative as an ovum donor when a relative may be available may value knowing her and knowing she comes from good genetic stock while caring less about preserving genetic continuity. They may feel relieved not having to deal with the social and relational confusion inherent in familial donation.

Couples choosing nonrelatives must identify the attributes that are important to them in a donor and the relationship they want to have with her. Their feelings about these matters may point to someone in particular, or conversely, prompt them to rule someone out.

Some couples prefer to ask a close and trusted friend with whom they have a special connection. Other recipients avoid asking a good friend, fearing that ovum donation could jeopardize their relationship if something went wrong, or if they did not become pregnant, or if the donor became attached to the child and viewed it as hers. Asking an acquaintance or a co-worker, or someone with whom they do not have a strong emotional connection, may feel less risky.

Motivations for Becoming a Known Donor

What motivates a relative or a friend to become a donor? This question puzzles many people—both inside and outside the field of reproductive medicine. Some wonder how people could put themselves through such grueling medical procedures. Others, who could not imagine watching their genetic child being raised by someone else, are troubled by the known aspect, but could imagine donating anonymously. Still others feel that under no circumstances could they ever donate their genetic material to another person, known or unknown.

As has been mentioned before, the donation of gametes can be viewed on a continuum. On one end are those who feel that giving away ova or sperm is the same as giving away blood. On the other end are those who feel that giving away gametes is tantamount to giving away a child. People have vastly different feelings and attachments to their own genetic material. Most people would agree that a gamete is neither a person nor a pint of blood; it is somewhere in between, but exactly where is a matter of individual interpretation. Because known donors are often women who would not have considered ovum donation on their own had a need not arisen with a relative or friend, they find themselves giving careful thought to the question: what exactly is a gamete?

Most potential donors place themselves toward the "blood" end of the continuum. Those who feel an intense connection to their genes, and feel that an egg is nearly equivalent to a person because of its potential to become a person, probably rule themselves out as donors. Women who agree to donate, especially if they are donating to someone they know, tend to regard the ovum, once it is out of their body—and even more so when it is fertilized with the recipient's husband's sperm—as no longer part of them. For them, the embryo takes on a life of its own, and although they recognize that many traits are genetically transmitted and the resulting offspring may resemble the genetic mother in both physical and emotional ways, they believe the genetic contribution is but a small piece in comparison to the gestational and rearing aspects of motherhood.

Most known donors are motivated primarily by empathy for the recipient. In many cases, especially those involving a sister, the donor has seen the anguish of the recipient and understands how important motherhood is to her. This understanding, together with her strong feelings of affection, convince her to donate. In many instances donors are motivated by their own joy and satisfaction in motherhood.

Sometimes a tragedy—frequently a brush with death—motivates a relative to donate her eggs. In these situations, donors have acknowledged that they probably would not have been able to make this choice if it were not for the tragic event in their family. For example, one woman, who had been treated for Hodgkins Disease and who had ovarian failure secondary to her chemotherapy, applied to an infertility program requesting that her older sister, who was 32 and had two children of her own, be her donor.

When interviewed, the older sister expressed a strong desire to donate to her sister but noted that prior to her sister's illness, she had been opposed to assisted reproductive technology, believing that childless couples should adopt. She spoke of how her views had changed when she watched her sister battle cancer and stated that she now felt that they had a shared purpose in their lives. Later, when her sister did become pregnant following her donation, the donor said that she felt "spirtually converted" by the experience, observing that she and her sister had never been closer.

The Request or Offer

Asking a friend or relative to donate eggs is not an easy task. Most recipients approach it with great trepidation, feeling that everything is at stake, never having imagined that they would be asking anyone for something that goes so far beyond familiar favors. Although recipients are fully prepared for the potential donor to say no, they feel vulnerable and know they will be devastated if she does. At the same time they may worry that she will feel forced to say yes. Often the donor agrees without hesitation. Perhaps she had already been thinking about offering to help in some way, but did not know or understand what she could do. Some known donors report thinking that the only way they could help was to be a surrogate. Heretofore unfamiliar with ovum donation, many donors are pleased when the process is explained to them. Not only are they able to help someone near and dear to them have a child, but they do not have to worry about the burdens of pregnancy and the emotional attachment that could develop as a result.

Frequently donors who know about ovum donation approach their relative or friend. Others make a general offer of help, not knowing exactly what they can do but being aware that reproductive technology can do wonders. In these situations recipients feel grateful and relieved. The fact that the donor offers before being asked is an indication that she is donating because she wants to, not because she feels unable to refuse the recipient.

Many who are asked to donate eggs, however, say no, for reasons ranging from not having the time, to fear of the procedures or side effects from the medications, to feeling that it would be too difficult to watch their genetic child being raised by someone else. Many who are asked wish they could say yes but realize that they could not do so without paying a steep emotional toll. This situation is painful for both people.

The recipient may experience a refusal as a personal rejection, an indication that her relative or friend must not care much about her. In their longing to have a child, infertile couples may not be able to fully appreciate that some people have feelings of ownership about their genes and imagine that giving away their ova would feel as if they were giving away their child. One such woman, diagnosed with premature ovarian failure, wept in the psychologist's office because neither of her two sisters (who had completed their families) would donate eggs. Their refusal made her feel unloved, though each said that if she needed a kidney or bone marrow (a far riskier procedure medically), they would donate in an instant, but that donating an egg would make them feel as if they were giving up their child.

Psychological Screening and Counseling

Couples who choose known ovum donation bring their relative or friend to the ART clinic where she, too, becomes a patient. They have already invested considerable emotional energy in the process of selecting her and asking her to donate, yet that is only the beginning. Donors must pass a medical screening before they are accepted, and most programs (77.6%, according to Braverman's survey) provide psychological screening as well. The physician and the mental health clinician must help all parties determine whether the proposed arrangement makes sense medically and psychologically and whether it seems to be in everyone's best interest, most importantly, the potential child's.

Most programs that have a mental health professional use a team model approach to patient care, with physicians, nurses, mental health providers, and sometimes administrators working collaboratively. The role of the mental health professional in ovum donation programs is to assess the emotional stability of both donor and recipient couples and to educate them about the complex psychological, social, ethical, and legal issues involved in this process. (The mental health clinician works similarly with participants in donor insemination, surrogacy and gestational care—see Chapters 5, 7, & 8).

The screening process also provides a forum in which to deal with the many concerns of both recipients and donors. Although approaches vary from clinic to clinic, commonly the mental health provider interviews the donor (and often her partner as well) separately from the recipient couple and usually prior to meeting with the latter. Many programs also conduct conjoint interviews with both couples once each has been seen alone. Although a large percentage of programs use psychological testing as part of the screening process, this practice appears more common in anonymous donor screening. The reason for this is that with known donors the recipient couples presumably know a great deal about their donor's stability, reliability and moods. By contrast, most anonymous donors come in as strangers about whom very little is known.

Considerations for Donors

Women who are asked to donate fall into three categories: those who refuse, those who tentatively agree and expect the medical and psychological screening process to help them make the decision, and those who readily agree. Potential donors who fall into this latter category typically still find it helpful to review the important social, emotional, and ethical issues with a trained clinician.

Program counselors frequently begin by interviewing the potential donor first. The clinician's job is to be everyone's advocate—including the unborn child's—and to help all parties make a decision that is in everyone's best interest. When clinicians meet with recipient couples, it is easy to empathize with them and to want to help them achieve their goal. Thus, if a clinician is already invested in a particular couple, having met them prior to meeting the donor, he or she may not be able to be objective when screening the potential known donor.

During the screening session, program counselors help a donor understand her concerns or conflicts about the process, and help her determine their significance. Frequently donors find that by voicing their concerns to someone who understands, they can make better sense of them. If the concerns prove serious, the counselor can help the prospective donor decide to say no, and can even intervene on her behalf. Most donors are not able to anticipate all the problems that could occur. An important part

of the counseling process, therefore, is to raise all the potential complications for her to ponder. Donors are asked to think about and to respond
to various "what if" questions, including the following examples:

- What if you decide to have (more) children and discover you are
  infertile?
- How will you feel if the child looks just like you or is just like you
  in some major way?
- What if the child is born with a serious birth defect?
- What kind of relationship do you wish to have with the recipient
  couple? The child?
- If the recipient couple dies, will you want guardianship of the child?

The responses will help everyone assess whether the woman is
prepared to donate and if it is in her best interest.

Inability to Separate

Donors may wonder about their ability to truly separate the genetic
aspects of motherhood from the gestational and nurturing aspects. When
this becomes a nagging concern rather than an occasional thought, it is
important for all involved to examine it. The mental health counselor
should encourage the prospective donor to explore her relationships with
her own children and to talk about her feelings. Some would-be donors
will discover that they see donating an egg as an act entirely different and
separate from having a child. Others, however, will reflect upon the ways
in which they feel connected to their children genetically and may indeed
wonder whether it will ultimately prove painful for them to donate.

Sometimes a prospective donor is unaware of her doubts, and the counselor must help her to identify them. For example, one potential donor
wondered aloud to the mental health counselor whether the baby would
take on the genetic traits of the mother who carried it for nine months,
rather than the donor's (i.e. *her*) traits. When the counselor explored this
with her, it became clear that this was the way that they donor was coping
with her wish to help her friend and with her discomfort with ovum donation: she was trying to convince herself that once the eggs were removed
from her body, they would bear no connection to her.

Feelings About the Recipient's Partner.

Donors may have concerns about the couple's relationship or about
whether they will be good parents. They may also have mixed feelings
about the recipient's spouse. Most known donors have a close and special
relationship with the recipient, but that closeness does not necessarily

extend to her partner. Negative feelings about partners are especially troublesome, because the child is being created from both of their genes and he will be the child's only parent should the mother die. This reality gives many donors reason to pause. Some potential donors conclude that they must put their feelings about the partner aside and proceed with donation. However, others decide that they have too much discomfort to be able to move ahead with the process.

Bonding

Like most other people, donors associate motherhood with gestation. This association allows them to believe that the pregnancy will transform the recipient into the "real" mother, and that the process of having eggs removed will cause the donors to relinquish emotional ties to their gametes. Nevertheless, it is common for potential donors to have nagging fears that it might be the genetic connection, after all, that causes bonding to occur. The clinician must help the potential donor explore the extent to which she feels attached to her genetic material.

Good Genes

Donors worry about passing on "good genes." They know that the recipient couple has positive feelings toward them, or they would not have been asked to donate in the first place. Donors are aware, however, that genes are randomly distributed, that each egg is genetically different, and that an offspring could inherit less desirable characteristics. They may still feel a strong sense of responsibility, however—even though they have no control—to donate a "perfect" egg. Donors worry about how they and the couple will feel if the child is born with a serious problem.

Obligations to the Child

Donors wonder whether the child will conceptualize the donor as the genetic mother or simply as a donor. The notion of being any kind of mother to someone they are not choosing to parent may seem frightening. Donors wonder whether they will be responsible in any way for the well-being of the offspring or have any obligation—legal, social, moral or emotional—toward him or her.

Most programs recommend that known donors and recipients seek counsel from an attorney who has experience in this area of law. A contract can spell out the rights and obligations of all parties. The contract may or may not be legally binding if it is challenged in the future by one of the parties. However, because many of the legal issues are tied in with the emotional and social issues, the process of meeting with an attorney can help all parties understand what is involved in the process of ovum donation.

Considerations for Recipient Couples

Although virtually all recipient couples begin the process of ovum donation with hope and excitement, most are not blinded by such a strong desire to become parents that they minimize potential complications. Counseling sessions allow the couple to express concerns and to explore the ramifications of the arrangement with a clinician. In addition, counselors must raise a host of "what if" questions, similar to those asked of potential donors, prompting the couple to look into the future and think about what, if any, outcome would cause them to regret this decision.

Inability to Separate

One concern recipients have is that the donor will not be able to separate emotionally from her egg and that, as pregnancy progresses, the growing fetus will feel like her child and that she will experience feelings of depression, longing, and emptiness, regretting having ever made the offer. Fortunately, this is uncommon, and most women who would have difficulty donating recognize this during the course of their counseling and avoid entering into a problematic experience.

Bonding

The experience of gestation has always been closely associated with the role of mothering, a connection that may explain why many infertile women readily embrace ovum donation. Nevertheless, most recipients wonder how they will feel carrying another woman's genetic child and whether they will bond to that child in utero. This question has another facet when they know the donor. They may wonder if, during pregnancy, they will look at the donor and feel that the baby belongs to her.

Still, most women know from experience that attachments can form easily through nurturing. Because they associate the maternal role with gestation and have faith in their ability to bond with a baby who did not come from their genes, we have found that this concern, though genuine, diminishes over time.

Authenticity

Recipient mothers wonder whether they will feel like the "real" mother of their child after birth and throughout his or her lifetime. If the donor is someone with whom they are in regular contact, such as a sister or a good friend, they may wonder if during Thanksgiving dinner, for example, they will look at their sister and feel like a fraud. They may wonder what others will think and feel and whether all who know will regard the donor as the true mother. They may wonder also whether their ability to claim the child as theirs will be even more threatened if he or she resembles the donor.

Concern for the Donor

Almost all recipients want the donation to be a positive experience for the donor, both at the time of the procedure and in years to come. Most are extremely sensitive to their potential donor's feelings, reassuring her frequently that there will be no hard feelings should she change her mind. Recipients frequently tell potential donors that they will always be grateful to them for even considering being their donor.

Situations occasionally arise when this is not the case. Invariably mental health professionals working with known donor pairs encounter prospective recipients who pressure potential donors. When this occurs, it is crucial that the clinician intervene and actively counsel both the potential donor and recipient about the inadvisability of moving forward. Sometimes the counselor can help the potential donor to speak up and voice her reservations. Other times it is simply best for the program to deny treatment to the recipient, explaining that the team cannot support their situation as it appears coercive. Some programs are willing to "fabricate" a medical or psychological excuse for the potential donor if she is fearful of the recipient's response.

There are also instances in which the potential donor *feels* pressured, even when this is not the recipient's intent. This is why it is so important that all participants be interviewed by a mental health counselor: these interviews provide an opportunity for donors to fully explore their feelings. Sometimes negative feelings about donating surface during these sessions and the mental health clinician helps the potential donor express them to the prospective recipient. Again, most recipients, although disappointed, are able to accept and support a donor's change of heart.

Fear of Obligation

Recipients worry that their donor may feel obligated to donate and that she may be afraid to tell them if she has a change of heart. As the screening process unfolds, many things may trigger a donor's ambivalence. The donor may be frightened of the medical process, rethink what it means to donate gametes, or be concerned about the confusing social and/or familial relationships that will occur.

When a family member is considering ovum donation, she may experience additional pressure—either overt or covert—from relatives who want to see the infertile couple become parents. Sometimes in their enthusiasm to embrace an option that seems like a "perfect" solution, relatives (frequently the parents of the sisters) may overlook potential complications.

Identity Confusion

Recipients wonder whether their offspring will eventually be confused about the manner of their conception, especially during adolescence when the search for identity is paramount and when teenagers commonly reject their parents. When third parties are involved in family building, especially when they are known, recipient parents may fear that their children are likely to form a stronger attachment to their genetic parent than to them. If the donor is a close friend or relative who frequently spends time with them, this concern may be especially troublesome.

Conjoint Counseling

Once both parties decide to proceed, a joint interview is useful; many counselors would say essential. It is a time for each party to share the concerns they discussed in their separate interviews—concerns that might affect the outcome. It is also an opportunity for the clinician to determine the extent to which the parties care about each other's well being, to ascertain how well they listen to each other, communicate, and problem solve —skills that will be necessary in their joint venture.

Shared Expectations

Any discrepancies, however slight, that arose during the individual sessions need to be brought up for joint discussion. The session provides an opportunity to assess the nature of these differences and to determine whether there is or can be agreement. The parties also have to agree about many issues including:

- Logistical arrangments during the medical process—rides to the clinic, for example, and who will give the donor her injections.
- Whether the donor will be reimbursed for her time or expenses or both.
- How many cycles the donor may be willing to undergo.
- What to do if an amniocentesis indicates a problem.
- Whether they will consider multifetal reduction in the case of a multiple gestation.

- Who will be told about the known ovum donation and when will they be told.
- How the process will be explained to the child.

Privacy and Openness.

It is our observation that almost all known donor ovum couples choose to be open with other people, most importantly their child. As we will discuss in the last chapter, it is our strong opinion that families formed with donor gametes must tell their offspring—preferably at an early age. Being open, however, does not mean that privacy must be completely forfeited. The only stakeholder who truly matters is the child! Those involved may decide to tell others selectively; who and under what circumstances must be negotiated among all parties. It is extremely important though, that everyone involved feel comfortable and agree with the chosen amount of openness or privacy.

Donor/Offspring Relationship

Clinicians who screen donors and their recipients must ask each of them what sort of relationship they would like the donor to have with the offspring. It is important that they agree about the nature of that relationship. For example, if a donor expects to have a very close relationship with the child—perhaps to become the godmother—and the recipient couple does not intend for her to have a major role in the child's life, the arrangement may not be workable. It is probably unrealistic, however, to expect that the donor's relationship with the child would be no different than her relationship with him/her had she not been the donor. Having had such a vital role in the creation of the child—a role she will never forget—the donor will undoubtedly have special feelings for this child. This attachment is a natural outgrowth of the experience they all shared together, and should not be viewed as an inability to separate genetics from motherhood (unless it becomes a pathological attachment). Being a special aunt to a special niece or nephew (or a special friend,etc.) can be an enriching experience for everyone.

Dyads within a Triad: Bonding and Separation

The addition of a third person in the complex technological procedures involved in making a baby drastically changes the ART dynamic. When there are three people involved, all of whom have an essential role in the creation of the child, it is inevitable that separate relationships occur between each pair.

Throughout the ART process, all parties involved in the triad go through various stages in relation to one other. The feelings that each person experiences are multifaceted, and the ties that develop intensify as the cycle progresses. The group begins as a triad, united in their common purpose. Yet as the drama unfolds, dyadic relationships emerge—husband and wife, the donor and recipient, and the donor and recipient husband. Each plays a prominent role during a particular stage. Depending on the stage, each person has the capacity to feel central to, or conversely, left out of the picture.

The bond that develops between the recipient and the donor is usually intense. These women are sharing in the preparations for an IVF cycle, but in a way the roles are reversed: the donor is undergoing ovulation induction and having her blood drawn and her ovaries monitored by ultrasound, while the recipient looks on, perhaps assisting with injections or rides to the clinic. If stimulation does not go well, and it sometimes does not, it is upsetting to all involved.

As the time for retrieval approaches, the husband-donor dyad comes into the foreground. Questions surface about the number of eggs that might be retrieved and whether they will fertilize. One recipient shared her feelings about this with the clinical social worker at her ART clinic:

> I felt like the odd woman out in the donor egg process, as my old friend from college was my donor, but this meant that *her* eggs would be fertilized by my husband's sperm. They are making the embryo/ baby while I wait; then I'll carry *their* embryo that I didn't contribute to conceiving.

If the retrieval has gone well and several eggs are obtained, all three— once again a united force—support one another while they await the results of fertilization.

When the Test Is Positive.

When the pregnancy test is positive, known donors are genuinely thrilled for the expectant couple. However, they may also experience a sense of letdown. After all, they have played a major role in the drama up until this point. Now they will be more peripheral to the process, as the couple dyad emerges as the central pair—the expectant parents.

Once a pregnancy has been confirmed, a process of separation and differentiation occurs among the members of the triad as the couple's attention turns to each other and to the child they are now expecting. Each needs to experience and take credit for his or her unique role in the ovum donation process. Recipients commonly have expressed a need to pull back from the donor when they are pregnant, giving themselves some time to bond with the growing fetus inside them. One recipient stated that she wanted to "get in touch with my own contribution to the pregnancy and creation of my child." Another woman expressed her need to pull back "in order to feel involved, not wanting to share the pregnancy with anyone else quite so soon."

When the Test Is Negative

When a known donor ovum cycle fails to result in pregnancy, all involved are extremely disappointed, especially if it was the couple's only chance for pregnancy. There is a tendency for each person to examine his or her role in the process, looking for an explanation. Donors commonly blame themselves, assuming their eggs were not good enough. If the cycle was cancelled due to poor stimulation, there is some truth to this assumption, though the donor did nothing intentional to cause the problem. When the cycle went well but the pregnancy test was negative, no one knows what may have gone wrong and therefore no one can be blamed. Questions may immediately arise about whether to try again.

Recipient couples need a lengthy period of time to grieve when the process does not work. Most put a great deal of hope into the cycle, having believed that the donor eggs were the remedy they needed. Depending on the financial resources of the couple and the willingness of the donor, they may attempt another cycle, but each person first needs to pull inward for a period of time.

Anonymous Ovum Donation

Although the medical process for ovum donation is the same whether the donor is known or anonymous, many of the social, psychological, and emotional issues are very different. Some couples who decide to use donated eggs feel certain that they prefer anonymous to known donation. They see this process as less complicated emotionally—in the present as well as in the future. Other couples would have preferred a known donor, but none is available. For the first group of couples anonymous donation is a second-choice path to parenthood; for the second group, it is a third choice. This distinction is significant because the latter group—those who prefer but who do not have a known donor—comes to anonymous ovum donation with additional losses that may touch old wounds, as shown by the following examples:

A potential recipient expressed great sadness to the clinical social worker about using an unknown donor. She had had a younger sister who had died in a car accident several years earlier. Now, in thinking about ovum donation, the recipient imagined that her sister would have been a wonderful donor and that she would have readily agreed to donate. As she spoke of this loss of her ideal donor, the recipient realized that she had never fully mourned her sister's death. With guidance from the clinician, she understood that she needed to work through this earlier loss and the ways in which it was connected to her infertility experience before she could proceed resolutely with anonymous ovum donation.

Another potential recipient told a clinical social worker that she felt hurt because her sister had refused to donate. This experience of being turned down rekindled earlier feelings of being disappointed by her sister, whom she had always considered selfish. The recipient felt certain that if the situation were reversed, she would gladly give eggs to her sister, because she had always been the one to give in their relationship. Her sister's refusal also caused the recipient to feel even less in control of her reproductive life; not only was she "forced" to use an anonymous donor but she had to reveal her infertility, and especially her need for ovum donation. With help, the recipient recognized that this experience meant she must let go of her hope for genetic continuity, as well as her hope that her relationship with her sister would live up to her expectations.

Choosing Anonymous Ovum Donation

Despite the understandable disappointment of couples who would prefer known donors, there are many others who prefer anonymous donation. Some of them may even have an appropriate donor but feel that anonymous donation offers them some clear advantages similar to those seen by couples who adopt confidentially.

Avoidance of Social and Relational Bewilderment

Many anonymous egg recipients would not want to have an ongoing relationship with the donor. They believe that if the child's genetic mother were involved in their lives, the child could be confused about who his or her "real" mother is. Furthermore, if the donor were a relative—a sister, for example—they believe the child would face the additional confusion of not knowing whether to relate to her as an aunt or as a mother.

Authenticity

Couples who have battled long-term infertility may experience a sense of insecurity about parenthood and a lack of entitlement about their right to be parents. Couples choosing anonymity believe this route will enhance their sense of authenticity and allow them to feel like the real parents. They fear that if the donor were part of their lives, the recipient's relationship with her child would be undermined.

Security

Some couples considering known ovum donation have fears that the genetic mother might try to claim the child as her own and take him or her away. Couples choosing anonymous donation feel protected by the anonymity, seeing it as creating a psychological barrier between them and the donor, enabling them to feel more secure as a family.

Privacy

Couples frequently choose anonymous donation because it affords them privacy. Although they might wish to know about the source of their donated gametes, they feel that using a known donor would compromise their privacy and force them to disclose to everyone how their child was conceived, thus interfering with the foundation and future of their family. Being private gives them control over the information regarding their child's conception.

Who Becomes an Anonymous Donor?

Couples considering anonymous ovum donation almost immediately question who the donors are. Many wonder why someone would put herself through a grueling procedure for someone she did not know. They may conclude that donors must be psychologically disturbed. Others assume that because compensation is usually involved, donors must be in financial difficulty. The truth is that most programs require donors to go through an extensive psychological and medical evaluation, and those with psychopathology are immediately screened out. In addition, many programs attempt to avoid accepting donors whose motivations are strictly financial.

228

Recruitment and Motivation

Most women who apply for anonymous ovum donation do so in response to an advertisement in their local newspaper, on a bulletin board (in settings that range from college campuses to supermarkets), or in medical centers. Other prospective donors learn about ovum donation because they had a friend who was a donor, because they know someone who works in an ART program, or because they saw a television program or heard a radio broadcast that piqued their interest.

The typical anonymous donor is a young woman in good health who has given careful consideration to the process. In many cases, donors are women in transition: students, mothers with young children who are not working outside the home, or women who are between jobs. Most are drawn to ovum donation for reasons of empathy or altruism. Some are drawn to it as a result of having suffered reproductive losses. The financial compensation is usually secondary.

Empathy and Altruism.

Often donors know someone who is or who has been infertile. If the infertile woman is a close friend or relative, the donor understands her heartache. Many donors have said that were it not for their relationship with their infertile friend (or relative), they would never have thought of donating eggs.

Other potential donors are mothers with young children who state unequivocally that motherhood has been the most rewarding experience of their lives. They feel deeply for those who desire children and are unable to have them and seek the opportunity to help such couples.

Donors who are primarily motivated out of altruism or empathy usually think of their eggs as genetic material—something to help start a life—not as a baby. They view their eggs as going to waste every month, and since they do not need them and someone else does, why not donate them? They believe that if they can do something of such importance for someone else, at little cost to themselves, that it is worth doing. Many donors include women who donate their blood regularly, are in bone marrow registries, or carry organ donor cards in their wallets. They feel that donating a life-giving part of themselves (that they do not need) is the *right* thing to do.

Reproductive Losses

Some donors may be attempting to "make up" for past reproductive losses, perhaps an elective abortion, about which they still have regretful feelings. One such donor, who had three children subsequent to her abortion at age seventeen, stated that one of her reasons for wanting to donate eggs was that she "took away a life and now wants to give back a life." Although this stated reason was initially a red flag to the counselor, it eventually became clear that the donation could be healing for the prospective donor. Rather than attempting to psychologically *undo* a past action, she might be able to *redo* it.

Women who have placed children for adoption sometimes apply to be ovum donors. Depending on the psychological assessment, it may or may not be wise for them to become ovum donors. On the one hand, they have already experienced a loss that is presumably much greater than the loss of an egg; they should know whether they can handle the long-term implications of egg donation. On the other hand, there is always the possibility that such a prospective donor, like some women who have undergone elective abortions, is still suffering from feelings of guilt or grief and is hoping that the altruistic act of donating eggs to an infertile couple will make up for the loss of their child who was adopted. Such women may be better helped by counseling and should not be allowed to donate unless they have come to terms with this loss and have reached a point of acceptance regarding the adoption plan that they made.

Adoptees have also applied to become ovum donors. Many programs will not accept them if important medical information is missing but will consider them as donors if they have access to their medical history. Although adoptees may have a variety of reasons for wanting to donate, they may also have unconscious motivations which need to be explored, having to do with their lack of a genetic link to their parents.

Psychological Screening and Counseling of Donors

The differences between screening sperm donors and egg donors are striking. Although the medical screening for sperm donors is thorough, the psychological screening is virtually nonexistent. Some feel this dual standard is sexist or paternalistic—that it reflects an inherent assumption that women are not capable of making a good decision without the help of a professional. Others believe that the screening processes for egg donors evolved from concerns raised about the lack of a similar process with their male counterparts. In other words, what is standard practice among sperm banks is far from what many mental health providers consider acceptable. Thus the sperm bank model is recognized to be a poor model for ovum donor programs.

Ovum donor programs tend to view the potential donor in one of two ways: as their patient or as a provider of gametes. Programs who regard donors as patients are generally concerned about both the medical and psychological well-being of the woman. They are concerned that the donor is well informed about the medical process and risks and that she understands the legal, ethical, social, and psychological implications of "giving away" her genetic material. In addition, such programs are concerned that the potential donor have reasons for donating that will enhance, rather than detract, from her self-esteem.

Clinics that view donors as providers of gametes—much as they view a pharmaceutical company as the provider of medications—are concerned primarily with the end result: whether they are providing infertile patients with good (and viable) gametes. They are not as concerned about the psychological state of the donor. They assume that she can make an appropriate decision about whether ovum donation is in her best interest, and she does not need a mental health professional to help her make that decision. These programs are usually concerned about thorough medical screening, and some may administer routine psychological assessment tests to rule out donors with serious psychopathology or personality problems. They probably have little personal contact with the potential donor and are not worried about the long-term psychological effects on her or on the family.

Most programs view the donor as their patient. In Braverman's survey, 77.6% of the eighty-two programs reporting stated that psychological screening was required. Of those programs requiring psychological screening, 78.4% used personal interviews as part or all of the screening process. Some of the programs requiring psychological screening used personality assessment tests (43.1%) and some used other standard psychological tests (27.5%). These statistics indicate that although most programs requiring screening include a personal interview with the donor, there are some programs that require only the use of standardized testing in their psychological assessment. Furthermore, most programs (58.6%) require partners of prospective donors to be seen as well. Depending on the time allotted to the counseling and screening process, clinicians may see the potential donor anywhere from one to three times.[42]

The purpose of psychological screening and counseling is threefold: to ensure that the woman is psychologically appropriate to be a donor (mature, responsible, and with no underlying psychopathology); to inform her of both the short- and long-term psychological risks of donating ovum; and to be sure the program is protected in the event of future litigation.

In attempting to determine psychological appropriateness, a family and individual history is usually taken, which includes questions about prior substance abuse, mental illness, and reproductive losses. This allows the clinician to form a picture of the potential donor and to understand what social and psychological forces have shaped her life and prompted her to apply for ovum donation. The information gathered, in combination with her motivations and current life situation, helps the clinician determine whether she is suited to undertake ovum donation at this time.

Another important part of the assessment interview is making sure that donors comprehend exactly what it is they are giving away. Referring to the "blood versus child" continuum, counselors must try to learn whether a potential donor views her gametes more as blood or more as the beginning of a person. Those who consider their eggs similar to a person usually screen themselves out as donors—if not before, then as a result of the interviews. However, if a potential donor claims that there is no difference between donating blood and donating eggs, it is the responsibility of the counselor to help her understand the distinction between them, and to explore what her genetic material does mean to her.

Program counselors must help prospective donors see the long- as well as the short-term implications of their donation. The counselor tries to anticipate potential events that might cause them to have regrets. One way this task can be accomplished is by asking a series of "what if" questions, similar to the questions asked of known donors. For example, if a potential anonymous donor has not completed her family, she must think about the possibility that something might happen in the future that would cause her to be infertile. If that unfortunate situation were to occur, would she regret having donated at a younger age?

Donors must think about the possibility that the offspring might want to find them someday. Legislation in the field of reproductive medicine is continually changing, and it is possible that one day all programs using donor gametes will be mandated to open their records. Prospective donors must also think about the possibility, though remote, of a medical emergency—that a child may need to find a match for an organ or bone marrow transplant, and the donor could be contacted.

Potential donors must consider whether to tell their future partner or future children that they had been an ovum donor—or their existing children, if they are already mothers. They must be made aware that their children will have half-siblings in the world whom they will probably never know. They must imagine themselves in the grocery store or in the local mall spotting a young child who resembles them at that age. Would the prospective donor wonder, for more than a passing moment, whether it was her child? Would the incident haunt her or would she be able to let it go?

An important consideration for all donors, regardless of whether their decision will be affected by it, is the reaction of their family. Recently a few "donor grandparents" have stepped forward to share feelings of sadness and loss about having grandchildren in the world whom they will never know. It is important for potential donors to understand that although they themselves may not feel a particular connection to the genetic material they are passing on, other family members may feel differently. Many donors do not plan to tell their family members, anticipating negative reations. In such cases, donors need to ponder the effect of keeping this secret from them, as well as the reasons they are doing so.

Potential donors must consider how they feel about revealing personal information. Many clinics ask donors to fill out a lengthy questionnaire that inquires about their social, psychological, physical, and medical history, and this information is offered to recipient couples if a pregnancy occurs. Potential anonymous donors must be comfortable with the idea of sharing extensive (though nonidentifying) information about themselves.

Each program has its own policy regarding disclosure of information about recipients to donors, including whether a pregnancy has occurred. Some programs refuse to give a donor any information about who is getting the eggs and refuse to inform the donor if a pregnancy occurs, believing that it is in her best interest not to know. These programs feel strongly that if the donor cannot live with uncertainty, she should not be a donor. Other programs leave the choice about receiving that information to the donor, believing that she knows what is best for her. Our initial impression is that most donors, when given the option, like to be informed; they prefer knowing the truth to living with uncertainty. They hope the news is good, and anticipate feeling joyful for the recipients and pleased about having made the pregnancy possible. Those who say they do not want to know may be ambivalent about the ovum donor process. It is important to explore their reasons for not wanting to know in the event that unconscious conflicts are revealed.

Of the eighty-two ovum donor programs that participated in Braverman's ovum donation survey, 60.3% stated that they had developed specific psychological criteria to reject ovum donors. Although it can be assumed that the remaining programs (39.7%) reject donors they feel are psychologically inappropriate, it is not clear on what basis—presumably a subjective one— they are rejected.[43] The Ovum Donation Task Force of the Mental Health Professional Group of the American Society for Reproductive Medicine has developed guidelines for accepting and rejecting ovum donors and we refer interested readers to these guidelines.

Legal protection is also a necessary reason for donor screening. Fortunately litigation in the area of reproductive medicine is rare, although there have been a handful of cases involving third parties and/or advanced technology that have received significant attention. In Chapter 2 we mentioned the case at the University of California-Irvine. Among the many charges that have been filed against the clinic are charges from former patients of unauthorized use of their eggs. As a result of these cases and others less widely publicized, ART programs recognize that something could go wrong that could cause irreparable damage to their reputation. Programs hope to minimize the chance of litigation by thoroughly screening both donors and recipients.

The Donor's Experience

When the medical process is completed, most donors report that it was not difficult. Their relative ease is probably due in part to the fact that women who fear needles and other invasive medical procedures either do not volunteer to be ovum donors or screen themselves out when they learn what the process entails. Some programs report that many of their donors volunteer to recycle, which serves as testimony that the process was not too trying. Other programs, however, have reported an unexpected number of donors who have had difficulty with the medical protocols.

During the screening interview, anonymous donors sometimes ask about the recipients, but their questions tend to be general. We have found, however, that as the process begins, donors become more curious about the couple receiving their eggs and frequently ask for more information about them. It is important that the mental health counselor be available to meet with them to help them distinguish whether they are simply curious or have serious reservations. The counselor can provide helpful observations and information, including the answers to some of the donor's questions about the recipients.

Some donors never ask about the recipients. It is enough for them to know that recipients are couples who want children and that the program agreed to treat them. They assume that anyone who wants children so badly would make good parents. Such donors seem to separate the process of donating gametes from the people receiving them. Some may fear that they would become too invested in the outcome if they knew more about the recipients. Others worry that the more information they have, the less anonymous the process is.

During the ovulatory phase of the cycle, when donors are receiving daily injections and must report to the clinic each day to be monitored, they receive a great deal of attention and appreciation from the staff. Most donors enjoy being in the spotlight; they know they are providing an invaluable service to infertile couples and, unless the medications are seriously affecting their moods, they usually report to the clinic in good spirits.

When the egg retrieval is completed and the donor's immediate obligation ends, some donors experience an unanticipated letdown. This may be due in part to hormonal changes, but it is probably also due to the loss of their special status as egg donor and the attention that it brings. The abrupt change in a donor's demeanor may be puzzling to staff if they have not prepared themselves for this possibility.

Many clinics ask donors to come in for an exit interview with either the counselor or a nurse after the retrieval is completed. This interview offers the donor an opportunity to say good-bye to the staff and to put closure on her experience. It also offers the program an opportunity to learn about her experience so they can better understand and work with future donors. Finally, the interview can help establish a system by which donors notify the programs of significant medical information in years to come.

The Recipients

Although some recipient couples were diagnosed early on with premature ovarian failure and consequently escaped months or years of invasive treatment, most recipients have spent what feels like an eternity attempting to have a family. Many have been through several unsuccessful attempts at *in vitro* fertilization; others have adopted a child(ren) and wish to enlarge their families. For all women embarking on ovum donation, however, regardless of where they have been in the world of reproductive medicine, ovum donation is their final attempt to bear—and give birth to—their child.

Psychological Screening and Counseling

It is probably obvious that couples who undergo ovum donation are screened much more thoroughly in IVF centers than couples who are using their own gametes to attempt pregnancy. In the early days of IVF it was fairly standard practice, however, to be screened psychologically before being allowed to cycle. Although this practice has been discontinued almost everywhere, clinics are more careful when it comes to procedures involving gamete donation.

The Role of the Mental Health Clinician

Although ART programs have widely diverging standards for accepting or rejecting donors, virtually all agree that not everyone is psychologically fit to be a donor. In counseling recipients, however, mental health clinicians, as well as the physicians with whom they work, struggle with a basic question about their role *vis a` vis* recipients: are they gatekeepers or consultants? If they are gatekeepers, their job includes screening potential recipients in or out of treatment. If they are consultants, their job is strictly to offer information to recipients, and to engage in a discussion with them about that information rather than to screen them.

Those who oppose gatekeeping point out that no one screens fertile couples; moreover, they are not in a position to judge who will be good parents. Counselors who argue this viewpoint also remind professionals that many couples who appear to have their lives in order and are model citizens make poor parents.

Those who feel that counselors should be gatekeepers point to adoption as the model from which they base their opinion. They feel that the best interest of the unborn child should be everyone's primary consideration. Some professionals also feel a moral obligation to the donor—and of course to the child—to ensure good parenting.

Most mental health clinicians appear to take a middle-of-the-road position, adopting liberal screening criteria. Unless a serious problem emerges in the counseling/screening interview or unless the recipients screen themselves out, the couple is approved for ovum donation. However, the definition of "serious" depends on the clinician and the clinic. Standards for acceptance or rejection vary greatly from program to program.

The Purpose of Counseling Recipients

The purpose of the counseling/screening interview is to assess the psychological readiness of the couple to undergo ovum donation and to help the couple anticipate both the short- and long-term social, psychological, and ethical implications of ovum donation. In the event that the counselor functions as gatekeeper, the task is also to determine whether the couple is accepted into the program. If the counselor is solely a clinical consultant, he or she can work more actively with the couple to help them decide whether ovum donation is in their best interest.

In assessing readiness for ovum donation, counselors attempt to understand how well each member of the couple—and the couple as a unit—functioned prior to infertility. They explore how the couple has coped with infertility and how it has affected their lives. Other questions investigate support systems, whether they have discussed ovum donation with anyone, and how and why they decided to pursue it.

The extent to which the couple has grieved the loss of having a biological child together can be an important barometer of their psychological readiness. Sometimes something emerges in the screening interview that reveals that the recipient continues to hold on to the wish for a biological child. For example, a prospective recipient will sometimes indicate that she has a belief—or hope—that the baby will "inherit" her genes in utero.

The second reason for screening recipients—to help them anticipate potential problems—can be done in many ways, including asking "what if" questions such as:

- What if your child wants to seek his or her genetic mother someday?
- What if laws change, and donor records can no longer be anonymous, and the donor wants to meet your child?
- What if laws change and your child's genetic half-siblings seek him/her out?

Counselors are also interested in whether the couple plans to be open with others about ovum donation and, most important, whether they plan to tell their child about how he or she was conceived.

Although an increasing number of couples recognize the need to tell their child the truth about his/her origins, some do not. Lingering feelings about infertility or fears that the child will be upset by the information, prompt some couples to feel that the truth is something they can easily hide from their child. Mental health clinicians are in a position to discuss the ramifications of secrecy on the child and on his nuclear family. Chapter 10 addresses this issue extensively.

Expectations about the Donor

Oocytes are difficult to obtain, and most programs do not have a large supply of donors. Even programs that allow recipients to make requests about donor characteristics, are often unable to honor these requests. Nevertheless, it is useful for counselors to discuss with prospective recipients their expectations of the donor. Such a discussion can help the clinician determine whether they are being realistic in their expectations, and if not, why not. Asking about the donor can also help the team members to be as responsive as possible to the couple's request.

Most recipient couples are very grateful to be able to receive donated ova and they try to have few expectations or requirements of a donor. Nonetheless, like parents through sperm donation, they hope that the donor will bear some physical (and ideally psychological) resemblance to them. Although many will tell the child the truth about his or her origins, they prefer a child that "fits in," because similarities will make it less likely that strangers will be asking bothersome and intrusive questions.

As with sperm donation, concerns about the donor extend beyond physical appearances. Aware of the significance of genetics, couples hope that the donor will resemble them in other ways as well. Although most seek personality and intellectual similarities, some couples focus on ethnic or religious connections. For example, one couple seeking ovum donation was so intent on finding a Jewish donor (regardless of physical or other characteristics) that the husband wrote a personal letter to every rabbi whose name was on a long list of Jewish clergy. When this search proved fruitless, he went on the internet, again in search of a "Jewish egg." While some would question his search and suggest that he was "not ready for ovum donation," there is a long history in both sperm donation and adoption of couples who wish to create or adopt children who share their ethnic history.

There are some instances, however, in which a couple's requests or requirements for a donor do reveal a lack of preparedness for ovum donation. One such instance occurred when a recipient expressed anxiety about the physical size of the donor. She stated that she feared that if the donor was too big, the baby would be too big, and her uterus might rupture. The prospective recipient continued to focus on ways she imagined the fetus could damage her. In this instance, a mental health counselor was able to help the woman identify her underlying fear that the child would feel like a stranger—that she might never be able to connect emotionally with him or her. After some additional counseling sessions outside the clinic setting, this couple realized that they were more comfortable with adoption.

Openness versus Secrecy

As we will discuss in Chapter 10, the question of openness vs. secrecy is a complicated one, involving profound ethical, legal, and psycho-social issues. Historically, sperm donation was almost always done secretly, however, this trend appears to be slowly changing, as people have come to recognize the hazards of secrecy. Nonetheless, according to anecdotal research, many more ovum donor than sperm donor couples seem to be choosing to be open with their children, as well as with others, about the origins of their child's conception. We can speculate about the reasons why this is so.

Until ovum donation became a reality appproximately a decade ago, gestation and motherhood were inseparable. Because the woman who gestates and bears a child has always been seen as that child's mother, most ovum recipients, though they may worry from time to time if they will feel like the *real* mother, assume they will bond with the child they carry. In this way, their experience is very different from the infertile man whose wife conceives with donor sperm: he must wait until after birth to establish a relationship with his child.

Additionally, women tend to be more open in our culture about their personal lives. They are accustomed to sharing problems with friends and family and looking to others for mutual support and advice. There may also be less stigma attached to being an infertile woman than to being an infertile man, perhaps because infertility, at least in the greater society, is assumed to be a woman's problem. Thus, women in general are more open about infertility than are their male counterparts, and so it stands to reason that they would be more open about ovum donation than men are about sperm donation.

There is another reason for what appears to be greater openness among ovum donor couples than among donor insemination couples. In the Donor Insemination chapter we noted that there may be sexual overtones for some couples electing to do donor insemination. The woman may feel as if she is having an affair or being adulterous, and her husband may have similar feelings. In ovum donation, sexual overtones seem to be absent. Because the woman is receiving an egg which, unlike sperm is not involved with lovemaking, neither she nor her husband are likely to feel that they are doing something that involves sexual transgression.

Finally, in meeting with recipient couples, the clinician must be certain that they recognize that gamete donation, similar in this way to adoption, is a lifelong process. The issues underlying this parenting alternative, as well as with others that involve third parties, are highly complicated and evoke intense feelings. A family created as a result of this technology will undoubtedly have hurdles to face. Thus, there is yet another purpose to screening and counseling recipients: to establish a comfortable relationship with a mental health professional. This contact is designed to lay the foundation for psychological support and assistance, should they feel a need for it in the future.

Matching Donors and Recipients

One of the most challenging aspects of ovum donation is the matching process. Depending upon the protocol of a given program, this task may be accomplished by one individual (usually the nurse or coordinator) or by a team. In either event, those involved in this modern form of matchmaking find themselves in an awkward position, feeling, at times, as if they are "playing God."

Actually, the word *match* is something of a misnomer, as that term implies a *fit*, or a *duplication*. Since everyone has a unique set of genes, there is no possibility of matching one person to another, although sperm banks, with their vast numbers of donors, create the illusion that it is possible. Thus couples involved in donor insemination are sometimes able to fool themselves into believing they have found a perfect match— a donor who seems just like the husband. When it comes to ovum donation—where eggs are scarce—such illusions are not possible.

Those involved in pairing donors and recipients—as individuals or as part of a team—take a variety of factors into consideration. They look at physical appearance, trying to avoid obvious mismatches, such as a five-foot blond recipient and a six-foot dark-haired donor. Matchmakers may also take educational background or intellectual attributes into consideration. They also attempt to take some personality characteristics into account, aware that many traits once thought to be the product of environment are now seen as inherited. Such knowledge increases the anxiety of the matchmakers. However, they are comforted by their awareness that there is never a guarantee that any trait—desirable or undesirable—will be passed on, as children are often very different from their genetic parents.

Some programs use pictures of donors and recipients to narrow the possibilities and to avoid confusing one person with another. Intuition, however, is probably the most important variable in selecting donor-recipient pairs. Many involved in this process attempt to use their "sixth sense" about who fits well with whom, to guide them in the selection process.

There are a few clinics in various parts of the country (often in university settings) that do have large pools of donors. Potential recipients are introduced to them via catalogs or scrapbooks. Such couples tend to feel more in control of the process, and like DI couples may be able to "convince themselves" they have found a perfect "match."

Because matching donors and recipients is a substantial responsibility, many programs are allowing recipients to participate. One way to do this is to find a tentative match (or perhaps two or three) and allow recipient couples to review information about the donor that includes a family medical history, physical attributes, interests, and talents. The recipients have the right to reject any or all of the donors offered, knowing that this may cause a delay, but that sooner or later there will be other donor profiles to review.

Couples who are involved in the selection process not only feel more in control but have an additional opportunity to think about what it means to accept a donated gamete. They must wrestle with questions such as whether they prefer a donor who has a family history of heart disease or a donor whose brother is alcoholic. The process also means that couples must face the fact that there is no perfect donor, just as they do not come with perfect genes. This knowledge may help them to have realistic expectations of their child.

A few clinics allow (even encourage) donor and recipient couples to meet. Many programs have found that these open arrangements are extremely satisfying to everyone. Elaine Gordon, a psychologist who works with several ART programs in southern California, commented that the people who appear to be the most comfortable with ovum donation—both donors and recipients—are the ones who participate in open arrangements. She believes that when ovum donation is open, everyone seems less anxious, and the process goes much more smoothly. As the cycle progresses, they tend to voice fewer complaints and appear comfortable with the protocols. When the process is open, she has found, everyone has a sense of peace as well as pride that what they are doing is right for them. Even when the pregnancy test is negative, recipient couples seem more resolved: their feelings are more sad than angry—the opposite of what they usually are for those who have not wanted to meet their donors.

Pregnancy through Anonymous Ovum Donation

Although ovum donation places relatively few physical demands on a recipient, it is immensely stressful from an emotional perspective. Most recipients go through the process with a great deal at stake. For some, the cycle represents their last hope for sharing pregnancy and childbirth, and for those unwilling or unable to consider adoption, it is their last chance for becoming parents together. Because so much is at stake and there is so little they can do about it, recipients are understandably anxious. During the first part of the cycle this anxiety focuses on their donor; recipients become increasingly curious about who she is and how she is doing. Although clinics try to schedule appointments so that donors and recipients will not meet in the waiting room, recipients find themselves looking around and wondering if the woman sitting across the room or the one who was leaving as she was arriving is her donor. Later, following transfer, the recipient's anxiety typically shifts to her own body and to what she can do to maximize her chances for successful implantation and pregnancy.

Although the overall pregnancy rates are substantially higher for ovum donation than for IVF with the recipient's gametes, many recipients have a negative pregnancy test. This news is especially painful for those who come to ovum donation with a history of reproductive loss such as cancer or premature ovarian failure. These women are even more prone to feel that their bodies are defective and have betrayed them once again. Recipients who did not become pregnant may feel a sense of failure and guilt. They know that substantial effort from several people went into producing and obtaining the eggs, as well as creating the embryos. It was truly a team effort, and recipients may feel that they have not only let down their husband but the donor and staff as well. The overriding feeling, however, is profound sadness and loss. Once again their bodies have let them down, and once again their wombs—and their hearts—are empty.

Some couples whose financial resources, emotional stamina, and desire enable them to attempt another cycle or two, do so. Sometimes this knowledge eases their grief. They know, however, that no matter how many cycles they can afford there is never a guarantee of a successful pregnancy.

A positive test beckons very different emotions, and about 40 to 50% of ovum donation recipients do become pregnant. For many recipients a positive pregnancy test is confirmation that their body is working properly. The news, however, is also received cautiously; couples who have been through long-term infertility know that there are always additional hurdles ahead—medical and emotional ones.

Because pregnancy after anonymous ovum donation is a recent development, there is little clinical expertise to draw upon. Based on our experience, however, a pregnancy that begins in this new way may bring special challenges for the couple—in particular, the woman.

Although they are thrilled to be expecting, in talking with women pregnant after anonymous ovum donation we have found that certain issues and feelings emerge. Many of these feelings are the same as the feelings described by women pregnant after IVF with their own gametes. They feel a heightened sense of vulnerability and loss—a sense that their pregnancy is extremely tenuous. Furthermore the feelings of defectiveness described by infertile women do not necessarily vanish after a positive pregnancy test—and sometimes not even after delivery. Additionally, mothers-to-be through ovum donation may have feelings that the baby they are carrying is a stranger, fearful about *who* s/he will be. (Although all pregnant women wonder who their baby will be, women pregnant with their own ova seem more curious than fearful.)

We have seen in this chapter that although ovum donation is the female counterpart of donor insemination, it is both medically and psychologically very different. Donor insemination has historically been surrounded by an aura of secrecy and shame leading to a denial of its occurance as well as prevalence. There has been little psychological counseling offered to DI couples, and virtually no psychological counseling offered to sperm donors.

By contrast, ovum donation is practiced in an atmosphere of far greater openness. Physicians are working collaboratively with mental health counselors to be sure that all those considering ovum donation understand the magnitude of this undertaking. Careful, cautious counseling plays a vital role in the process, helping prospective donors and recipients to carefully examine the lifelong social, psychological and ethical challenges of this family building option.

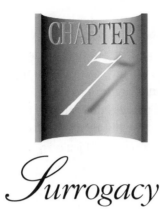

Surrogacy

Although it has a prominent place in this book about assisted reproductive options, surrogacy is not new, nor is it an outgrowth of the recent advances in reproductive medicine. Rather, surrogacy, the first-known form of third-party reproduction, dates back to biblical times. Then, as now, it raised complex social and emotional issues.

The history of surrogacy begins with Abraham and Sarah, the first infertile couple mentioned in Western literature:

> Now Sarah, Abraham's wife, bore him no children and she had a handmaid, an Egyptian, whose name was Hagar. And Sarah said unto Abraham, "Behold now, the Lord hath restrained me from bearing: I pray thee, go unto my maid: it may be that I may obtain children by her." And Abraham hearkened to the voice of Sarah.
>
> Genesis 16:1-2

Abraham's decision to follow his wife's advice and to have her handmaiden bear his child provided a solution to their childlessness. Hagar, history's first-known surrogate mother, conceived and gave birth to Abraham's first son, Ishmael. This event, however, did not resolve the pain of infertility for Abraham and Sarah. Instead, Sarah reacted with unexpected bitterness toward Hagar's pregnancy, saying to her husband, "The wrong done me is your fault!"

The Bible goes on to chronicle the problems that continued between Sarah and Hagar. These extended to Sarah's relationship with Abraham and continued even after Sarah gave birth to a long awaited child, Isaac. Thus, even after Sarah's own prayers had been answered, she remained bitter and said to her husband, "Cast out that slavewoman and her son, for the son of that slave shall not share in the inheritance with my son Isaac."

The story of Abraham and Sarah is prophetic. It introduces the idea that surrogacy is a complicated process that offers no easy solution to the pain of infertility. Sarah was the first, but by no means the last, woman to find that she had unanticipated reactions of jealousy and resentment to the pregnancy and childbirth experience of another woman, even one who was bearing a child for her. Similarly, Hagar was not the only surrogate to discover that surrogacy could bring an unanticipated and problematic outcome.

Who Considers Using Surrogacy

Most people who consider becoming parents through surrogacy are married, childless couples. Many are veterans of years of unsuccessful infertility treatments or of repeated pregnancy losses. Others are couples in which the woman has suffered a serious illness that rendered her unable to bear children. Some come to surrogacy as a third choice, having already endured failed attempts at gestational care or perhaps, adoption "fall throughs."

Surrogacy is attractive to couples because it offers them the chance to have a child who is the genetic offspring of the father. This is especially important to those men—and women—who feel deeply about carrying on genetic and generational ties. Although they have been criticized for their "machismo" and male egotism, most couples exploring surrogacy do not focus on maintaining some sort of patriarchal order. Rather, they are moved by what is, for them, a matter of the heart: the longing to perpetuate a family heritage. Sometimes this longing is tied to feelings about specific family members, especially loved ones who have died. Other times, it is tied to feelings about their religious or cultural history. For example, some offspring of Holocaust survivors feel a strong need to do what they can to keep a family line alive.

Some couples who explore surrogacy have taken a careful and serious look at adoption and have concluded that surrogacy offers them more opportunity for control. Having surrendered so much control during their infertility experience, they welcome the opportunity to select their child's birthmother and look forward to having a relationship with her throughout her pregnancy and during labor and delivery. Indeed, according to Dr. Hilary Hanafin, psychologist at the Center for Surrogate Parenting and Egg Donation, 85% of the couples working with her center are present at the delivery. Although changes in adoption have offered expectant parents increased opportunities to participate in pregnancy, labor and delivery, some couples still prefer surrogacy because it offers them the assurance that they will be involved for the entire pregnancy.

There are couples who pursue surrogacy because they are frightened of adoption or they perceive adoption as unavailable to them. Those who fear adoption often rely on information that they have read in the popular press or have seen on TV. Most focus on health concerns or on fears that the birthparents will change their minds. Couples who perceive themselves as unable to adopt also tend to draw conclusions from scanty information or herseay. Some are concerned that they are too old or have not been married long enough. Others have read or been told that adoption takes many years to accomplish. For each of these groups—and others—surrogacy seems like a safer, more secure and predictable option.

Most couples who consider surrogacy begin with only a vague sense of what is involved. Fortunately, there are resources available to them that can de-mystify the process and help them determine whether surrogacy is truly the best alternative path to parenthood for them.

The most comprehensive source of information for prospective parents through surrogacy is the Organization of Parents through Surrogacy (OPTS), a volunteer staffed, non-profit organization that has representatives throughout the United States. OPTS volunteers help couples begin to explore surrogacy and they are available to respond to questions and concerns as people make their way through the surrogacy process. OPTS can be reached on the web at www.opts.com.

Another valuable resource for couples considering surrogacy is The American Surrogacy Center (TASC), an internet site. Through TASC, interested individuals can access nine internet support and discussion groups that involve surrogacy.

The vast majority of couples who consider surrogacy do so for medical reasons. In fact, responsible surrogacy practitioners work only with couples who have medical problems (or "aging eggs") which make pregnancy impossible or inadvisable. However, this is not always the public perception of families involved in surrogacy. Critics charge that some women use surrogacy for reasons of "convenience"—they allegedly want to avoid the discomforts or physical limitations of pregnancy. Critics further allege that these are wealthy women and that their payment to surrogates, who are usually not wealthy, represents the exploitation of one group of women by another.

Although surrogacy poses some serious ethical dilemmas, which we will try to address throughout this chapter, avoidance of pregnancy has not, in our experience, been one of them. Wealthy women have the same desires and longings to conceive, carry and give birth to their bio-genetic children as non-wealthy women do. Although their financial security may be what makes commercial surrogacy available and accessible to them, it is not the reason that they become involved in this path to parenthood.

The Development of Twentieth Century Contractual Surrogacy

Throughout history, there have been informal surrogacy arrangements between couples and women who were friends, acquaintances, or family members. These have usually involved little if any remuneration beyond expenses and have been assumed to have been motivated almost exclusively by close feelings between people who knew each other well.

It was not until the mid 1970s that contractual surrogacy became available to infertile couples. In 1977, the late Noel Keane, a Michigan attorney, made public the fact that he had advertised in college newspapers and found a woman who agreed to conceive and carry a baby for a childless couple. His announcement met with extensive publicity, including television and media appearances and magazine features. It was also followed by announcements from other lawyers, as well as from physicians and small business people, that they, too, could assist couples to become parents through contractual surrogacy.

The arrival of contractual surrogacy at much the same time that IVF was being developed and adoption was changing dramatically created a social climate of great controversy, curiosity and interest. People had new opportunites to consider with IVF and they were forced to look at adoption in new ways, as fewer caucasian babies became available for adoption and as the practice of adoption began to shift from anonymity and secrecy and to increased contact and exchange of information between birth and adoptive parents. Each of these changes—in reproductive medicine and in adoption, had an impact upon surrogacy.

IVF: Impact on Surrogacy

The arrival of *in vitro* fertilization in 1978, just two years after contractual surrogacy began, altered the course of surrogacy. Many couples who might otherwise have pursued surrogacy because of what was formerly a conclusive infertility diagnosis such as blocked fallopian tubes, instead turned to IVF, a treatment which, if successful, offered them the possibility of experiencing a pregnancy and having a child genetically connected to both of them. In addition to offering the couple a full genetic and gestational connection to their child, IVF also eliminated the legal questions associated with surrogacy.

In vitro fertilization led to the development of two other advances in reproductive medicine that had special appeal to certain couples who might otherwise consider surrogacy: ovum donation and gestational care. Once eggs could be fertilized outside the body, there was no reason that genetic and gestational motherhood could not be separated in those instances in which a woman had lost part of her reproductive function. In other words, IVF made it possible for a woman who could not produce eggs to become pregnant with an egg that was retrieved from another woman and fertilized *in vitro* (with her mate's sperm). IVF also made it possible for a woman who could produce eggs but could not carry a pregnancy to have her eggs retrieved, fertilized *in vitro* (again, with her partner's sperm), and then transferred to the uterus of a gestational carrier.

Ovum donation, the transfer of eggs from one woman to another, first became available in 1984. Couples who would otherwise have pursued surrogacy due to premature ovarian failure or "aging eggs," were now candidates for ovum donation. Many saw this option as having several advantages over traditional surrogacy: the couple could share a pregnancy together, make all the decisions regarding prenatal and obstetrical care, and avoid the legal questions involved with surrogacy. The child born to them would not have to be adopted. Futhermore, they saw it as a family building option that offered them more privacy than they were likely to feel with surrogacy. Finally, the financial costs were lower.

Gestational care, the subject of Chapter 8, commonly referred to as gestational surrogacy or host-uterus surrogacy, first became available in 1986.

This option, viewed by some as but a minor variation of surrogacy, represented a significant opportunity for infertile couples. Unlike other alternative reproductive options—donor insemination, ovum donation, and traditional surrogacy—which all involve the donation of gametes, gestational care offered infertile couples the chance to have a full biogenetic child. Many saw it as raising far fewer ethical questions than other alternative paths to parenthood.

Had the ARTs, including ovum donation and gestational care, not come along on the heels of surrogacy, perhaps more couples would have pursued parenthood through surrogacy. Undoubtedly these new options diverted people's attention; they saw clear advantages to choosing IVF and some advantages, depending on their medical condition, to choosing either ovum donation or gestational care. The result was that relatively few couples pursued surrogacy.

Changes in Adoption: The Impact On Surrogacy

The decrease in the number of infants available for adoption was another change that affected surrogacy. This decrease was influenced by the increased availability of birth control, by the 1973 U.S. Supreme Court decision of *Roe v. Wade* in which abortion was legalized, and by the gradual lifting of the social stigma regarding single motherhood.

The late 1970s and the 1980s brought increased awareness of and sensitivity to the experiences of adoptees and birthparents. The notion that birthparents were easily able to place their children in the hands of adoption agencies and then move on in their lives without looking back was recognized as a falsehood. An accompanying assumption—that adoptees who were raised by loving parents would have no need to know about their birthparents—was also deemed untrue. A new appreciation for the significance of genetic ties, the need to know from where one comes, and for the longings of birthparents for the children they bore replaced these old myths.

This new appreciation raised the awareness of adoption professionals to the profound losses shared by all members of the adoption triad: the birthparents, the adoptee, and the adoptive parents. Increased understanding of these losses prompted many people to look more cautiously at surrogacy and to view the surrogacy triad as very similar to the adoption triad. Dr. Michael Grodin, professor of medicine and ethics at Boston University School of Medicine, has drawn several comparisons between adoption and surrogacy. He raises concerns about couples and surrogates entering into an agreement regarding the placement of the child prior to that child's conception. Agreements of this nature have the potential, Grodin cautions, to complicate a child's identity formation. Adoption is always complicated, even when parenting arrangements are "resolved at birth," and the child's later concerns about lineage, as well as about biological and social parentage, can become paramount.[44]

Another way that changes in adoption affected surrogacy involved the use of language. Prior to the 1980s, the language surrounding adoption promoted negative feelings about the adoption process and about all members of the adoption triangle. Adoptees were labeled "adopted children" even as adults. Birthparents were referred to as "real parents" (suggesting that the adoptive parents were not real) or "natural parents" (implying that the adoptive parents were not natural). Children were said to have been "given up," "given away," "put up," or "surrendered" for adoption. A movement towards using more positive—and more appropriate—adoption language began with Marietta Spencer, a Minnesota social worker, who introduced the concept of Positive Adoption Language (PAL). Her pioneering efforts have been carried on by Patricia Irwin Johnston, a nationally respected professional in the field of adoption, who has written extensively on adoption. PAL raises people's consciousness by replacing the old terminology with more respectful adoption language. For example, that birthparents make "adoption plans" and families are "built" through adoption.[45]

Heightened appreciation for the power of language has caused people to question the language of surrogacy as well. Supporters and critics of surrogacy alike have challenged the use of the word *surrogate* to describe the role of the woman who conceives, carries, and delivers a child. Critics of the practice have asked why she is not simply termed *the mother* or pejoratively referred to as *the breeder*.[46] Supporters of surrogacy have struggled to find more constructive language, such as *pre-birthmother* or *birthing mother*.

The language of surrogacy is complicated by the fact that there are now two very different reproductive options—both frequently identified as surrogacy—one in which the surrogate bears her genetic child, and the other in which she bears the genetic child of another couple. These options are not the same either psychologically or genetically and have very different impacts on the families involved. For this reason we have

251

chosen to separate these alternative family building options into two chapters. Chapter 8, Gestational Care, will discuss the process whereby one woman carries the genetic child of another couple.

In addition to changes in language, the 1980s brought increased openness in adoption. The former practice of confidential adoption in which the birthparents and the adoptive parents received little, if any information about each other, was replaced in most agencies by a greater willingness and desire for all parties to share information with one another. The practice of open adoption emerged, whereby the two sets of parents would meet, exchange identifying information about each other, and agree to stay in contact. There are also many adoptions that participants describe as "semi-open"—they meet, exchange some information and maintain limited contact, often through an agency. Some proponents of open adoption are critical of these "semi-open" arrangements, stating that an adoption is either open or it is confidential—there cannot be middle ground.

The shift toward contact between birth and adoptive parents has extended to the practice of surrogacy. We need only compare "Elizabeth Kane's" account of her experience as a surrogate in *Birthmother* (Harcourt, Brace and Jovanovich, 1988) with a 1993 cover story from *People* magazine. As an early surrogate, Kane was given a pseudonym and allowed to have only minimal contact with the contracting couple. By contrast, the *People* story depicts the close relationship that developed between a television star and her look-alike surrogate. As this story implies, contact between contracting couples and surrogates has come to be supported, encouraged, and facilitated by many programs.[47]

Contracts and Money

Noel Keane's 1977 arrangement introduced both the idea of a surrogacy contract and the concept of payment for surrogacy. This payment, intended to serve as compensation to the surrogate for her expenses and inconveniences before, during and immediately following pregnancy, became a tremendous source of controversy, raising several concerns.

Is Surrogacy "Baby Selling?"

"Baby selling"—in which birthparents offer to transfer their parental rights to an expected or already born child for adoption by a couple neither of whom is genetically connected to the child in exchange for money—is illegal in all states. Would contractual surrogacy—where a woman agrees, for a significant fee, to be impregnated with the sperm of a contracting man and to transfer her subsquent maternal rights to the genetic father's wife upon the birth of a child—also be considered baby selling? Birthparents in adoption are not allowed to accept any money beyond reimbursement of medical, counseling, legal and living expenses. These basic expenses are seen as a service for children already conceived by parents unprepared to parent. Donor insemination, while a service for infertile couples, involved such small amounts of money for the sperm donor as not to engender baby-selling concerns.

Supporters and opponents of surrogacy have argued both sides of the baby selling question. Supporters argue that the child will be raised by his/her bio-genetic father, who is certainly not "buying" his own baby. They liken surrogacy to sperm donation and support the infertile couples' right to have a child that has half their genetic background. Opponents counter that the contractual nature of the agreement makes surrogacy a form of breeding for profit. Michele Harrison, assistant profession of psychiatry at the University of Pittsburgh School of Medicine, is one such outspoken critic of surrogacy:

> The last time in the history of the United States that human beings were bred for transfer of ownership was during slavery. Slave women bore babies, some of whom were fathered by the slave owners themselves. Not since slavery have we attempted to institutionalize the forced removal of infants from their mothers—except in cases of abuse or clear lack of fitness.[48]

Does Surrogacy Exploit Women?

The question of exploitation also arises in reference to the payment involved in contractual surrogacy. Critics worry that poor women will be enticed by financial gain and will enter surrogacy arrangements solely for the money. One such outspoken critic is Gena Corea, who calls surrogates "breeders" and identifies surrogacy practitioners as "breeder businesses." In her book, *The Mother Machine*, Corea presents a lengthy indictment of surrogacy, offering several examples of how surrogacy exploits women. She points out all the physical and emotional risks that a woman under-takes to receive a mere $10,000 (the standard fee at the time her book *The Mother Machine* was published in 1985).[49] One of the many quotes that she uses to support her arguments comes from a psychologist screening candidates for a surrogacy program. She quotes Dr. Howard Adelman as saying:

I believe candidates with an element of financial need are the safest. If a woman is on unemployment and has children to care for, she is not likely to change her mind and want to keep the baby she is being paid to have for somebody else.[50]

Supporters of surrogacy argue that the fees paid to surrogates are too small to be enticing, considering the amount of time, risk and effort involved. However, critics counter-argue that the size of the payment is relative: it seems insignificant to middle and upper-middle class women, but is substantial—and therefore attractive—to poor women. They add that it is sexist to expect women to do so much for no payment and wonder what the fee would be to a man were the situation reversed.

In an effort to address the issue of coercion and to avoid the risk of exploitation, some people have suggested that there be minimum income guidelines for surrogates. However, many supporters of surrogacy object to this idea, saying that it would discriminate unfairly against poor women. Each of these arguments finds itself on a slippery slope supporting one side of the payment debate while inadvertently supporting the other.

In 1986, a group of former surrogates formed the National Association of Surrogate Mothers. As advocates for surrogacy, they explained their reasons for participating in surrogacy, described the positive experiences that they had had, and addressed the ethical issues of reproductive freedom. They explained that they saw surrogacy, like abortion, as an issue of choice.

Is it in a Child's Best Interest to Be Created through Contractual Surrogacy?

Perhaps the most difficult question to address and examine with regards to surrogacy involves the question of the best interests of an unborn— indeed, an unconceived—child. Again, supporters and critics of surrogacy take strong positions on either side of this compelling question.

OPTS members are vocal in emphasizing their belief that a child born through surrogacy is a deeply wanted child and will therefore be loved and cherished. They argue further that being wanted and loved are key ingredients in a child's emotional development. As one parent through surrogacy said,

Our child will always feel secure knowing that we wanted him so much and that we went to such great lengths to have him. I look at all the children whose parents don't seem to care at all about them and know that he will feel very lucky.

254

Critics of surrogacy counter this argument by noting that love is not necessarily enough. They remind others of the pain involved in adoption and note that many adoptees report feeling a profound sense of loss, even when they have devoted, loving parents. Critics worry that children born of surrogacy will feel a similar sense of loss, wondering why they are not being raised by their biological mothers and feeling a sense of disconnection and loneliness. They wonder how a child will feel about him/her self, knowing he/she was the product of a contractual arrangement. Furthermore, they question whether the contractual arrangement will become a tragic family legacy, bringing pain not only to the child born of surrogacy but to his/her descendents for generations to come.

Legal and Ethical Concerns

Beyond issues of reimbursement, legal and ethical concerns about the contract's enforcability have also been raised.

Can a Woman be Held to a Pre-Birth (pre-conception) Agreement to Place her Child with Another Mother?

Critics of surrogacy argue that asking a woman to make a pre-conception agreement to place a child is another form of exploitation. They point out that this is fundamentally different from adoption, in which a birthmother always has a right to change her mind after birth (a surrogate also has this right but the expectation is that she will adhere to her contract). In fact, in most states, birthmothers must wait at least a few days postpartum before surrendering parental rights and in some states, there is a designated period of time during which a birthmother can change her mind.

Surrogacy supporters argue that a pre-conception contract is not a matter of exploitation but rather of a woman's reproductive freedom. They say that it is insulting to suggest that women are incapable of making an agreement and holding to it. Faye Johnson of OPTS states

> In order for a woman to become a surrogate she most often goes through a rigorous application process, including psychological tests and physical examinations. Often she must travel, take time off of work, and attend meetings with lawyers and psychologists. Some women will have to go through several months of inseminations before conceiving. When I think of all that's involved, I have a hard time believing that this is a woman who doesn't know what she is doing! I have an even

255

harder time with people who think that they know what is best for her and who imply that she is incapable of making informed decisions for herself.[51]

William Handel, Esq., founder and director of the Center for Surrogate Parenting and Egg Donation, Inc. in Beverly Hills, California, also objects to the notion that a woman entering into a surrogacy contract is being exploited. Handel emphasizes that surrogacy contracts, which he has worked hard to develop, go to considerable lengths to protect the rights of all women participating in surrogacy. Today's contracts, unlike earlier ones which placed emphasis on producing a baby (an illegal transaction), compensate women for their time and energy and clearly stipulate that consent to relinquishment is not a precondition for payment.

Despite these changes in the contracts, critics of surrogacy still argue that it is unreasonable to expect a woman to know how she will feel about placing a child whom she conceives and gestates before she is even pregnant.

What If the Surrogate Does Not Want to Relinquish the Child?

There have been very few reported instances of surrogates who changed their minds and wanted to parent the child they bore through surrogacy. Nonetheless, this can happen and the reality of the pain involved was made public by the now infamous "Baby M" case.

The Baby M case pitted Mary Beth Whitehead, a married, working class mother of two and a surrogate mother, against her contracting couple, Bill Stern, a research scientist, and his wife, Betsy, a pediatrician. Dr. Stern, who suffered from multiple sclerosis, and turned to surrogacy because pregnancy could exacerbate the symptoms of her illness.

The Sterns and Whiteheads entered into a surrogacy agreement through Noel Keane's program. In preparation for the program, Ms. Whitehead underwent a psychological evaluation with Dr. Joan Einwohner. Her report, which was never shared with either the Sterns or Ms. Whitehead, expressed concerns about accepting Ms. Whitehead in the program. Dr. Einwohner was specifically troubled by the fact that Ms. Whitehead indicated that she wanted to have more children and thus questioned whether she would be able to relinquish the child she bore.

Unaware that the psychological evaluation had raised serious questions, the Sterns and Ms. Whitehead went ahead with their surrogacy plan. The pregnancy was healthy and uneventful, but by the third trimester, it became clear that Ms. Whitehead was having difficulty emotionally with the process. This difficulty intensified when she gave birth to a baby girl, whom she named Sara (the Sterns named her Melissa).

Although Mary Beth Whitehead initially placed the baby with the Sterns, she changed her mind within weeks and began efforts to gain custody. These efforts took the case into the courtroom, where it drew tremendous media attention. Some of that attention focused on the obvious class differences between the Sterns and the Whiteheads, with some criticizing Betsy Stern for being a career woman and others scorning Mary Beth Whitehead for the choices she had made.

In addition to court-appointed psychologists and psychiatrists, who were called in to make a determination about what was in the best interest of the child, the Baby M case attracted several advocacy groups. These included a group of feminists and the Concerned United Birthparents, (CUB), an advocacy group for birthmothers. Both groups, as well as others critical of surrogacy, defended Ms. Whitehead's right to change her mind after birth and to parent the child born to her. They were opposed by equally passionate adoptive parents' groups and others who sought to defend Mr. Stern's right to parent his child, as well as Betsy Stern's rights as an adoptive mother.

The Baby M case was initially tried by Judge Sorkow, who decided the case on the basis of what he found to be in the child's best interest. He terminated Ms. Whitehead's parental rights and awarded custody to the Sterns stating:

> The Sterns and Whiteheads have different life styles, social
> values and standards. The rancor is too great. This court
> doubts that they can isolate their personal animosity and
> 'all of a sudden' cooperate for the child's benefit.[52]

The New Jersey Supreme Court reached its ruling on the Baby M case in February, 1988. It reversed Judge Sorkow's opinion and stated that existing adoption laws applied to surrogacy arrangements. Consequently, the birthmother—in this case, Mary Beth Whitehead—could not receive payment and could not be held to a prebirth decision to surrender her parental rights. The court then designated her the baby's legal mother but awarded custody to the Sterns.

Although it raised many difficult issues, the one that was of most concern to everyone interested in the Baby M case was that of the best interests of the child. Melissa/Sara was clearly a wanted and loved child.

However, the battle between her birthmother and her biological father and his wife graphically illustrated that a surrogacy contract does not protect anyone in those instances in which a surrogate changes her mind.

To emphasize how rare it is for a surrogate to change her mind. Handel points out that if there were a lot of surrogates changing their minds then Mary Beth Whitehead's decision would not have received such attention. Others agree, saying that it is much more common for the surrogate to worry that the couple will change their minds and leave her with the baby.

Ironically, the case that was most significant in establishing the rights of the expectant parents involved a gestational carrier and not a surrogate: *Johnson v. Calvert.* Anna Johnson, a gestational carrier for Mark and Crispina Calvert, attempted to gain custody of the child she bore. This case became relevant to surrogacy because the court used language that blurred any distinction between surrogacy and gestational care. Rather than focus on the fact that the surrogate is carrying her genetic child and a gestational carrier is not, the California Supreme Court looked at intent. In so doing it ruled that it was the *intended* parents whose rights should be upheld. In a statement that set precedent in favor of the contracting couple, Justice Edward Panelli recognized payment to the surrogate as "compensation for her services in gestating the fetus and undergoing labor, rather than giving up her parental rights."

Does the Contracting Couple Have any Legal Right to Intervene in the Surrogate's Prenatal Care and Decisionmaking?

The American College of Obstetricians and Gynecologists (ACOG) has attempted to address the reproductive rights and freedoms of a surrogate in its 1990 opinion on surrogacy. ACOG affirms a woman's right to enter a surrogacy agreement, but stresses that certain measures must be taken to protect her reproductive freedoms during and after pregnancy:

1 She should have the right to make decisions during the pregnancy.

2 She should be the source of consent with respect to clinical intervention and management of the pregnancy.

3 The contract should include provisions for such contingencies as: the pre-natal diagnosis of a genetic or chromosomal abnormality, the inability or unwillingness of the surrogate to carry the pregnancy to term, the death of a member of the commissioning couple or the dissolution of their marriage during pregnancy, the birth of a handicapped infant and the decision of the surrogate to retain custody of the infant.[53]

Frank Chervenak, director of ultrasound and ethics at New York Hospital, and Laurence McCullough, of Baylor College of Medicine, also support a woman's right to participate in surrogacy as long as she is protected during her pregnancy. They regard the fetus as a patient and oppose any provisions in the surrogacy agreement that would require or forbid diagnostic or obstetrical management during the course of the pregnancy. They write:

> Thus any provisions in a surrogacy contract calling for antenatal diagnosis or abortion before viability or restricting either are ethically unfounded. That is, the commissioning couple is under an ethical obligation to the pregnant woman to respect her autonomy, based on her right to control her pregnancy before viability.[54]

The Need for Legislation and Guidelines

When we look back on the history of contractual surrogacy, it is clear that early practitioners provided surrogacy services in a legal and ethical vacuum. Sadly, but not surprisingly, experiences such as the Baby M case revealed the dangers of operating without legislation and guidelines for practice. In recent years, responsible practioners, as well as many participants in surrogacy, have attempted to develop and implement legislation and guidelines. As of this writing, there has been limited progress.

The Need for Legislation

Although several states have enacted laws concerning surrogacy, most of this legislation focuses on the contract, without establishing standards for practice. Several states (Indiana, Kentucky, Louisiana, Nebraska, North Dakota, New York, and Utah) have voided paid surrogacy contracts and some have voided unpaid contracts as well. In July, 1995 the Minister for Health Canada called for a voluntary ban on commercial preconception surrogacy arrangements, however no such ban was enacted. Hence, couples in both the U.S. and Canada remain free to enter into surrogacy contracts, but must be aware that their agreements may not be upheld if contested.

Other existing surrogacy legislation addresses: 1) payment to surrogacy practitioners (with several states prohibiting compensation for facilitating surrogacy arrangements); 2) the question of who are the legal parents of the child (with some states assuming that the contracting couple are the legal parents of the child and others assuming that the surrogate and her husband are the child's legal parents); 3) the provision of medical and psychological screening of surrogates and couples, and requirment that contracts be submitted to a judge prior to any attempt at pregnancy. Clearly there is need for further legislation that addresses four essential issues: who should practice surrogacy, who builds families using surrogates, who can become a surrogate and what if the surrogate doesn't want to relinquish the child?

Who Should Practice Surrogacy?

The original surrogacy practitioners were primarily lawyers and physicians who entered the field without backgrounds in psychology or child welfare. Although their intentions may have been honorable—a desire to help infertile couples create families—they were probably naive about the emotional and social complications that might arise. This naivete, together with the fact that there were clear financial incentives attracting lawyers and physicians to contractual surrogacy, mandated that that guidelines be established for who can arrange and facilitate surrogacy arrangements. As of this writing, a variety of recommendations have been made, but no widely accepted standards for practice are in place.

In its policy statement on surrogacy, the American College of Obstetricians and Gynecologists (ACOG) recommends that "surrogate parenting arrangements be overseen by private, nonprofit agencies with credentials similar to those of adoption agencies."[55] ACOG is referring to the fact that adoption agencies must abide by clearly delineated state laws in determining who can adopt a child and in providing counseling and other services to birthparents. Hagar Associates, in Topeka, Kansas, for example, is a fully licensed adoption agency, and it applies the guidelines of adoption practice to surrogacy.

Currently, there are no restrictions upon who can facilitate surrogacy. Although it seems clear that prospective parents, prospective surrogates and above all, unborn children, deserve the protections that come with regulation, no such protections have been established. Sadly, surrogacy can still be practiced by individuals with inadequate training in child welfare and psychology, who may be motivated primarily by financial gain. Practitioners in the field must therefore self-regulate and participants in surrogacy must protect themselves. Until clear standards for practice are set and enforced, responsible practitioners and prospective participants are wise to seek the advice and consultation of OPTS whenever possible. It is our hope, also, that they will turn to experienced adoption agencies for guidance.

Who Can Be a Surrogate?

Perhaps the most challenging policy-making question regarding surrogacy is whether there should be restrictions on which women—if any—can be contractual surrogates. Efforts to resolve this question inevitably lead to the clash of two of the central principles of medical ethics: autonomy and beneficence.

There are those who believe that any woman should have the right to participate in contractual surrogacy, provided she meets the medical and psychological standards of the surrogacy program to which she applies. These proponents of *autonomy* believe that women can make responsible decisions about their own bodies and that efforts to restrict them from surrogacy would impinge upon fundamental freedoms, in this case, reproductive freedoms.

Beneficence, like autonomy, has a central place in medical ethics, referring to efforts to protect the rights and well-being of individuals. Those who approach surrogacy from the perspective of *beneficence* feel that there are a number of compelling reasons for restricting participation in contractual surrogacy. These reasons include:

1. *The belief that informed consent is impossible with regards to surrogacy.* Can any woman truly know how she will feel about relinquishing a child that she has not yet conceived, let alone carried and delivered? Can she possibly forsee feelings that she will have about this decision in years to come? If the answer to these questions—and several other critical ones—is no, then she is not giving true informed consent.

2. *The belief that payment contaminates the situation, making it impossible for women—especially those in financial need—to make decisions that are based on their best interests and those of all of their children.* Although a woman may have other reasons for participating in surrogacy, it is difficult to distinguish the role that these reasons play in her decision. She is undoubtedly being enticed—at least to some degree—by payment.

3. *The belief that it can never be in a child's best interest to be brought into the world through contractual surrogacy.* Although some would argue that surrogacy offers life to someone who would otherwise not

exist, others say that the contractual arrangement and the intended relinquishment by the biological mother bring with them a life time of heartache and pain.

Proponents of both autonomy and beneficence agree that it is unethical to restrict some women, but not others, from surrogacy. For example, what if efforts to eliminate financial motivation led to the disqualification of poor women from surrogacy? Should they not have the right to profit from surrogacy if wealthier women have this opportunity? What if women who had previously had abortions were eliminated because their application for surrogacy might well be an effort to repair or repent a past wrongdoing? Should they not be permitted to try to work out feelings about abortions through surrogacy when other women might be entering surrogacy contracts in the hope of repairing other hurts, losses or transgressions?

Hence, we see that although there may appear to be many compelling reasons why women should not participate in contractual surrogacy, it would be discriminatory to permit participation by some groups and not by others. For this reason, counselors, lawyers, physicians and all others involved in surrogacy must see themselves as having a personal mandate to do all they can to ensure that every woman who becomes a contractual surrogate has fully explored—to the very best of her abilities—the current and future implications of this decision for herself, her existing family, and most of all, the child that she is agreeing to conceive, carry, deliver and relinquish at birth.

Surrogacy in Practice

Couples who decide to pursue parenting through surrogacy find that there are many different ways to go about it. There are a range of programs, most of which reflect the backgrounds and training of those who run them. Some programs are run by lawyers, others social workers, and still others, by individuals who had personal experience with surrogacy.

As we mentioned earlier in this chapter, couples interested in surrogacy should begin by contacting OPTS (the Organization of Parents Through Surrogacy), an independent, volunteer-staffed organization that has no ties to a particular program or practitioner. Hence, it can provide couples with a range of options, with objective information and observations about each. OPTS members serve as telephone counselors, providing couples with first-hand accounts of their experiences with surrogacy. OPTS can be found on the World Wide Web at www.opts.com. In addition, most surrogacy practitioners have their own web sites which can be found easily through a search. New information about all aspects of surrogacy is added daily.

As with all other questions regarding infertility and its resolution, couples exploring surrogacy should contact RESOLVE, by calling the national office of RESOLVE in Somerville, Mass. at 617-623-0744. RESOLVE telephone counselors can direct callers to publications and to other RESOLVE members who have become parents through surrogacy.

Couples who prefer predictability in terms of cost, time frame, and outcome, will probably find that they are more comfortable working with a large, comprehensive surrogacy program (this is similar to adoption—some couples prefer the conveniences of a full service agency, while others prefer to pursue adoption independently.) These programs offer a wide range of services, including locating and screening surrogates, psychological counseling for couples and surrogates, legal counsel, and medical expertise. Larger programs also have the benefit of experience; having worked with many other couples and surrogates, they know how to help prospective participants determine if surrogacy is right for them and they know what can be done to make the process easier for all parties.

Some couples find that they are more comfortable working with a smaller program. Although there may be less history to inform them and probably fewer surrogates to work with, couples appreciate the personal connection they feel with a small staff that is involved with only a few surrogates and couples.

Some couples prefer to undertake surrogacy individually. This increasingly popular path may begin with a lawyer, physician, or other individual who locates potential surrogates and who works with other professionals, but who does not offer a full-service program. Alternatively, it may begin with the couple locating a surrogate on their own, either from among family, friends or acquaintances, or through advertising or other networking. In either event, couples undertaking an independent surrogacy arrangement will need to have legal counsel, as well as medical and psychological services for themselves and their surrogate. Although independent arrangements go well in most instances, they may involve more risks than participation in an experienced program. These risks include the possibility of unexpected medical or legal expenses (an advantage of working with a program that provides all the services at a set fee is that costs can be predicted), the possibility of insurance problems, and the chance that the surrogate or the couple will be insufficiently screened or prepared for the psychological challenges of surrogacy. Since there are very few mental health professionals who are experienced with surrogacy, a couple working independently might have difficulty locating a counselor who is skilled in this area.

OPTS cautions people about undertaking individual arrangements in an effort to cut costs. They may save the money that would otherwise go to administrative costs, but the legal, psychological, and medical expenses in surrogacy add up rapidly, even when all is going smoothly. Couples who enter a pay-as-you-go situation may be surprised by how many unanticipated costs they encounter.

For many couples, financial considerations are a key factor in their decision making. Some want to compare surrogacy costs with those of adoption, since they are also investigating that option. Others are more concerned about the ethical issues associated with surrogacy and want to make sure that they will not become involved in a process that could in any way resemble baby selling.

Although there are variations in the cost of surrogacy, the range is approximately $25,000 to $50,000. The surrogate generally receives $10,000 to $15,000 compensation for her time and effort; the remainder of the fee covers legal and psychological services to both the couple and the surrogate, medical insurance and clothing allowance for the surrogate, and the administrative costs of the surrogacy program. The surrogate also receives reimbursement for extra day-care costs, lost wages, and travel expenses. Additionally, the couple should factor in the amount of lost wages and travel expenses that they will themselves incur.

Couples selecting a surrogacy program can be confused about expenses since some programs present itemized charges and others are inclusive. Therefore, it is important that couples considering surrogacy take a careful look at what their total costs will be. For example, since medical complications can occur, it is critical that a couple understand the extent and limits of the surrogate's medical insurance policy.

Although there are many ways of approaching surrogacy, there are four steps that all couples must take prior to attempting conception:

1. Undergoing psychological and medical assessment of their preparedness for surrogacy.

2. Locating a surrogate.

3. Arranging medical and psychological evaluation for their prospective surrogate.

4. Arranging a legal consultation for themselves and their surrogate.

Evaluation of Prospective Parents

Couples considering parenthood through surrogacy generally undergo less evaluation and screening than do prospective surrogates. This discrepancy is by design: many practitioners do not wish to be gatekeepers. They feel that it is unfair to make infertile couples prove they will be fit parents when fertile couples are put to no such test.

Although it is true that fertile couples do not have to prove themselves in order to become parents, there is well-established precedent in adoption for the assessment of prospective parents. Adoption workers assess the emotional, medical, marital, vocational and financial stability of the intended parents, and most surrogacy practitioners feel the criteria should be applied to couples seeking to parent through surrogacy. Beyond these considerations, a couple's understanding of the special challenges of this path to parenthood are explored.

Adoption agencies see it as their mandate to act in "the best interest of the child" and surrogacy practitioners must do the same. Certainly the longings of couples to parent are compelling, but psychologists must attempt to keep the feelings, rights and well-being of unborn children in the foreground. Applying the "best interest" standard to surrogacy means determining that the prospective parents are likely to provide the child with a stable and loving home and that they are expected to live to raise the child to adulthood.

A surrogacy program can also be a licensed adoption agency and conduct a formal home study with all couples who apply to them. In its policy statement on surrogacy, the American College of Obstetricians and Gynecologists firmly supports this approach:

> For the near future, surrogate parenting arrangements should be overseen by private nonprofit agencies with credentials similar to those of adoption agencies. Such agencies should seek to ensure that the interests of all involved parties are adequately protected. The agencies should conduct confidential counseling and screening of candidate surrogates and

candidate commissioning parents. Their primary goal should
be to promote the welfare of the future child, as well as the
welfare of any existing children of the surrogate.[56]

Critics of surrogacy would take issue with this approach, arguing that
it is never in the best interest of a child to be conceived and carried "for
the explicit purpose of relinquishing the child to another at birth."[57]

Medical Criteria

Since the surrogate will be artificially inseminated with the contracting
husband's semen, it is essential that he be screened for sexually transmitted
diseases. The would be father should also have a complete semen analysis,
since it is important to have a current assessment of his fertility.

Both members of the contracting couple should have physical exams
to confirm that they are in good health. Just as they have a right to know
about the health of the surrogate, she has a right to know of any existing
or suspected medical problems with the contracting couple. The risk in
not providing her with pertinent medical information is that she may feel
cheated or misled if she later learns of a medical problem.

Finally, some couples participating in surrogacy programs are encouraged to have the husband undergo consultation with a geneticist to assess
the potential for birth defects. This is often recommended even when
there is no known risk of congenital abnormalities.

Psychological Criteria

The purpose of a psychological evaluation of prospective parents is to
identify those who should not become parents through surrogacy either
because they are likely to be unfit parents, or because they are not adequately prepared for the undertaking. The former group includes people
who exhibit serious psychopathology and those who have substance abuse
problems. The latter group includes couples who remain unresolved about
their infertility experience, who have not clearly thought through their
reasons for pursuing surrogacy, or who are unprepared for the future
challenges that surrogacy brings. Although some of these couples may
eventually be suited for surrogacy, the mental health clinician needs to
help them understand that they are not yet ready to move ahead with
this option. Some will be bringing medical efforts to a close; others will
need to grieve their infertility more actively.

As with a prospective surrogate, the clinician will try to determine
whether a couple is prepared to do surrogacy and the extent to which

they are in agreement about the process. Couples are seen together and separately. In the individual sessions, the psychologist can get a sense of how each partner feels about surrogacy: are they equally enthusiastic about pursuing this option, or has one member pushed the other to do something that he or she questions? For example, a woman feeling guilty about her infertility and fearing that her husband will want to leave her might urge him to try surrogacy, anticipating that this "solution" will assuage his disappointment, as well as her guilt.

The decisions surrounding surrogacy can try even the most stable marriages. Conjoint meetings can provide important information about the strength of a relationship. The clinician can see how they communicate and resolve conflicts and can get a clearer sense of their shared history, especially concerning their infertility and how they have coped with this crisis. Some relationships are so conflict-ridden that couples should be turned away from a surrogacy program. Equally important is to help essentially stable couples anticipate, understand, and prepare for their potential vulnerabilities in the surrogacy process.

The clinician should review a long series of "what ifs" with all couples considering surrogacy. These unlikely but plausible outcomes remind couples that even the most carefully laid plans can go astray. Having experienced disappointment and frustration, it is important that they be reminded that this undertaking cannot promise to spare them further loss. The following are some of the "what ifs" that all couples should consider:

- What if their surrogate does not become pregnant or has a miscarriage?
- What if their surrogate undergoes pre-natal testing and a problem is identified?
- What if they do not like the way that a surrogate is taking care of herself during the pregnancy?
- What if the surrogate develops closer bonds with the baby than anticipated?
- What if the surrogate seeks custody?
- What if the surrogate seeks more contact with the child?
- What if the surrogate's feelings change in years to come and she approaches them wanting more or less contact than they had anticipated?
- What if the child wants more or less contact with the surrogate than all had anticipated?
- What if the child experiences psychological difficulties as a result of this arrangement?

- What if the couple is criticized by members of their family or their community regarding this decision?
- What if the decision to have a child by surrogacy causes tension between husband and wife?

The couple, like the surrogate, is entering into uncharted waters. Therefore, they too need psychological exploration and guidance. An important part of the screening process is to help the couple assess their relationships with family and friends with regard to surrogacy. They need to confront the fact that many people are critical of surrogacy and to consider how their decision may affect their relationships with family, friends and the community at large.

The counselor needs to explore the couple's expectations regarding the child. What if the child is different from the child they have imagined they will parent? How might they feel if the child is born with a medical problem? What if the child bears a strong resemblance to the surrogate and very little to the biological father?

Finally, the counselor should attempt to get a clear sense of the couple's expectations of the surrogacy process. It is important that they think through the kind of relationship they wish to have with their surrogate and the degree of involvement they want with her pregnancy. Dr. Hanafin has found, for example, that some couples are "hypervigilant" and have difficulty trusting as they go through the process. They tend to have so many questions and worries that they create tension in the relationship with the surrogate. Other couples tend to be more removed, preferring to let the surrogate manage her own pregnancy and wishing to remain more distant from her. Both groups can be challenging to work with, but Dr. Hanafin has found that it is usually the more distant couples who experience the most tension. Their aloofness can be upsetting to their surrogate, leaving her feeling depleted and unappreciated. Given that a relationship with a surrogate lasts at least ten months, and often, considerably longer, couples need to be comfortable with some form of contact.

Who Becomes a Surrogate?

Women seeking to become surrogates often speak positively of their personal experiences with pregnancy, labor, and delivery. They say that they felt "happy" and "fulfilled" during pregnancy and enjoyed uncomplicated deliveries. Many add that as much as they like being pregnant, they are not prepared to add another child to their family at this time.

Prospective surrogates also speak of their compassion for infertile couples. Often they have had a friend or relative who has gone through infertility or pregnancy losses. Having been exposed to the pain that a childless couple endures, these women feel inspired to help. They see bearing a child as a way that they can help and have personal satisfaction at the same time.

Dr. Hanafin found that many of the surrogates she studied said that they loved being mothers and that they decided to become surrogates because they could not imagine life without children. Others added that they felt they had not yet done anything remarkable or made an impact, and this was an opportunity to do something of major significance—something that would surely make a lifetime difference for someone else. Some said that they had been very young when they had experienced their first, and often unplanned, pregnancy. They look forward now to the opportunity to plan a pregnancy and to undertake it with more understanding of the process, a greater degree of control, and a sense of wisdom and maturity. Dr. Hanafin and others have found that there are women who have borne children yet were once told that they were infertile. Having lived with the fear, but having been spared the reality of infertility, some say that they feel a responsibility to help those who have not been so fortunate. Similarly, we have spoken with surrogates who did experience infertility or pregnancy loss before successfully building their families. These experiences had a lasting impact on them; they were drawn to surrogacy hoping to reduce the pain of a childless couple.

Although these are all admirable motivations for participating in surrogacy, it is important to acknowledge that women seeking surrogacy also present with other less altruistic motivations. It is not unusual for women to reveal a combination of reasons for seeking participation in surrogacy, often including some reasons that are controversial or problematic.

One such reason for seeking to become a surrogate is financial gain. As we discussed earlier in this chapter, questions arise about "baby-selling." In addition, there are ethical concerns about a woman feeling that she can—or must—"rent her womb." Hence, it seems crucial that financial gain not be a woman's only reason for seeking surrogacy, but more often than not, it is one reason among several. In many instances, a difficult determination must be made as to the relative weight of financial reward and other factors in a woman's decision to apply for surrogacy.

When asked how they can carry a child for nine months and then place it with another couple, many surrogates respond by saying that they do not regard the child as their own. Some refer to the bond they feel with their husbands and state that in order for a child to be theirs, it has to be a child that they conceived with their husband. They say that being inseminated with another man's sperm is a very different process, and they consider the resulting child to be his child and that of his infertile wife. Many add that the egg from which the child was conceived would have otherwise been wasted and they believe they are putting it to good use by bringing a child to an infertile couple. As one former surrogate said, "The child could only exist because of the union and love of the infertile couple. It was created in their spirit, dreams and hard work. It was always meant to be their baby."

Many women approach surrogacy believing that they can create a baby for another couple and that they, the couple, and the child will feel comfortable with this decision in both the near and distant futures. Such women should be encouraged to familiarize themselves with adoption literature, and, specifically, with the accounts by both birthmothers and adoptees about their feelings towards "birthbonds." Only after a woman has given careful consideration to the potential strength of birthbonds and has acknowledged that the child she bears may have longings for her (and that she may also have longings for the child), can she be truly ready to make an informed decision about surrogacy.

Another question that prospective surrogates must confront involves bonding. Those who believe that a strong, unbreakable connection between mother and child begins in utero, often ask how surrogates can give up the babies they carried. Dr. Hanafin has found that most surrogates report that a form of bonding does occur, but that it is primarily with the expectant parents, not with the unborn child. One surrogate describes her experience with the couple:

> It is hard for me to find words to describe the relationship
> that developed between us. It didn't happen all at once, but
> grew over time and with the pregnancy. And although it hap-
> pened among the four of us, it was most powerful between

us—the two women. The bonds forged over our many phone calls, our lunches out, and most of all, our visits to the doctor are strong, solid, and lasting.[58]

Cristie Montgomery, a former surrogate who later facilitated other surrogacy arrangements, focuses on the meaning of the word expecting. She observes that in surrogate pregnancies, it is not the surrogate who is expecting, but the woman who intends to raise the child.

It is possible that this strong connection to the "expecting couple" serves as a coping strategy so that surrogates are able to diminish their connection to the child. If so, the strategy may not work over an extended period of time. Indeed, the surrogate may be convinced before, during, and even after the pregnancy, that *she* was truly not expecting, but that perception may change over time. Potential surrogates must dig deep into their psyches making sure that they are not hiding their real feelings from themselves.

Concerns have been raised about the emotional stability of women who choose to be surrogates. For this reason, responsible practitioners require psychological testing, in addition to an extensive clinical interview.

Critics have also suggested that all women who apply for surrogacy are "breeders" who are allowing themselves to be exploited. Dr. Hanafin, who has worked with hundreds of surrogates, takes issue with this. She states that the women she has known are "strong, bright, clear-thinking, empathic, responsible individuals who have initiative." She says that most of these women "have established a clear sense of themselves by the time they are in their mid to late twenties and combine this sense of self with an ability to be other-centered." In fact, Dr. Hanafin is cautious about accepting a woman who seems "too other centered" because she feels that these women may not be able to make good decisions for themselves. However, she emphasizes that, in her experience, these women have been in the minority.

Many women who initially express interest in surrogacy do not go on to carry a baby for another couple. Some drop out when they realize all that is involved or when they encounter serious opposition in their families. Others screen themselves out later in the process when they find that the experience is more stressful and demanding than they had imagined it to be. Finally, many are turned down by programs because something trouble-some surfaces in their clinical interview, the psychological testing, or their medical exam.

271

Locating a Surrogate

Couples who decide to locate a surrogate on their own do so in various ways: perhaps by word of mouth; through an internet search; responding to (or placing) an ad in a newpaper or magazine. Most find that if they are persistent, they are able to find a woman who seems suited to work with them as a surrogate. Many such women say that they had actually been considering surrogacy for a long time, but had not known how to go about it until they came across the notice on the web or the printed advertisement.

Couples going through established programs or working with lawyers who help to arrange surrogacy do not have to advertise on their own. Spared the stresses and strains of telephone calls or letters from strangers, they review profiles of women who have been accepted by their program. The information that contracting couples receive about the surrogates varies among practitioners, but all provide couples with some social, psychological, and medical background on the surrogate, as well as with a physical description.

How couples and surrogates decide to work together varies considerably, depending on whether the couple is going through a program or working it out on their own. A couple working independently will probably select their first-choice surrogate before she has undergone medical or psychological evaluation. Therefore, it is possible that they will face a significant disappointment early in the process: they may choose a woman, feel enthusiastic about working with her, and then be advised against going further for medical or psychological reasons.

By contrast, couples working with programs that locate surrogates usually consider only women who have already been cleared medically and psychologically. Hence, they are spared time and effort, as well as the potential frustration and disappointment that would arise if the surrogate they selected was not accepted into the program.

Although most couples and surrogates appreciate having the opportunity to choose each other, there is often a psychologist or other skilled person involved in the matching process. For example, Dr. Hanafin advises that couples meet surrogates with whom they are likely to work well. She emphasizes the importance of shared values, similar personalities and belief systems and she suggests looking for people who seem to approach situations in similar ways.

Cristie Montgomery, a former surrogate, observes that "there is someone for everyone." She cautions against trying to put people together who have little in common and says that even when a surrogate or a couple has a concern or request that seems highly unusual or even odd, there is usually someone who feels comfortable working with them.

An important part of the matching process involves determining that surrogates and couples have shared expectations regarding the pregnancy, labor and delivery, and contact following birth. For example, couples who expect frequent communication with their surrogate during pregnancy need to work with a surrogate who has a similar expectation. Similarly, those who expect to stay in touch with their surrogate in years to come need to be matched with a woman who agrees that their relationship will not end with the birth of the child.

Special attention also needs to be paid to the possibility that there can be something wrong with the fetus. Before a couple and a surrogate can agree to work together, they must be in agreement about whether the surrogate will undergo an amniocentesis and if so, under what circumstances, if any, they would decide to abort the fetus. They must discuss the possibility that other medical or psychological situations could arise that might prompt the surrogate to seek an abortion. For example, she could develop a medical problem, the treatment of which is complicated by pregnancy. Although not all such circumstances can be anticipated, it is important that the couple and the surrogate—together with their counselor—attempt to anticipate how they will handle unexpected outcomes.

Evaluation of Surrogates

Surrogacy programs vary in the criteria that they use for acceptance into their programs. We are including criteria here that we feel represents minimal standards for responsible surrogacy practice.

Medical Criteria

A prospective surrogate should be a nonsmoker over the age of 25, who has proven fertility evidenced by the fact that she has had at least one child. She must be in good general and reproductive health, with no evidence of genetic or sexually transmitted diseases. Extensive family histories are taken in order to assess the risk of serious hereditary disorders.

Psychological Criteria

Psychological assessment of a prospective surrogate takes her life circumstances, her motivation, and her determination into account. She should have had at least one child, whom she is parenting (and ideally have completed her family), have a strong support system, and should have a stable lifestyle that can withstand the challenges of surrogacy.

While determination is often a positive factor, indicating that a woman believes strongly in this endeavor, it may also prompt a surrogate to try to camouflage things about herself that she fears might cause her to be rejected. The clinician faces the challenge of developing an alliance with a prospective surrogate that will enable her to examine the process honestly and to carefully think through whether surrogacy is truly in her best interest and that of her family, now and in the future. The psychological assessment addresses two central questions:

Is she an emotionally stable individual?
Is she psychologically prepared to be a surrogate?

Since surrogacy involves complex and challenging physical and emotional tasks, some of which will extend years beyond the pregnancy, women who serve as surrogates should be emotionally stable and resilient. Being a surrogate is not a time-limited experience. It is an experience that she will never forget and that will remain part of her history—and that of her family—regardless of whether she continues to have contact with the child and the child's family. A surrogate will always be the genetic and gestational mother of someone she did not parent—someone who may want further contact with her for a variety of reasons.

The MMPI-2, a widely accepted psychological assessment tool, is often used to evaluate prospective surrogates. Some clinicians administer both the MMPI-2 and the Rorschach, another well known and widely respected psychological test. The Rorschach, a projective psychological test, gives a great deal of insight into an individual's personality, as well as her emotional and intellectual processes. In addition, it can predict the extent to which people respond objectively to their environment as opposed to their own unconscious process, and may help identify those individuals who can remain calm and clear thinking should unexpected difficulties arise.

In addition to testing, a psychologist will assess the extent and nature of the potential surrogate's coping skills. Discussions about her history, including mental health issues, sexual relationships, reproduction, drug and/or alcohol use, and social connections, can provide important information about her stability and about how she copes with the vicissitudes of life.

In determining preparedness, it is crucial that the clinician try to understand why a woman wants to be a surrogate and how she feels it will affect her life. The clinician must determine whether part of her motivation may be an attempt to "undo" prior losses, especially reproductive ones. For example, women may turn to surrogacy because of unresolved feelings about past abortions or having placed a baby for adoption. In fact, a study done by Dr. Philip Parker, a psychiatrist who studied the profiles of surrogates in the 1980s, found that 35% of the surrogates reported that they had had an abortion or placed a child for adoption.[59]

Although there is no objective list of "good" or "bad" reasons to become a surrogate, psychological exploration can help determine if a woman's reasons are likely to be good or bad for her. It is important that a woman try to anticipate how she will feel in years to come, after she has completed her surrogacy experience. In other words, it is crucial that her reasons for wanting to be a surrogate are likely to be later validated in her life. Otherwise, her experience as a surrogate may make her more vulnerable to future psychic injury.

Preparation for Surrogacy

A woman may be a responsible and stable individual and still be unprepared for surrogacy. Therefore, it is critical that time be spent exploring her understanding of surrogacy and her reasons for wanting to undertake this process. The psychotherapist must determine if surrogacy is something that she has thought carefully about and whether she has considered some of the ways in which the experience might prove difficult for her and for her family, not only in the coming months but in years to come. If she has not thought about potential difficulties, it is important to understand why not and to get assurance that she is capable of exploring these issues in depth. Information as to whether she is naive, ill informed, or acting impulsively is essential, since these are all reasons for excluding her from surrogacy.

Part of the counselor's role is to try to talk a prospective surrogate out of surrogacy. As paradoxical as this sounds, hearing arguments about potential pitfalls can help the prospective surrogate decide whether surrogacy would be a mistake that could have long-term negative repercussions for her. Or she may conclude that she can live with (and face) any problems that might ensue from the arrangement. In other words, while hoping for a positive outcome, she must be well prepared for potential difficulty. The clinician must be supportive of her right to change her mind, helping the prospective surrogate to see herself as acting responsibly and maturely should she decide not to go ahead with surrogacy.

Some of the questions that a mental health counselor should ask a surrogate to examine include the following:

1. *In years to come, will I look back and feel that the child I birthed was mine? If so, will I have regrets? Will I feel I have wronged myself, or worse still, the child?* Although no one has a crystal ball with which to predict the future, it is crucial that a surrogate consider the extent to which she might bond with the baby during pregnancy—a baby to whom she is genetically and gestationally connected—and therefore experience intense feelings of loss upon placement. If she has had other children, it will be helpful to think about when and how she bonded with them—primarily in the gestational stage or during infancy? She must try to imagine herself as an older woman and think about whether she will wonder about the child or about grandchildren she may never know.

2. *Is there something that could happen in my life that might change the rightness of this decision?* Life is unpredictable. In order to help protect herself from looking back later with regret, the surrogate, with help from the clinician, should attempt to think of circumstances that might prompt her to regret her decision. For example, if one of her children became seriously ill or died, would she regret having been a surrogate? Would this sort of tragic event cause her to look back, reexamine her earlier decision, and feel she made a serious mistake?

3. *Am I prepared to handle the potential social and emotional consequences of my decision to become a surrogate?* Even the most informed surrogates may not have considered the complexity of the undertaking. Consequently, it is crucial that the psychotherapist assume an educational as well as an evaluative role, introducing a series of "what if" questions to the surrogate such as:

   • What if she conceives and then miscarries?
   • What if she has an ectopic pregnancy (which could compromise her future fertility)?
   • What if she gives birth to a handicapped child?

276

- What if she discovers after an aminiocentesis that she is carrying a child with a genetic disorder?
- What if she discovers herself forming a strong attachment to the child in utero or at birth?
- What if she later regrets her decision to undertake this pregnancy or to relinquish the child?
- What if something unanticipated happens in the lives of the intended parents—divorce, serious illness, death—that prompts her to have misgivings about her decision?
- What if the parents change the terms of the agreement in years to come and want less—or more—contact than she had counted on?
- What if the child approaches her in years to come seeking more of a relationship than she had planned for? What if the child is angry with her and challenges her decision?

The surrogate must consider that the pregnancy could place significant stress on her marriage, her relationships with her children, her work and/or her relationships with colleagues and friends. Her responses to each of these possibilities can indicate the extent to which she has thought through this undertaking.

The psychotherapist must look specifically at the social context in which the prospective surrogate lives. Since surrogacy is stressful in many ways, it is essential that she have an active and reliable support network available to her. Although a large program with a varied staff and several other surrogates can provide some of that support, it helps for her to have people in her personal life who value what she is doing. This support is even more important for the surrogate working on her own or with a small program.

In her 1989 study, Kathy Forest studied thirty-two surrogate mothers following their pregnancies. Her findings underscore the importance of social support, especially from husbands, during and after a surrogacy experience. The women she interviewed spoke of the importance of support from family and friends. It was essential to them because there were times during their pregnancies when they felt ostracized.[60]

The psychological evaluation includes the surrogate's husband or partner in order to confirm that he not only understands why she wants to become a surrogate but is able to be supportive of her decision. He is asked whether he has considered the possible ramifications of the decision in terms of their marriage and family life, and he must be reminded of

277

possible health risks that pregnancy entails, as well as the possibility of a multiple gestation, a pregnancy loss, or an obstetrical emergency. He is reminded that he will probably face questions and criticisms from others who will query him as to how or why he agreed to his wife's decision to conceive and carry a baby for another couple. He is further alerted to the fact that some of these comments may involve negative insinuations about the insemination process and may make insulting references to the fact that his wife conceived with another man's sperm. Finally, he should be asked to consider how he might feel toward the baby, who will be the half-sibling of his children, as well as his wife's genetic offspring.

4. *How will my children, my parents, siblings and other relatives understand my actions now and in the future?* A prospective surrogate should consider how her children understand her decision to have a baby for another couple. It is important that she remind herself that their reactions to the idea of a surrogate pregnancy may differ from their feelings once pregnancy has been established. Similarly, they may have unanticipated reactions following the birth of a child, as well as in years to come. Although they may see it now as an act of kindness and a way to help childless couples, they may also feel that their sibling was given away.

A prospective surrogate should consider her children's experience not only from the perspective of loss (the loss of a sibling) but also from the perspective of their security. Might this experience raise uncertainties for them about their own permanency in the family? It is essential that she consider how this decision may compromise or blur their sense of safety and belonging.

The prospective surrogate needs to discuss whether she intends for her children to have any ongoing contact with their half-sibling, and, if so, it needs to be confirmed with the contracting couple. Dr. Hanafin has known couples who have felt strongly that their children should remain in touch with the surrogate's children, seeing this contact as an important part of their development. By contrast, other couples have wanted distance, feeling that the contact would be confusing to their child. It would indeed be unfortunate if children wanted and expected to see their half-sibling and were refused the opportunity to do so.

In helping the surrogate assess her children's needs, the clinician should explore their social context. She should discuss with the surrogate and her partner how they will coach their children to tell their friends, schoolmates, and teachers about their mother's pregnancy and how they will support and guide the children, should they encounter unkind or unsettling questions and comments.

The surrogate must also consider how her parents, siblings and other members of her extended family—including in-laws—may react to surrogacy. She is making a decision which will alter the boundaries of their family and hence, it may prompt negative or uncertain feelings. She should do what she can to address the questions and concerns of family members before moving forward.

5. *How will I feel when the pregnancy is over—when life returns to normal?* Psychological preparation for surrogacy involves reminding a woman that a surrogate pregnancy is a time-limited event and that when it is over she will no longer receive the attention she received for nine months. It is crucial that she be prepared for the let down she may feel when the pregnancy is over. Careful discussion and consideration of what it means to be in the limelight, and then out of it, may help her to avoid feeling cheated by the experience, especially when she is also dealing with separation from the couple and the baby, as well as with postpartum hormonal changes.

The counselor can help the surrogate look at the larger context in which she lives. She must consider whether she lives in a community that is likely to be respectful of her decision and her privacy or whether her neighbors and community associates are likely to be judgmental and antagonistic. She must think about what it will be like for her to guide and support her family when they are confronted by negative attitudes and opinions about her decision.

Legal Counsel

Participants in surrogacy need legal counsel. Often a lawyer is an integral part of the program they choose, but many participants still seek independent legal counsel. Independent legal consultation offers surrogates and couples the additional assurance that they are not being coerced or otherwise misled. Couples participating in a surrogacy program in another state may need to hire a lawyer in their home state to do the legal work to ensure that the wife will be the child's legal parent. In most instances, this involves a stepparent adoption shortly after the child's birth.

Although most states do not have statutes that prevent couples and women from entering into surrogacy contracts together, there are some states including Arizona, Indiana, Kentucky, Michigan, New York, Utah and Washington) that do. This does not mean that people are prevented from entering into surrogacy arrangements in these states, but it does mean that any existing contracts will be considered void if the surrogate changes her mind. Furthermore, it is unlikely that a court of law in any of the other states will hold a contract binding if the surrogate changes her mind. As are other aspects of surrogacy, this situation is similar to adoption in that a woman who agrees, prior to birth, to place her baby with a couple is free to change her mind after giving birth. In other words, prebirth placement contracts are not legally binding.

If this is the case—that a contract is good only as long as both parties are in agreement—one might wonder why so many people go to the trouble and expense of entering into surrogacy contracts. Susan Crockin, a Massachusetts lawyer specializing in reproductive law, sheds some light on why such contracts can be extremely helpful regardless of whether they will ultimately hold up in court. Crockin observes that the process of legal negotiation forces people to think through each aspect of their decision and helps them to determine the degree to which they are truly in agreement. Entering into a contract emphasizes the seriousness of the endeavor and alerts people to some of the disappointments that they may encounter.

Pregnancy and Birth through Surrogacy

Although the decision to move ahead and attempt pregnancy through surrogacy feels like the end of an arduous journey, participants recognize that they have a long way to go. Their shared goal will not be complete until the surrogate has conceived, carried and delivered a child. For some that process proves remarkably uneventful; for others it is yet another difficult journey.

Attempting Pregnancy

Once a surrogate and a couple have entered into an agreement and the surrogate has been tested to confirm that she is not already pregnant, inseminations begin. Depending on where the couple and the surrogate live, this can be a complicated process. In some instances, the couple delivers the semen to the surrogate, who inseminates herself. Other arrangements span long distances and involve freezing and shipping sperm (although the use of frozen semen lowered the pregnancy rate in the past, many programs are now using a special test yolk buffer for the transport of semen and report improved pregnancy rates).

Although husbands have been tested for HIV, the only way to be certain that the sperm is disease free at the time of insemination is to freeze it and retest the man several months later. This is not commonly done, since it will delay the process, but some surrogates insist upon it.

For an infertile couple who has gone through years of medical treatments, working with a surrogate means a shift in their expectations about pregnancy. Having come to assume failure, they are now in a position to expect success; the presumption is that the surrogate is fertile. Infertile couples, however, have a long history of being disappointed, so many approach surrogacy very cautiously, afraid of being too optimistic.

Many surrogates do become pregnant easily. When this happens, couples have a range of reactions. Some are startled, having been conditioned to failure. Others may experience a tinge of sadness, feeling that the wife's infertility now stands in stark contrast to the husband and the surrogate's fertility. None of these reactions is unusual, and overriding them are feelings of happiness and enthusiasm.

One of the advantages of having psychological support throughout the surrogacy process is that the counselor can offer helpful advice to both couples and surrogate and can serve as an intermediary in times of question or stress. The counselor can help all participants determine how they prefer to maintain contact, how often it should occur and how they should deal with geographical distance or proximity. For example, in arrangements in which there is considerable geographical distance between the couple and the surrogate, participants may decide to plan visits at certain intervals or milestones during the pregnancy. By contrast, participants living near each other may need to set up some boundaries and guidelines so that that no one feels that things are "too close." The counselor can also help participants identify ways to celebrate both the pregnancy and the birth.

When the surrogate does not conceive after a reasonable length of time (often six attempts), everyone is upset. They wonder whether the problem is in the insemination process itself (e.g., improper handling or preparation of semen or poor timing) or whether there is an undiagnosed male factor. They may begin to wonder about the possibility that the surrogate herself has impaired fertility, since prior fertility is predictive, but never a guarantee of future fertility. The couple then faces a dilemma: should they investigate possible problems in the surrogate, or the would-be father, or both, or seek out another surrogate? The latter decision is certain to bring with it some feelings of guilt on the part of the couple. The surrogate may share some of these feelings, particularly guilt over not having come through for them.

It is helpful to have an experienced person who can offer support and guidance to all parties. Efforts can be made to minimize the feelings of failure that are inevitable in both surrogate and couple. At a time of disappointment, they may need to be reminded that they did all that they could to make the process work.

The Pregnancy

Most surrogates do become pregnant. Following conception, couples and surrogates enter into a new phase of their relationship. This time can be full of great excitement and satisfaction, but it also brings additional concerns. It is important that the couples, the surrogates, and their partners have psychological support available throughout the pregnancy.

The stresses that arise in a surrogate pregnancy vary and cannot be predicted. However, one that is usually present, especially in the first trimester, is the fear of pregnancy loss. Although most surrogates are not at increased risk for pregnancy loss, miscarriage is a universally common occurrence. Hence, it is only natural that couples and their surrogates, who have all worked hard together to achieve pregnancy, will fear its loss.

One surrogate, who experienced a miscarriage when she was building her own family, and another in her surrogacy experience, contrasted the losses in this way. She reported that although both losses were deeply felt, the loss that occurred in her surrogate pregnancy was for her less profound. She observed that since it was the couple that was "expecting," it was they who seemed to feel the full impact of the loss. She observed further that much of the sadness she felt, following the surrogacy miscarriage, involved the couple and her feelings of concern and caring for them.

Fear of pregnancy loss is not the only concern that arises during a surrogate's pregnancy. Surrogates are likely to have other questions and they should be counseled to take these concerns to their physicians, nurses or counselors. These concerns may include medical questions such as whether they can take a medication during pregnancy or what to do if they think they have been exposed to an infectious disease such as chicken pox. They may also have interpersonal concerns, either involving the intended parents or family members and friends. Taking questions to professionals, rather than to the couple, avoids raising anxieties unnecessarily. Similarly, when the couple feels a concern—or has a question—they should take it to their counselor. He/she can help them determine what—if anything—to do about it. The alternative—to contact the surrogate—would likely cause her to feel that they were trying to control or "micromanage" her pregnancy.

Although media attention has focused on the fear some couples have that their surrogate will change her mind and try to keep the baby, a surrogate may be frightened that the opposite nightmare will occur: the couple could change their minds and leave her with a baby she is not prepared to parent. Hence, it is very important that couples not only be in frequent contact with their surrogates throughout the pregnancy, but that they also let them know how much they look forward to the baby's arrival. For example, discussion about furnishing a nursery offers reassuring evidence that they are eager to provide a home for their new baby.

Like other expectant parents, couples may worry that something will go wrong. Although in all likelihood the baby will be born healthy, those who have experienced infertility are conditioned to disappointment and loss. Having worked so hard to achieve this pregnancy, they are vulnerable to further heartache. Once again it is important that couples not discuss these fears at length with their surrogate, who is already coping with the normal physical and emotional challenges of pregnancy. In addition to the ongoing availability of an experienced clinician, some programs have organized peer support for surrogates.

Some programs attempt to create a network for surrogates and ask former surrogates to contact women who are newly pregnant through their center. These arrangements can help validate the feelings and experiences of current surrogates. At the same time, they offer former participants a way to remain involved with the program and the process.

The amount of contact that a couple and surrogate have during pregnancy varies from one couple-surrogate pair to another. There are also variations among programs; some programs promote contact, others discourage it, and still others allow the preferences of both parties to determine the amount of contact they will have. What is most important is that couples and surrogates have shared expectations and that all are comfortable with the level of contact that they maintain.

What If the Surrogate Wants to Parent the Child?

Although it occurs infrequently, there are instances in which the surrogate has "second thoughts" about relinquishment. Sometimes these "second thoughts" are just that: fleeting moments during pregnancy—or immediately following delivery—that quickly pass. There are, however, very rare instances in which a surrogate feels a sustained and compelling need to parent the child she is carrying. In this unfortunate situation she should contact her counselor as soon as possible so that the two of them can explore the significance of her feelings.

In the event that the surrogate has truly changed her mind and wants to parent the child, many legal (and emotional) questions arise. A couple can contest custody with the surrogate and depending upon the state they live in and the courts involved, they may—or may not—be granted custody. However, it is likely to be a lengthy, expensive and painful battle that—at best—awards them custody of a child who is sought by his/her birth-mother. Our readers need only recall the lengthy and painful battle over Jessica DeBoer/Anna Schmidt to realize the hardship that comes to all involved in such a legal contest.

We encourage any couple who finds themselves in such a distressing situation to try to contain their hurt and anguish, and to work—as best they can—towards establishing a positive on-going relationship with the surrogate regardless of the outcome of the legal battle. Needless to say, this will involve a great deal of strength, courage and restraint on their part, but their efforts are likely to prove rewarding in the long run.

The Birth

Most couples want to be present at their child's birth. This event gives the couple the opportunity to bond from the beginning, and their surrogate the opportunity to participate in and feel gratified by their joy. Although unexpected events, such as a very early or rapid labor, or an unavoidable travel hindrance, sometimes conspire to prevent new parents from being in the delivery room, most make every effort to be there.

Both couples and surrogates often welcome practical help regarding their hospital stay, since this is a new and unfamiliar experience for each of them. They need information about stepparent adoption (in many states this is the requisite procedure so that the adoptive mother can assume parental rights), circumcision, birth certificates, pediatrician contacts, and car seats.

Many couples and their surrogates also appreciate guidance regarding their evolving relationship, especially if something unexpected occurs, such as an obstetrical problem or a birth defect. However, since even couples and surrogates for whom all goes smoothly are in uncharted territory, it is helpful to have advice from their agency. The Center for Surrogate Parenting and Egg Donation offers its couples a series of recommendations regarding the days and weeks following birth:

1. Couples should spend at least several hours at the hospital with their surrogate and baby. This time provides them with an important opportunity to share their joy with their surrogate and allows the surrogate to see—first hand—how much the baby means to them.

2. New parents should introduce themselves to the hospital staff. Although there may be some people who are unfamiliar with surrogacy—or possibly even antagonistic to it—experience has demonstrated that many hospital staff members are eager to be helpful and inclusive.

3. Couples should stay in the town in which the baby is born for a minimum of two days. This helps the surrogate to have a chance to get some closure on the experience. During this time she needs not only to see them with the baby, but also to have her children see them with the baby.

4. Couples should give their surrogate a gift before leaving. This gift should be something that will last and which will provide her with an on-going reminder of their gratitude.

5 Couples and surrogates should make a specific plan about when they will next be in contact. This plan may include telephone calls or in person visits, depending on geography as well as personal styles and preferences.

After Delivery

Psychologists working with surrogates and couples have observed changing relationships between them in the period following delivery. Although most agree that bonds have formed between the surrogate and the couple, these bonds take different forms. Some couples and their surrogates have frequent telephone contact, especially in the first few weeks. Others need to establish some distance, possibly sending a note or some photographs regularly. Some new mothers turn to their surrogates (who are experienced mothers) for information and guidance; others need to be independent in order to establish their authenticity as mothers. What is most important during this time, as during the pregnancy, is that the couples and surrogates are in agreement regarding contact. When they are not, one or the other is likely to feel disappointed or even abandoned.

Although most couples and surrogates experience loss as they move away from the intense experience that they have shared, many also feel a mutual need to decrease their contact after the first year. At that point, the relationship usually takes the form of a correspondence, with letters and photos exchanged once or twice yearly. However, some couples and surrogates develop and maintain a much closer ongoing relationship.

Perhaps the most important determinant of whether the couple and surrogate maintain a relationship that includes visits and family get-togethers is the extent to which the surrogate and her children want to know the couple and their child. This issue must be discussed in advance, so that the couple, the surrogate, and the surrogate's husband have shared expectations about ongoing contact between the children. Some see contact as important for the well-being of their children; others feel that an ongoing relationship would be confusing.

Regardless of the degree of contact between them, following delivery most surrogates and couples move to a new phase in their lives. For the couple, there is the adjustment to parenthood; they are delighted to have a child to love and nurture. Some parents proudly tell strangers of their child's unique beginning. Others attempt to maintain more privacy by saying little or nothing about the circumstances of their baby's birth. Some even say that their baby was adopted, feeling that this half-truth is the best way to protect themselves and their child from intrusive questions.

For the surrogate, the months following delivery offer both opportunities and challenges. One opportunity is that she now has more time and energy to focus fully on her own family. Some decide to take some time for themselves and pursue advanced schooling or train for a new career. Perhaps these pursuits help them cope with feelings of separation and loss from the baby, the couple and the program. Effective coping strategies are critical at this time, since surrogates are experiencing post-partum physical and emotional changes. In addition, some face the additional stress that comes from criticism of their participation in surrogacy. For the thirty-two former surrogates studied by Forest in 1989, social ostracism and negative media attention were the most difficult aspects of the surrogacy experience.[61]

Some surrogates cope with their feelings of loss following pregnancy by remaining involved in surrogacy, either as volunteers or as paid staff members in surrogacy programs. Others remain involved with surrogacy in other ways, including planning a second pregnancy with the same couple or even seeking another opportunity with a different couple.

The willingess of some surrogates to have a second child is attractive to many couples. When the relationship has been good, as it often is, couples are eager to attempt another pregnancy. As one mother through surrogacy described it, "we felt that our surrogate walked on water and hoped to have another baby with her."

For the surrogate, the decision about whether to have a second baby often depends on timing. Her life schedule and theirs may be in synchrony, making this something she can and would like to do. However, there are also instances in which the parents are eager to expand their family and their surrogate is not able or ready to undertake another pregnancy.

When a couple desiring a second child works with a new surrogate, or when a surrogate enters into an agreement with a second couple, each can experience some disappointment. Couples and surrogates report having such happy associations and memories of their first surrogate pregnancy that a second experience—with a new couple or surrogate—can be a letdown. However, Hilary Hanafin has also known surrogates who found their first experience somewhat mediocre and decide to have a second surrogacy pregnancy, hoping that it will be more satisfying.

In one survey of its members OPTS found:

- 100% of their respondents remain in contact with their surrogates, the most frequent contact being photos and letters on birthdays and holidays.
- 83% of their respondents had seen their surrogate since the birth of their child, and all had included their children (and hers) in the visits.
- 67% said that contact was initiated equally between the surrogate and the couple.
- 42% rated that contact "very comfortable" (another 33% said it was "comfortable" and 25% said that they had some ambivalence about it).
- 67% reported that there was nothing that troubled them about having contact.

Among the concerns that were reported were feeling awkward with their surrogate's family; viewing their surrogate as needy; and having to say good-bye again.[62]

Parenthood through surrogacy is a challenging experience that does not end with the birth of a child. First, there are the normal demands of parenthood. Much as they looked forward to the opportunity to raise a child, couples inevitably find that it is difficult. A cuddly baby soon becomes a curious toddler, who then turns into a demanding two year old. The years pass quickly. Before they know it, parents are on the daily roller coaster ride of adolescence, looking back upon the bygone days of the terrible twos as but a blissful dream.

Along with the normal demands of parenthood are the special challenges of parenting through surrogacy. Questions about privacy, disclosure, and how to help the child make sense of his/her origins (see Chapter 10), are continuous challenges that face couples who choose this option.

Finally, couples must grapple with issues of affiliation and advocacy. Some parents through surrogacy choose to maintain as much privacy as possible and do not openly identify themselves with surrogacy; some feel a need to affiliate with others who have taken the same road to parenthood; and some feel a responsibility to work to help make surrogacy an option for other prospective parents.

Although we believe that most people who enter into surrogacy arrangements do so with the best of intentions and maintain these positive feelings throughout the experience, we remain concerned about what it will mean for them—and for all their children—in the future. We wonder if a woman can truly anticipate how she will feel after she has conceived, carried, birthed and relinquished her bio-genetic child, and, to some extent, we worry about how she will feel later in life, when she looks back upon this experience. We wonder, also, if she can truly predict and understand how her other children will feel about this arrangement, not only in the near future, but throughout their lives. Our thoughts turn with caution also to the children conceived through surrogacy. Although deeply loved and cherished, they may feel confused about their identity. We urge those couples considering surrogacy to consider it carefully, attempting to project into the future and to anticipate the long term struggles and challenges.

$\mathcal{G}$estational Care

The development of *in vitro* fertilization brought a host of new possibilities for infertile couples. As we have discussed several times in earlier chapters, once eggs could be fertilized outside a woman's body, genetic and gestational parenthood could be separated. For that segment of infertile women who had lost part of their reproductive capacity, the separation of reproductive functions meant exciting new options. One new outgrowth of this ability to separate the various components of motherhood was ovum donation. Another was gestational care, a technology that allowed women with functioning ovaries but who were unable to carry a pregnancy, to have their IVF-created embryo(s) transferred to the uterus of another woman.

We begin examining the process by which one woman carries another couple's baby with a dilemma: how best to refer to it. Some people feel strongly that it should be identified as a form of surrogacy, since one woman is carrying a baby for another couple. (And in that sense, the word *surrogate*, which according to the *American Heritage Dictionary*, means "one that takes the place of another; a substitute," may be more appropriate here than it is in "traditional" surrogacy). Those approaching it from this perspective commonly use the terms *gestational surrogacy* or, less commonly, *host-uterus* or *IVF surrogacy*. Others believe that this process is not surrogacy, as the public has come to know (and in some cases, dislike) surrogacy, and therefore it should not be identified as such. Those who share this perspective focus on the fact that the intended parents are the genetic parents and that the woman who carries the child will not be placing her genetic child in a step-parent adoption (as she would be with surrogacy). Hence, they refer to the woman who carries the baby as a *gestational carrier*, a term that emphasizes her physical (non genetic) contribution.

As clinicians, we have given a great deal of thought to each of these perspectives in order to determine what language to use. We decided to call the process *gestational care* and to refer to the woman who carries the pregnancy as the *gestational carrier*. We recognize that the term *gestational care* will be unfamiliar to most readers, but we use it because we believe it accurately describes the process. However, when we quote practitioners who use the term *gestational surrogacy*, we will respectfully use their original language.

The developments of *in vitro* fertilization and commercial surrogacy coincided historically, and because of this historical coincidence, couples who might otherwise have turned to surrogacy had other options. For many women who had been unable to conceive, particularly those with tubal disease, IVF was a miraculous treatment. When it worked, IVF enabled the women to become pregnant themselves, eliminating the need for a surrogate.

A second and smaller group of couples who initially considered or pursued traditional surrogacy were those in which the women had functioning ovaries, but were unable—because of medical illness, prior surgery, or congenital abnormality—to carry a pregnancy. For them, the concurrent arrivals of surrogacy and IVF represented a new and exciting possibility: they could make embryos via *in vitro* fertilization and have them transferred into the uterus of another woman. This possibility, which existed from the beginning of IVF, became a reality in the mid-1980s with the birth of the first baby through a gestational care pregnancy. From this point forward, gestational care has offered a woman who is unable to go through pregnancy, labor, and delivery the opportunity to mother a child who is her genetic offspring.

Early in its development, gestational care was seen as a slight variation of traditional surrogacy, and in the eyes of many, it still is. Because the process involves one woman carrying a baby for another, many practitioners involved in traditional surrogacy arrangements have become involved in gestational care arrangements as well. Although the medical complexities of the process require that they develop close working relationships with physicians and with clinics that offer *in vitro* fertilization, many of the other essential aspects of a practice that involved legal, social and psychological services were already in place.

Although gestational care became closely associated with traditional surrogacy early in its history, reproductive endocrinologists, nurses, and mental health professionals who work with gestational care in medical settings view them very differently. One such group, Pennsylvania Reproductive Associates in Philadelphia, began a Gestational Carrier Program in 1988. By incorporating the necessary legal and psychological services into their medical team, they were able to offer IVF with embryo transfer to another woman's uterus as part of their medical treatment program.

The discussion that follows looks at the social, ethical, and legal questions associated with gestational care. As we examine these questions, it becomes clear that some of the controversy has arisen because gestational care inherited the complicated, sometimes troubled, ethical legacy of surrogacy. It is also clear that this process prompts some new, unique, and very different questions, focusing primarily on what it means for one woman to carry the genetic child of another couple.

A Social and Ethical Perspective

As we have noted throughout this book, people have different feelings about the importance of genetic versus gestational ties. There are those who believe that the most important link between parent and child is a genetic one, because genes are the bloodline connecting the present generation with generations past. Others emphasize the significance of the bond that develops between a woman and the child she is carrying; they see the gestational aspect of reproduction as equal to or even more important than the role of genetics.

The identity of gestational care has been shaped not only by its origins in two fields (IVF and surrogacy) but also by the complex and conflicting views concerning genetic and gestational bonds. Those who focus primarily on genetic ties tend to see gestational care as linked to the ARTs. They regard the use of a gestational carrier as an important aid for certain reproductive problems that afflict women, in particular uterine problems.

Representative of the view that gestational care is a form of assistance for infertile couples rather than a form of surrogacy, is the group at Pennsylvania Reproductive Associates. They draw clear distinctions between their Gestational Carrier Program and the practice of traditional surrogacy:

The importance of a genetic distinction has been reaffirmed through clinical experience. Women evaluated as potential gestational carriers report that they can accept carrying a child that is biologically unrelated to them, and they feel that they would have great emotional difficulty relinquishing a child that is, in part, biologically theirs. Being genetically inert, the carriers report that they are able to separate themselves emotionally from the baby and decrease the attachment process throughout the pregnancy.[63]

Many involved in programs that offer traditional surrogacy as well as gestational care do not share the views of these clinicians. Although they acknowledge the genetic differences between the two processes, they emphasize what they have in common: one woman carries a baby for another. In either situation, the women involved must separate pregnancy from motherhood. In both cases it is the infertile woman and her mate (the contracting couple) who are the expectant parents, not the woman who carries the baby.

Practitioners involved with traditional surrogacy as well as gestational care report that some of the couples they work with focus on genetic ties, and others emphasize the importance of gestation. Sometimes when gestational care does not result in a pregnancy, couples do turn to traditional surrogacy. Other couples turn comfortably to adoption or to childfree living.

However they feel about genetic and gestational ties, couples involved with gestational care must come to terms with the reality that they are entrusting their child's prebirth care to another woman, sometimes a stranger, and that she is providing her body to nurture its growth and development. Embryos are very precious, especially when there is a finite number, as when a couple has undergone IVF in order to freeze embryos prior to the woman's cancer treatment. And since pregnancy is often a complicated process that can involve physical risk, there is also the possibility for conflict of interest between the couple and the gestational carrier. For example, a woman could develop serious medical problems during the pregnancy and require surgery that could harm the fetus. Less serious but also worrisome conflicts can arise if the couple, understandably anxious over the safety and well-being of their growing child, attempts to control the gestational carrier's behavior and/or life-style during pregnancy. These are but a few of the situations that can arise when a woman agrees to carry another couple's baby.

Mental health providers, physicians, lawyers, and ethicists involved in the new reproductive technologies have attempted to address the serious questions that surround gestational care. What are the rights during pregnancy and after of a woman who agrees to carry and deliver a baby for another couple? Is she a "mother" in any sense of the word, or is her role more akin to a prebirth caretaker or a nanny? What are the rights of the couple who agree to entrust her with their embryo? Do they have any jurisdiction over her body during pregnancy and, if so, what is it?

The American College of Obstetricians and Gynecologists (ACOG) has issued a policy statement emphasizing the significance of the woman who carries the child and affirming her rights as the mother:

> The woman who carries the child 1) Should be the sole
> source of consent for all questions regarding the prenatal care
> and delivery and 2) should have a specified time period after
> the birth of the infant during which she can decide whether
> or not to carry out her original intention to place the infant
> for adoption.[64]

George Annas, professor of health law at Boston University School of Medicine and Public Health and a respected expert in the field of reproductive law, makes this point even more emphatically. In an article that clearly identifies the woman who carries and delivers the child as mother—regardless of whether she is genetically connected to it—he writes:

> The woman who gives birth to the child should irrebuttably
> be considered the child's legal mother. She could agree to
> give the child up for adoption, but only after its birth, and
> in accordance with the state's adoption laws.[65]

Nancy Reame, a professor in the School of Nursing and Reproductive Sciences at the University of Michigan, grapples with some of the complexities of a gestational care pregnancy. She acknowledges the ACOG guidelines and notes that they may help to protect a woman's rights regarding her own health care. However, she points out some of the pitfalls of allowing the gestational carrier to be the decision maker:

> The autonomy of the gestational surrogate mother may
> compromise the rights and responsibilities of the genetic

parents.... For example, the gestational surrogate would have the right to abort an unrelated fetus if she no longer wished to carry the pregnancy. Alternatively, she could be responsible for the custody of a child with birth defects rejected by its biological parents.[66]

Thus one can see that although these statements reflect similar beliefs regarding prenatal decisions, they reflect different sentiments regarding who is the "real" mother.

The practitioners at Pennsylvania Reproductive Associates, as well as many others involved in gestational care, feel that a gestational carrier's rights to make decisions related to her pregnancy can be protected and respected without her having to be designated as the mother. What they do instead is to prepare contracts that carefully delineate her rights: the right to make decisions about her obstetrical care and the right to make decisions regarding her body during pregnancy (nutrition, activity level, rest, travel). The physician, psychologist, and nurse who are the team members, take the following position: Once the pregnancy is established, the carrier, in consultation with her physician, should be the sole source of consent for medical decisions and delivery.

Similarly, Dr. Hilary Hanafin, of the Center for Surrogate Parenting and Egg Donation emphasizes that the woman who is pregnant and her physician have the right to make medical decisions during pregnancy even if the fetus is not genetically related to her. However, Dr. Hanafin believes that every effort must be made in advance to anticipate potentially difficult obstetrical decisions and to confirm that couples and their gestational surrogates are in agreement about how to handle these decisions.

A Legal Perspective

From a legal perspective, a positive contribution from the field of surrogacy has been the development and evolution of a surrogacy contract. The original surrogacy contracts focused on the baby who was to result from the agreement rather than on the services being provided by the surrogate. More recent contracts have emphasized the time, effort, and physical and emotional wear and tear involved in surrogate pregnancies and have compensated the woman for her efforts rather than for the baby (baby selling is illegal in all states). This evolution is especially relevant to gestational carriers, who are clearly providing a service rather than a 'product,' since the embryo (product) was already created and belongs to the genetic parents. Compensation for time and effort is also critical because it is possible that a woman will spend a great deal of time and effort simply trying to become pregnant. (The odds of a pregnancy per cycle are approximately the same as they are for IVF, based on the age of the genetic mother.)

Lawyers whose practices include traditional surrogacy bring crucial experience to gestational care. The family building option of gestational care has also forced them to address some new issues, including the rights of the couple and the surrogate during the pregnancy and following delivery. Another question that arises with a gestational care pregnancy concerns identifying the legal parents at birth. Whereas traditional surrogacy usually requires stepparent adoption—the surrogate is initially the child's legal mother, having provided her ovum as well as her uterus—gestational care programs have developed some effective ways of establishing the parental rights and responsibilities of the biological parents that do not involve adoption.

William Handel, director of the Center for Surrogate Parenting and Egg Donation reportedly handled the first gestational care case in which the genetic mother's name was placed on the birth certificate. Handel files maternity and paternity suits on behalf of his clients, the genetic parents prior to delivery. Just as a father can file a paternity suit in instances in which he has not been recognized as his child's father, so also can genetic parents file prebirth maternity and paternity suits to "prove" that they are the child's genetic parents. Since the gestational carriers are not seeking parental rights, these suits are uncontested, and they have proven to be an effective vehicle for enabling the genetic parents to be designated the unborn child's parents as early as the last trimester of pregnancy.

Similarly, Steven Litz, of Surrogate Mothers Inc., in Indiana, petitions the court when the gestational carrier is six months pregnant, seeking that a legal relationship be established between the genetic parents and their unborn child. Lawyers in other programs have developed similar mechanisms for ensuring that the biological parents are deemed the legal parents at the earliest point possible. This legal effort protects the couple as parents and protects the woman who is pregnant from any parenting obligations since she has never intended to parent the child she is carrying. Legal agreements also protect the child from the possibility of being in legal limbo.

Although various attorneys have sometimes been able to establish the parental rights of the genetic parents prior to birth, at other times they have been unsuccessful. One New York court refused to acknowledge a "maternity action" filed in an attempt to establish that the genetic mother of twins born to a gestational carrier was the children's legal mother. This refusal occurred despite the fact that the genetic and gestational parents were in agreement. The court concluded that New York law did not allow an order establishing maternity; therefore the state legislature, not its courts, must be asked to expand the law to cover technological advances.[67]

Gestational care has also inherited some of the legal baggage that has burdened surrogacy arrangements. Effective legislation has been sorely lacking for both options, leaving the practice of both largely unguided and unregulated. To the extent that laws have been passed, they are largely restrictive, and most fail to distinguish between the role of a gestational carrier and a traditional surrogate. A law that initially passed in the California legislature in September, 1992, but was subsequently vetoed by the governor, would have been an important exception. It attempted to make distinctions between the two options by stating explicitly that a child born of a gestational care agreement is the legal child of the contracting couple.

For the most part, gestational care arrangements have been spared the dramatic court cases that have been so damaging to traditional surrogacy. There has, however, been one well-publicized case, *Johnson v. Calvert*. Anna Johnson, who carried a baby for Mark and Crispina Calvert, attempted to gain custody of the baby following delivery. The initial ruling, in October 1990, was that Ms. Johnson had no parental rights. On appeal, the California Supreme Court reached similar conclusions in February 1993. In May of 1993 the California Supreme Court made a second ruling and went much further in its support of the Calverts. It focused on the question of intent and said that the people who "intended" to raise the child should be designated as the parents.[68]

Although the *Johnson v. Calvert* case advanced the cause of gestational care by setting valuable legal precedent, it also had negative repercussions because it brought unwanted media attention to this option. The fact that Ms. Johnson sued for custody indicated that even a gestational carrier who is not genetically related to the offspring might change her mind and want to parent the child she carried.

Gestational Care Couples

Many couples are introduced to the idea of gestational care when they are in crisis. Having endured an illness or surgery that resulted in the inability to become pregnant, many women receive offers from a close friend or family member who is willing to carry a child for them. Some of these offers, although made with sincerity, are later withdrawn when altruistic volunteers learn all that is involved in gestational care. Similarly, some couples who may initially respond to the offer with enthusiasm decide against pursuing the process because of its medical uncertainty, high costs and psychological and/or legal complexities.

Couples and their volunteer gestational carriers may be advised against the process by physicians, psychologists, or family and friends. For example, if the prospective mother is close to (or over) age 40 she may be advised against gestational care because her advanced age makes success unlikely. There are also many couples, as well as gestational carriers, who a psychologist or other mental health professional feels are unprepared or ill suited for this unusual undertaking.

Not all couples with medical need, as well as emotional desire, for a gestational care pregnancy have a family member or friend who is willing or able to help them. Others may know a willing volunteer but conclude that the closeness of their relationship may in fact be detrimental to the process. Some couples decide that it is important enough to them to have a genetic child that they are willing to enter into an agreement with a stranger.

As we have noted, people feel differently about the importance of genetic ties. Hence, some couples might consider working with a gestational carrier but eventually decide against it, concluding that what is most important is for them to become parents. They then turn to adoption as a more expedient (and more certain) path to parenthood. For them, gestational care is appealing but too costly, too time-consuming, and, most important, too much of a long shot.

Other couples look at the challenges involved in gestational care and decide that the option is worth pursuing. Some base their decision on their feelings about bloodlines: they want a child who is genetically connected to them and to those who came before them. Others focus more on the idea of known versus unknown genes, fearing that adoption is too risky. Still others, especially cancer survivors, experience a powerful longing to have a genetic connection to their child as a way of ameliorating the pain or despair associated with their illness or surgery. Having faced their mortality, they view genetic continuity as a way to live on.

Couples who have a genetic child and then suffer a subsequent reproductive injury are also among those drawn to gestational care. Feeling blessed with an adored child who came from their genes, and having previously had the experience of pregnancy, many of these couples regard gestational care as a perfect solution. They conclude that they can handle the high costs ($35,000 or more, assuming they have neither a volunteer carrier nor insurance coverage) and low odds for success (again age is a major determinent.)

Seeking Gestational Care Services

There are a variety of ways that couples can arrange to work with a gestational carrier. Those who have a family member or friend who has volunteered to help them usually begin by contacting a reproductive medicine center that offers ART. Whereas at one time couples had to work through a surrogacy program or through one of a handful of medical centers that offered this option, this is no longer the case. In fact, as more and more couples have become aware of this option, and more physicians are comfortable participating in it, gestational care has become an option with widespread availability.

Couples who do not have a volunteer carrier are more likely to work with a surrogacy program that offers both surrogacy and gestational care, or with a reproductive medical clinic that offers comprehensive services that include help with finding a carrier. More and more couples, however, are locating their own carriers through advertisements in the media or through the internet.

What is critical is not the style and format of the program, but that they have medical, legal and psychological services in place. Those who seek care through an ART medical practice should confirm that the clinic has had experience with this option, has medical protocols in place, and offers psychological services or referrals to a qualified clinician. Those who seek care through a surrogacy program should confirm that they have a working relationship with a highly skilled ART team.

Fees for surrogacy are high—totaling around $35,000, which includes compensation to the surrogate. Gestational care can be much more expensive, however, because of the complicated medical procedures that are involved with each cycle, and because it often takes more than one or two cycles to establish an ongoing pregnancy. Although there are some one-time costs, such as administrative, legal and psychological fees, (and the bulk of the carrier's fee) the medical costs of IVF are repeated each cycle (as of this writing, a few insurance carriers, in states with mandated coverage for infertility, are paying for at least some of the costs associated with gestational care). It is therefore essential that couples understand what they will be paying for and when. For example, they need to determine what their costs will be for subsequent cycles if the first does not work, and for cryopreservation if they have extra embryos. It is also critical that the gestational care program or practitioner be knowledgeable about what insurance companies, if any, are willing to pay medical expenses in a gestational care pregnancy.

Medical Indications

As with surrogacy, couples who use established programs must go through extensive screening procedures before they are accepted into a gestational care program. To our knowledge there are no practitioners who believe it is ethical to undertake gestational care for reasons of convenience. Thus couples considering this option must demonstrate medical need, which can be established in a number of ways.

In the first category are women who have no uterus—either resulting from congenital absence of the uterus or removal due to cancer or other gynecological or obstetrical problems. Thus they have suffered the loss of part of their reproductive capacity. If at least one ovary is intact, the potential to have a genetic child remains.

A second category includes women who have been diagnosed with cancer and are about to undergo a chemotherapy regimen that will destroy or severely damage their ovarian function. Prior to chemotherapy they may elect to undergo IVF in order to cryopreserve embryos. Since pregnancy may no longer be possible, or may be contraindicated (at least for several years after treatment,) such couples may opt for gestational care.

Many cancer survivors see gestational care as an important ingredient in their recovery. Having come face-to-face with death, they see having a child, and especially a child genetically related to them, as a link to their future. Many also see gestational care as a way of reducing the losses they have experienced; even in the face of significant losses, they have been able to salvage their ability to reproduce.

Some gestational care situations resulting from cancer treatment pose profound ethical dilemmas involving the best interests of the unborn offspring. If a woman's long term prognosis is poor, many practitioners believe it is unfair to bring a child into the world whose mother is likely to die before s/he is an adult. On the other hand, since there are no guarantees for anyone's future, other professionals feel that it is unfair (and discriminatory) to exclude a couple from becoming parents on the basis of medical history, especially if the other parent is in good health.

One couple's story poignantly captures the dilemmas that can arise for caregivers and couples alike. The couple contacted the IVF program in which they had embryos stored from a successful cycle that occurred three years before. They told the staff that when their son—born after a successful IVF cycle—was a year old, the mother was diagnosed with a serious form of cancer and given a poor prognosis. The couple had a friend who was willing to be their gestational carrier and they were determined to have their embryos transferred to her. Both the husband and wife said they hoped to witness the birth of their second child before the wife died. She needed to attempt to give the embryos life in order to die in peace. The medical team was in an ethical quandary: they felt tremendous empathy for the couple and wanted to grant them this request, yet they did not believe that it would be in the unborn child's best interest to do so. The team felt that it was tragic enough that their already born son would soon lose his mother. The center decided not to do this procedure and explained their reasons to the couple (who of course, had the right to take their request —and their embryos—to another program).

When a couple has only a finite number of cryopreserved embryos, there is additional pressure on all involved. These couples have no further opportunities for genetic parenthood; transfer of their existing embryos presents their last chance for a child who is genetically connected to each of them. Thus they and their gestational carrier approach the treatment cycle with keen awareness that the stakes are high.

Women with structural problems of the uterus or with severe uterine scarring (Asherman's syndrome) following a pregnancy loss, an elective abortion, or (occasionally) after a normal pregnancy, fall into a third category of medical need. Scarring makes it difficult for an embryo to implant. Frequently, however, minor surgery can correct the condition. When it does not, a couple may attempt gestational care. Similarly, women who have malformation of the uterus, often as a result of DES exposure, may be unable to carry a pregnancy safely to viability.

Couples in this category who choose gestational care usually do so after several unsuccessful IVF attempts or after many early pregnancy losses, or both. Repeated pregnancy loss appears to confirm their inability to carry a pregnancy to term, providing probable justification for the theory that the couple's problem resides in the woman's uterus, not in the embryos. Faced with the irony of being able to create healthy embryos but lacking the ability to gestate them, some couples welcome gestational care as the solution for their infertility problem.

Other women, who fall into a fourth category, have been advised not to attempt pregnancy for medical reasons. Heart problems or a chronic illness such as multiple sclerosis, for example, may contraindicate pregnancy. Usually such women are able to become pregnant, but pregnancy is likely to compromise their health. Gestational care offers them and their partners the opportunity to reproduce without undergoing the potential risks of pregnancy.

There is a fifth and final group of couples who are considered by some physicians (though not others) to be candidates for gestational care pregnancies: those for whom several attempts at IVF have failed, despite the fact that the couple produced healthy embryos and the woman's uterus appears to be normal. When IVF repeatedly fails to result in pregnancy, some physicians conclude that the problem must reside in the uterus and that some unknown or untreatable factor is preventing implantation. They suggest that these couples might benefit from having their embryos transferred into another woman's uterus. Other physicians disagree with this rationale, believing it is inappropriate to direct people to this alternative rather than helping them to grieve and move on other options such as adoption.

An interesting case example illustrates an additional reason why gestational care is rarely a "solution" to failed IVF attempts. A couple had turned to gestational care after several failed IVF attempts that were eventually attributed to uterine problems. However, since they had produced several embryos, they decided to maximize their efforts by having the better embryos transferred to the gestational carrier and the ones that appeared less optimal transferred to the mother. The unanticipated result was that both women became pregnant and delivered siblings two days apart. This story, although unusual, seems to support those who believe that gestational care should be reserved only for women with a known uterine problem. Nevertheless, it is important to remember that many explanations for infertility are undocumented; they are educated guesses at best, yet they frequently determine treatment.

Psycho-social Assessment of Couples

Although some mental health professionals only meet with the couple together, others recommend also meeting with each partner individually. Sessions together offer couples an opportunity to hear each other's perspective and to confirm that they are in agreement; individual sessions offer each of them a chance to speak in private with a counselor and to voice any concerns that they might be reluctant to share with their partner. In combination these meetings should address several questions.

Are both partners in agreement regarding this choice? Arranging for gestational care is an expensive and difficult undertaking, with significant potential for disappointment. The clinician must determine whether the couple has considered other parenting options and whether each understands how they arrived at the decision to undertake gestational care.

If the couple plans to undergo gestational care with a family member, it is essential that they explore the full implications of this decision. Whatever the outcome, the process that they are embarking upon together is likely to affect family relationships for years to come. They need to discuss with each other their feelings about the prospective gestational carrier and consider issues that might arise as a consequence of their decision.

Has the couple considered how stressful the process is likely to be, and are they prepared for possible disappointment? Attempting gestational care, like other alternative paths, means that couples must reembark on the emotional roller coaster that for many became all too familiar during their infertility treatments. The chances of ending up with a child through this option depends in large part on the woman's age; however, no matter how young she is, the odds are always against a pregnancy occurring—in any one cycle. Couples must acknowledge the series of obstacles that may lie ahead. There could be problems with egg retrieval, fertilization, transfer, implantation, or pregnancy loss. The most likely scenario is that everything will go smoothly but no pregnancy will occur. Each step along the way will be intensely stressful, with the threat of loss or disappointment always lurking.

Has the couple anticipated at least some of the challenges that could arise during a pregnancy involving a gestational carrier? No one can anticipate all the questions and issues that might surface during a pregnancy. Nonetheless, it is important that couples consider some of the issues that have arisen for other couples and think about what they would do if they found themselves in similar situations.

Mental health professionals stress the need for couples to discuss their feelings about amniocentesis, as well as about what they would want to do if the results indicated a problem. Accordingly, they need to be in agreement about the conditions under which they would terminate a pregnancy or engage in multifetal reduction. Only after they agree as a couple can the program make sure they are matched with a woman who shares their views on these key issues.

Has the couple grieved the loss of pregnancy and childbirth? It is essential that couples, in their eagerness to seize the possibility of having a genetic child, not overlook all that they have been through. Since the need for gestational care was often the result of a traumatic experience, such as a life-threatening illness or emergency surgery, it is important that couples have taken time to grieve. If they neglect this task, they are likely to be all the more vulnerable to the frustrations and disappointments that arise in the process.

Pregnancy is more important to some people than to others. In general, women experience a far greater loss than do their partners when pregnancy is not possible, although some men do look forward to seeing their wife pregnant and to sharing the experience with her. It is vital that couples talk together about what it means to each of them to lose the opportunity to share a pregnancy. Even if gestational care succeeds, there will be loss involved. The dimensions of that loss, including the process of conception itself, need to be identified and acknowledged.

Have they talked about their plans to family or friends and if so, what was their reaction? Couples attempting gestational care will have to make some decisions about whom they tell and what they tell them. Those who are working with a friend or family member may have more difficulty maintaining privacy. Couples who decide to work with a stranger can more easily postpone telling others about their decision. Some wait to see if pregnancy is achieved, feeling that the wait spares them from having to give progress reports on their efforts. Others are open from the start; they do not want to be forced to hide their plans or account for the time lost at work from medical appointments.

Prospective parents must consider whether they are emotionally equipped to embark on a family-building option that is so controversial. They can try to anticipate how family and friends will react, but they should remind themselves that many people are misinformed about gestational care, confusing it with surrogacy. Others who understand the difference may still feel strongly that no woman should carry a baby for someone else, regardless of the medical reasons. On the other hand, many couples who tell their families that they have decided to attempt gestational care are pleasantly surprised by the support they receive, finding their families are comfortable, perhaps even familiar, with this parenting option.

Have they have thought about how their child may feel about his or her conception and birth? Thinking about how and when a child might understand and integrate information about his or her origins is crucial. There is no reason to hide the truth—ever. Furthermore, the child could easily learn about it from a family member or friend, and feel betrayed by his/her parents for having kept it a secret. Finding and talking with others who have undergone this process can help them sort out the questions and decisions they will face. Chapter 10 includes a discussion about openness in third party parenting and about how and when to discuss it with children. Although couples who turn to gestational care will parent their genetic child, much of the discussion involving secrecy pertains to all forms of third party reproduction and is thus applicable here.

Has the couple considered how many times they will attempt a pregnancy through gestational care and what alternatives they will pursue if it does not occur? Because gestational care is so expensive, as well as invasive, many couples attempt only one or two cycles. Furthermore, although most of the medical treatment involves the genetic mother (who undergoes IVF) the carrier is involved as well. Most couples feel that it is one thing to impose on their own time, and another to inconvenience their carrier for a prolonged duration.

In preparation for the likelihood of disappointment, couples may want to consider other options. Some may think about moving on to surrogacy, feeling that "half a genetic connection is preferable to no genetic connection." (Sometimes they may be drawn to surrogacy because they have grown fond of the carrier and she has offered to become a surrogate for them.) Others will decide on adoption as their next choice. And still others may opt for child free living.

Have they explored the potential legal issues? Although there have been few legal disputes to date regarding gestational care, couples nevertheless need to work with a lawyer who is experienced in this process and can draw up a contract. The contract is unlikely to be upheld in court, since a woman cannot legally relinquish a child prior to birth. However, it may hold psychological if not legal weight, as did the case of *Johnson v. Calvert* that we discussed earlier in this chapter (the judge based his decision primarily on intention). Furthermore, the process of entering into an agreement provides an important opportunity for couples and gestational carriers to discuss critical and potentially devastating issues, such as failed pregnancy attempts, amniocentesis, elective abortion, multifetal reduction, and birth anomalies.

Gestational Carriers

Some women offer to undertake a gestational care pregnancy because they want to help a friend or family member in need. Often they are sisters, but sometimes they are cousins, sisters-in-law, or friends. Most are women who never before imagined that they would carry a baby for someone else. Now, moved by a tragedy in the life of a loved one, they see an opportunity to help out in a most meaningful way.

Other women decide on their own, unrelated to any desire to help a loved one, that they want to carry a baby for a childless couple. Dr. Hilary Hanafin, psychologist at the Center for Surrogate Parenting and Egg Donation, has worked with a large number of these women, some of whom were traditional surrogates and some gestational carriers. In her experience, the motivation of surrogates and gestational carriers is similar: they want to do something that matters for others and that adds meaning to their own lives. Many have had friends or family members who were infertile and feel strongly that helping a couple realize their dream of parenthood is one of the most meaningful contributions they could make.

Surrogates and gestational carriers are women who enjoy pregnancy, labor, and delivery. Although their families are complete, they look forward to experiencing these pleasures again. For them, the prospect of carrying a child for another couple is a real opportunity: they can enjoy a pregnancy but be spared the parenting responsibilities that follow.

Although both surrogates and gestational carriers are typically women who have enjoyed pregnancy and may look forward to re-experiencing it, there are many women who only agree to be gestational carriers but would not become surrogates. They want to carry a baby for someone else as long as it is not their own genetic baby. They are clear that if they provided the egg in addition to the gestational environment, the child would be theirs. Dr. Andrea Braverman, psychologist at Pennsylvania Reproductive Associates, reports that the majority of women in her gestational carrier program feel this way. Only on rare occasions have gestational carriers later served as surrogates for couples. In her experience, this change of heart has happened only after a couple and the carrier have gone through failed ART attempts together and have developed close bonds.

Other practitioners report different experiences: women apply to their programs interested in either traditional or gestational surrogacy. Such women have apparently concluded that the children they give birth to in these situations—whether conceived with their eggs or as the result of an embryo transfer—are not their children.

Awareness of these different points of view—one that a genetic tie (or lack of one) makes all the difference in the world, and the other that it is almost irrelevant—helps us to understand why some potential surrogates/gestational carriers offer one option and not the other, while others do not draw a distinction between them. It also helps us to understand why some women—those who would carry a child only if it was the other couple's embryo—apply to programs that are medically based and do not offer traditional surrogacy. Conversely, those who feel less strongly about their genetic material but more strongly about the gestational bond are more likely to become involved with surrogacy programs that offer both options.

Beyond genetic considerations, there are additional reasons why some women who consider carrying a baby for another couple prefer gestational care and others prefer surrogacy. Those who are willing to carry a child only if it is the couple's genetic offspring may make this decision based on the perceived needs of their own children. They may feel that they minimize the risk of their children's feeling that a sister or brother is being given away, if the child they carry is biologically unrelated.

Some women choose to be gestational carriers because they feel that they are less likely to be seen as baby sellers or as exploited women who are giving up their children. Lori Capone, a former gestational surrogate and an articulate spokesperson, has addressed some of these issues:

I did not receive compensation for selling my child—she was never mine—and her parents did not purchase her from me. I received monetary compensation for going through the physical and emotional trials of pregnancy. Certainly no one can begrudge me that. I had a difficult pregnancy and a complicated birth culminating in an emergency Caesarean section. Forgive my lack of altruism, but I feel I did deserve compensation for the physical labor involved. It's different when you bear your own child because having your own child is compensation enough.[69]

It is important to note here that not all women who draw a distinction between surrogacy and gestational care prefer the latter option. Some conclude that surrogacy is more likely to be successful, since it does not require *in vitro* fertilization and embryo transfer. They may also prefer its relative simplicity—the surrogate does not have to have her cycle closely monitored in anticipation of embryo transfer—and she does not face a high risk of multiple gestation.

Another medical reason why some women prefer surrogacy to gestational care relates to convenience and efficacy. Artificial insemination (the means by which a surrogate conceives) is a simple procedure that a woman can perform on her own, if she chooses. Pregnancy is usually achieved within six normal menstrual cycles. By contrast, gestational care, which relies on *in vitro* fertilization with embryo transfer, is a complicated procedure, requiring carefully coordinated monitoring of both women's menstrual cycles. In the best medical centers, this process has a 40 to 50% chance of pregnancy per cycle, assuming the genetic mother is under age thirty-five and is producing healthy eggs. However, in less experienced centers or with older genetic mothers, chances for pregnancy are lower.

Medical Assessment

Although the gestational carrier will not be passing on her genes to the child that she carries, she will be undergoing pregnancy, labor, and delivery, and so it is important that her general health, as well as her fertility, be determined. The medical assessment and screening of a gestational carrier is similar in many ways to that of a surrogate (see Surrogacy Chapter).

Medical evaluation looks for any evidence of a uterine problem that might interfere with implantation or with carrying a pregnancy. Since most programs require that a woman have at least one child before undertaking gestational care—and surrogacy as well—(this requirement is usually for psychological reasons—so she knows what it means to be pregnant and to bond with a child in utero), she therefore has a medical history that provides useful information about any prior pregnancy. For example, a program might decide not to work with a woman who has a history of recurrent miscarriages, premature delivery, or some other obstetrical problem that could compromise a future pregnancy. In all other respects, the medical screening is similar to that of traditional surrogates.

Psycho-social Assessment

The psychological evaluation includes a careful examination of a candidate's emotional stability and her readiness to become a carrier. In addition to many of the questions that are addressed in the evaluation of a prospective surrogate (see Chapter 7), a clinician attempts to sort through a number of other issues.

Coercion

Some women volunteer to carry a baby for relatives or good friends and then find that they have second thoughts about doing so. In this case, the potential carrier may not know how to withdraw from the situation, knowing how much is at stake for the couple, and not wanting to break their hearts. Such women are likely to feel duty bound, especially if there is family support and encouragement. The notion of reneging may seem unthinkable. Sometimes what initially felt like support, however, may begin to feel like pressure, or even coercion, especially if gifts or financial incentives are offered.

A mental health clinician working with prospective gestational carriers must give them every opportunity to change their minds. A woman who has serious doubts may need help figuring out how and when to tell the couple that she has decided against it. The clinician can assist her with this task, explaining to the couple why it is probably not in her best interest—and accordingly not in theirs—to proceed. Having a 'valid' reason from a professional can reduce feelings of regret or guilt that burden the prospective gestational carrier. Furthermore, couples usually pay close attention to the feelings and reactions of their gestational carrier and may sense when the woman has had a change of heart or is confused about whether she should continue the process. Having a clinician who will step in and clarify what is going on may be a relief to them.

Willingness to Gestate a Multiple Pregnancy

The process of ovulation induction that occurs in an IVF cycle carries with it a 25 to 30% chance of multiple gestation. Consequently, every prospective gestational carrier must consider how she might react to learning that she is carrying more than one fetus, and possibly more than two.

Psychologists working in reproductive medicine know that many women discount the possibility of a multiple pregnancy. Consequently, it is imperative that the psychological assessment and preparation of the carrier address this possibility. The woman and the contracting couple must agree on how such a pregnancy would be handled. Otherwise, potential gestational carriers may blind themselves to the realities of their undertaking and later find themselves unprepared to deal with the challenges of a multiple gestation.

A prospective gestational carrier needs to give special consideration to the prospect of multifetal reduction. Before discussing it with the couple the potential carrier must sort through her own feelings about this matter. She must then decide whether she would be willing to undergo a reduction and if so—or if not—whether she is prepared to live with the outcome (e.g., guilt following the procedure or, alternatively, guilt and sorrow if she refuses it and the babies are born very prematurely). As in surrogacy programs, every effort is made to pair gestational carriers with couples who have the same views on this subject. A woman opposed to abortion under any circumstances would be matched only with a couple who had similar feelings.

Sometimes, however, even the most carefully thought out plans bring unanticipated results, as in the following case. A 32-year-old woman and her husband had a year old son. The mother had had an emergency c-section while delivering her son and ended up with a partial hysterectomy. They located a gestational carrier through a local program, choosing a woman who had four children and had had four easy pregnancies and births. Neither the couple nor the carrier felt comfortable with multi-fetal reduction and so they elected to transfer only two embryos, hoping for a singleton (or possibly a twin pregnancy). Everyone wanted to avoid a triplet pregnancy, primarily out of concern for the carrier who had many responsibilities and hoped to be active during her pregnancy.

The carrier became pregnant with a singleton on the first cycle, but unfortunately miscarried. Since they had cryopreserved embryos, and since the pregnancy rates are lower with frozen embryos, they decided to transfer three on the next cycle. Sadly she did not get pregnant. After much discussion among themselves and with their physician, they elected to put back three embryos on the next (fresh) cycle, which was to be their last, primarily for financial reasons. The carrier herself had said, "go for it." Everyone was delighted when the initial pregnancy test was positive—but shocked a few weeks later when the ultrasound showed three strong heartbeats. Fortunately the pregnancy had a very positive outcome; she delivered healthy triplets at 35 weeks, and everyone was thrilled—but the carrier and her family were inconvenienced far more than they had anticipated.

Dealing with Negativity

Most of the world—particularly those who are not in the field of reproductive technology—does not distinguish between surrogacy and gestational care. Furthermore, surrogacy is not a widely supported family building option. Many people are critical of women who carry a baby for nine months and then hand it to someone else, even if that baby was not genetically hers. Consequently, a potential carrier needs to be prepared for the probability that she will be criticized by family, friends, or neighbors. It is also possible that her children will be taunted as a result of her becoming a gestational carrier. On the other hand, it is also likely that many people will support her decision—even applaud it. She needs to be prepared for both possibilities and know that she can remain strong in the face of criticism.

Bonding during Gestation

Although she may feel clear that the child will belong to the genetic parents, the gestational carrier needs to try to understand how she perceives her role and how she is likely to feel toward the baby she is carrying. She must believe in her ability to separate the gestational from the genetic and rearing aspects of motherhood. It may help to reflect on her earlier pregnancies and remember the extent to which she bonded with her babies in utero. If she bonded deeply during pregnancy, she needs to consider whether gestational care is likely to be different. This issue may be more complicated for women who volunteer to carry for family members. Since they will be genetically connected to the baby they carry, and can expect to have an ongoing relationship with the child, they will probably welcome attachment, yet they must be reasonably certain ahead of time that they will feel like the aunt, for example, and not like the mother.

Conjoint Counseling

Although it is difficult to know ahead of time exactly how their relationship will evolve, it is important that all parties to gestational care sit down with one another before proceeding. The purpose of this meeting is to determine that they are in agreement about all aspects of the process and about how they will conduct their relationship. The meeting should be facilitated by a mental health practitioner—ideally the same person who met separately with both parties. In that way, the clinician can bring up any issues that had previously come up and about which there may be disagreement. These meetings can also help everyone anticipate the challenges that lie ahead and formulate a game plan for how they will procede.

Agreements between strangers call for different arrangements regarding their relationship during and after the pregnancy. It is important that they acknowledge the deeply personal and intimate experience they are sharing. They should find it helpful to talk together about their feelings regarding privacy, including such matters as participation together in physical exams or ultrasound procedures. It will be important also, to discuss how they each feel regarding the extent to which they desire contact—either by phone or in person. It is important for the carrier to reflect upon her own need for support and to plan to communicate her needs as they evolve. There is no single way for a couple and a gestational carrier to conduct their relationship, but there are ways of going about it that would be right or wrong for certain individuals.

Family members and friends working together already have a relationship, in many cases one that is longstanding. That relationship, however, is likely to be changed—or challenged—by this process. Conjoint meetings can help clarify issues that arise and provide an opportunity for everyone to voice concerns before they become problematic. These meetings are important in helping everyone determine how they will deal with family members and friends during the pregnancy and in years to come. Regardless of whether the couple and carrier had a prior relationship, however, if there is likely to be any tension between them, it will probably surface during the joint meeting. The clinician will be able to help them determine whether they can work through their differences then and in the future.

The Gestational Care Experience

Like ovum donation, in which one woman's fertilized eggs are transferred to another woman's uterus, gestational care involves coordinating
two women's cycles. In the case of gestational care, this is usually accomplished by giving the carrier Lupron and then beginning her on Estrace
at the time that the intended genetic mother begins her treatment cycle.
The success of this effort is assessed by frequent blood tests during the
week prior to anticipated embryo transfer.

If the gestational carrier's cycle has been successfully synchronized
with the genetic mother's cycle, embryos are transferred two days after
fertilization. However, if the women's cycles are not adequately "in sync",
the embryos will be cryopreserved for use at a more optimal time.

Some couples and their carriers plan on cryopreservation from the
start. They do so in an effort to reduce the need for the carrier to take medications, instead having her undergo embryo transfer at the optimal point
in her natural cycle. Although attractive to many because it is a more "natural" process, this technique does reduce the chance of pregnancy to some
degree, depending on the individual program's success with cryopreservation (some programs have substantially greater success freezing and
thawing embryos than do others).

The decision about how many embryos to transfer is especially difficult
with gestational care. On the one hand, couples and their carriers are very
eager to achieve pregnancy as promptly as possible, since this is a costly,
time consuming and demanding endeavor. For this reason, they are
tempted to transfer a maximum number of embryos, probably three or
four (depending upon embryo quality, the genetic mother's age and the
pregnancy history of the carrier). However, there are also compelling
reasons to avoid high level multiple gestations: neither the carrier nor
the couple wish to face decisions regarding multifetal reduction, nor the
challenges for all concerned of prolonged bedrest or of prematurity.

What makes the question of numbers so complicated is that it is especially difficult to predict success in gestational care. If the genetic mother
is young, the genetic father is fertile, and the carrier has a history of easy
conceptions and uneventful pregnancies, the process *should* work.
However, what no one knows in advance—unless the carrier has had her

children through IVF—is how easily she becomes pregnant after embryo transfer. It is entirely possible that she may be very fertile when she conceives in vivo and somewhat less fertile following *in vitro* fertilization.

The period after embryo transfer is stressful in any IVF cycle, but often more so when it involves a gestational carrier. The high costs of gestational care prevent many couples from trying more than two or three times. Thus for many couples, a negative pregnancy test following embryo transfer may well represent their last chance at genetic parenthood.

Beyond financial stress—and the limits that this places on future options—there is considerable emotional stress. With gestational care, there are three or four adults involved, presumably all hoping to achieve a pregnancy. Each is not only concerned with his/her feelings, but also with the emotions of the other participants. The carrier, for example, wants the couple to be happy and does not want to disappoint them. She may wonder what she might do—or not do—to maximize the chance that an embryo(s) will "take." The couple, by contrast, may be worried about her well-being—will she become so discouraged or exhausted that she won't be willing to try again? They may struggle with feelings of helplessness as they "wait it out", knowing there is now virtually nothing they can do to help ensure pregnancy. Hence the days following embryo transfer pass very slowly. Typically, the carrier, who has been pregnant before, watches for familiar signs and signals of pregnancy. The couple, feeling somewhat helpless, try to cope quietly with their anxiety and to resist the temptation to ask her how she is feeling.

If a pregnancy is achieved—and the odds per transfer cycle can be about 40% (in good programs and with good candidates)—everyone is thrilled.[70] New challenges quickly arise, however: the threat of miscarriage, the risk that the pregnancy will be ectopic, or the risk of abnormalities.

Confirmation of a gestational care pregnancy means that a couple and their carrier may face both the joys and potential complications of a multiple gestation. Most couples, eager to become parents, welcome the possibility of two babies "for the price of one," especially if they have a finite number of embryos, or if it is their only/last attempt. Unfortunately, however, a multiple gestation is a more risky pregnancy bringing with it significant medical and emotional challenges.

Although every gestational carrier is informed about the possibility of a multiple gestation prior to undergoing the procedure, some are still unprepared for its ramifications. These may include miscarriage or prematurity, or prolonged bed rest. The latter is especially difficult for a woman with young children. The carrier is also likely to gain a substantial amount of weight, something that is uncomfortable and limiting. Finally, there will occasionally be a gestational carrier who, with the genetic parents, faces the difficult question of multifetal reduction. Although she will have been prepared for this decision in advance, the reality of the undertaking may be far more formidable than she anticipated.

The Pregnancy

Ongoing support during pregnancy is essential for carriers and couples throughout the process. This support can take a variety of forms—support groups, individual meetings, phone calls from the mental health clinician—depending on the needs and preferences of those involved and upon whether the carrier is a close relative or friend of the couple or a stranger. What is most critical is that all participants have access to a clinician who understands their situation and with whom they have, or can build, a relationship. It is not always possible, usually due to geography, for the clinician associated with the program to follow everyone carefully, though s/he can always be available by telephone, if not in person.

As we stated previously, during the counseling sessions prior to the procedure, the couple and their carrier can discuss how they would like their relationship to proceed, including how much contact they want to maintain and how involved they will be in the pregnancy. Experienced practitioners stress the benefits of a close and mutually supportive relationship between couples and their carriers. The relationship between the two women is especially important, and whenever possible, the mother-to-be should attend doctor's appointments with the carrier. If geography prevents regular visits, both parties can keep in touch frequently by telephone. As with surrogacy, the most problematic situations tend to be the ones in which the couple remains emotionally distant from the carrier.

The Birth Experience

The arrival of any baby is a wonderous event. The arrival of a baby through gestational care is truly a miracle of modern science. Couples and carriers who have undertaken a pregnancy together look forward to delivery as a time of shared celebration.

Most couples make every effort to attend the birth of their child. They must be prepared, however, for the possibility that something may not go as planned. The baby may come early or labor may progress very rapidly, causing the parents-to-be to miss the delivery. One mother we spoke with had traveled two hours each way, throughout her carrier's pregnancy, in order to attend all medical appointments. She and her husband were prepared to leave for the hospital, with plenty of time to spare, as soon as they got the call that the carrier was in labor. Their plans failed them however, when a tractor trailer jackknifed on the highway, and they were stuck in a five-hour traffic jam.

Most couples and their carrier spend some time together following delivery. They have forged a strong bond, and it is important to maintain it in the hours that follow the birth. Gestational carriers take great pride and delight in seeing the new parents with their baby. Their expressions of joy and appreciation help carriers reaffirm the rightness of their decision.

Couples report few difficulties with hospital staff. Rather, they say that staff frequently go out of their way to be helpful, to accommodate the new parents, and to adjust to this new form of parenthood. However, not everyone in the hospital setting will be familiar with or supportive of gestational care. Personnel may say or do unkind things, and hospitals may have rules and regulations that prove restrictive to the new parents.

As we mentioned earlier, some lawyers experienced with gestational care have developed procedures for assigning parental rights to the biological parents. These procedures depend, in part, on the state in which the gestational carrier gives birth, and in part on the hospital. Each couple must make sure that their lawyer is familiar with the laws that will apply in the hospital where their gestational carrier gives birth and that he or she has taken appropriate steps to ensure proper preparation of the birth certificate.

After the Baby Arrives

After the baby has arrived, the new parents and the gestational carrier generally spend some time—usually a day or two—together. If she is a family member or close friend, these visits may be part of a larger family celebration. At least one visit should include the carrier's children during which they should see the new parents holding their baby. That way they have a visual image to take away with them—an image that reinforces the reason why their mother became a carrier in the first place.

Couples who work with a gestational carrier that they did not know prior to this arrangement face a different sort of leave taking. Theirs is a relationship that was established for a specific purpose and now that goal has been achieved. Most likely the participants have grown close over the past several months, but they must now find ways to separate comfortably and graciously, all the while laying the ground work for on-going contact—or perhaps more. Many begin this process with a visit in the hospital and continue it with a parting celebration somewhere else, typically a restaurant. This ritual is especially important if the couple lives at a distance and will be leaving the city in which the gestational carrier gave birth. Most couples and carriers view it as a special time—a time to bring closure to this uniquely intense experience and to cement an everlasting bond.

The weeks and months following birth involve certain challenges. The separation can feel both awkward and uncomfortable to both carriers and couples. Some say that they were not sure when, how, or whether to contact each other. Both carriers and couples describe trying to balance their fears of being intrusive with their need to stay connected. Each may wait and hope that the other will call. For this reason, Dr. Hanafin recommends that couples and their gestational carriers make a plan for their next contact before they separate. Knowledge that they will speak by telephone or exchange letters within a week or two makes it easier for each to say good-bye.

Although there may be some sadness upon separation, everyone involved is also motivated to move on. The carrier has family to return to; the pregnancy, while satisfying, was distracting and required considerable time and energy. The couple, blessed with a child who never would have existed without the miracles of modern science, return to their lives.

Gestational care remains a new and relatively uncommon path to parenthood, reserved for those with particular medical indications and who can afford the high costs this treatment incurs. As with all third party arrangements, gestational care involves complicated social, ethical, emotional and legal issues. Those couples and carriers who pursue gestational care should do so with full awareness of the challenges that lie ahead.

Our sense is that couples and gestational carriers who decide to work together are strengthened by their common goal of bringing life to a child who would not otherwise exist, and bringing genetic parenthood to a couple who has suffered reproductive loss. It is a goal that celebrates the advances in modern reproductive medicine. One gestational carrier described her experience in this way:

I had the chance to help people become parents who should have had a child long ago. For me, that was a very wonderful thing to be able to do. Every time they send me a picture of her, I feel filled with pride. There are many things I haven't done in my life so far, but I have helped bring someone into the world who was trying very hard to be born.

CHAPTER

9

$\mathscr{E}$mbryo Adoption

Embryo adoption is the process whereby an embryo, created from the egg of a woman and the sperm of a man, is gestated in the womb of another woman to be raised by her and her partner, neither of whom provided the gametes. Although we refer to this process as adoption, we use that term strictly in a *social* sense rather than in a *legal* one. Like traditional adoption, the couple who raises the child has no genetic connections to him or her, but unlike traditional adoption, the couple does not have to go through a legal process in order to be declared the child's legal parents. Instead of legally adopting the child after birth, however, as is the case in all other adoptions, the couple biologically adopts during the early embryonic stage—at the point of embryo transfer.

Embryo adoption is an option for couples who want to share a pregnancy experience and have neither eggs nor sperm to contribute to that process. Embryo adoption is an option for single women desiring a pregnancy who do not have a designated sperm donor and are unable to use their own eggs. It is also an option for couples in which only one member is infertile but who want to have an equal genetic (i.e. non-genetic) relationship to their child.

From a medical-technical standpoint there are two ways to accomplish the process of embryo adoption. The first is for the couple to receive a pre-existing cryopreserved embryo(s) that has been donated by its genetic parents. The second is for a woman to undergo an ovum donation cycle in which donated eggs from one source are inseminated with separately obtained donor sperm. Although both methods result in an offspring who is not genetically connected to the parents, from an ethical, emotional, and social policy perspective, these two avenues to embryo adoption are decidedly different.

We call the first option, which results from the donation of an existing embryo, *embryo donation*, and the second option—the intentional creation of a child through donated eggs and donated sperm—*embryo creation*. In both cases, the offspring has no genetic connection to his would-be parents; we thus decided to place both options under the general heading of *embryo adoption*. We do recognize, however, that in a sense the use of the word *adoption* may be somewhat misleading, as traditional adoption has never involved the intentional creation of children for the purpose of being adopted. Thus embryo donation, which finds homes/ wombs for existing embryos, bears a greater resemblance to adoption than does embryo creation.

Embryo donation, like traditional adoption, began as a perceived solution to a problem. IVF programs and some of their patients were troubled by the prospect of having extracorporeal embryos that couples/individuals no longer wanted stored in their facility. This question was of particular relevance to people who had moral or religious objections to discarding embryos. The idea of donating those embryos to other infertile couples was appealing in much the same way as traditional adoption is appealing; it offered a legitimate and altruistic use for these surplus embryos and the opportunity for pregnancy and parenthood to childless couples. Embryo donation was attractive to ART programs from a legal perspective as well: by offering embryo donation they could avoid violating laws in states that prohibited experimenting on or discarding embryos.

As we will discuss later in this chapter, embryo donation has not proven to be the popular option that physicians and programs anticipated. There are fewer embryos available for donation than anticipated, for two reasons. First, most couples use their frozen embryos, either following an unsuccessful cycle or, later, after the birth of a child(ren) to expand their families. Second, many couples who once indicated they would willingly donate embryos later conclude that they are not comfortable with this choice.

Because of the apparent scarcity of embryos available for donation, and because some couples/individuals lack viable eggs and sperm, some clinics are now offering IVF cycles in which male and female donor gametes are used. To some this process may be considered a logical extension of single gamete donation; to others it is tantamount to creating children for adoption.

Although from a genetic and social standpoint offspring of created embryos are the same as the offspring of donated embryos, (they are not genetically related to either parent) the differences in their origins are substantial. In one instance the couple gestates and raises a child that began as an embryo intended for the genetic parents but is now destined not to be born. In the second instance, couples are intentionally taking gametes from two separate donors and creating an embryo for the sole purpose of "prebirth adoption."

Embryo adoptions are clearly new paths to parenthood, bringing with them complex psychological, social, emotional, and ethical considerations. We have neither experience nor psychosocial research to draw upon. Thus we must borrow insights from the fields of adoption and gamete donation as we discuss this option.

Reasons for Choosing Embryo Adoption

Many people, both outside and inside the field of infertility, wonder why a couple would choose embryo adoption rather than adopting a child who is already born. There are many reasons why this alternative is appealing.

For couples who have experienced long-term infertility, embryo adoption offers the opportunity to be pregnant and give birth, as well as the opportunity to parent. Through pregnancy, embryo adoption offers the couple a chance to bond with their child prior to birth. In addition, the woman has control over her child's prenatal environment, thereby eliminating potential problems caused by unhealthy gestational conditions.

For couples who have adjusted to infertility treatment and who are willing to undergo more medical procedures, embryo adoption may be preferable to tackling what they perceive as a complicated and often daunting new world—that of adoption. Furthermore, depending on the clinic and on whether the couple's health insurance policy covers the procedure, embryo adoption may be much more affordable than adoption after birth. Embryo adoption also offers the couple the guarantee of known paternity (not always the case with traditional adoption), assuming that the clinic shares medical, social, and psychological information about the genetic father in the case of embryo donation, and the sperm bank provides the same information about the sperm donor in the case of embryo creation. Embryo adoption also offers couples privacy. Traditional adoption, by definition, is always public, whereas embryo adoption can be private, allowing the couple to reveal it when and to whom they choose.

Embryo donation is appealing to couples who have problems with the idea of intentionally creating children/embryos to adopt. They prefer knowing that the embryo they adopt was conceived by a couple who longed to be parents and went to great lengths to achieve that goal. Embryo donation may be appealing to couples who believe that the blending of genes from the donating couple, whom they may imagine to be a close, loving pair, are in some way preferable to the imagined genes of birthparents who did not intend to create a child togther.

Embryo creation, on the other hand, is preferable to couples who believe it can offer them greater genetic selection. Although they realize that ovum donors are scarce and that donor selection may be limited, they know they can carefully select the sperm donor. This process of combining their choice of gametes may give them a greater sense of control, as well as the illusion that they are "designing" an ideal child. Couples who are attracted to embryo creation may also feel more emotionally secure that no one will come after their child, whereas with embryo donation the couple may fear that the genetic parents will someday try to claim him.

Ethical Issues in Embryo Adoption

Some in the field of reproductive technology believe that the ethical issues are the same for both created and donated embryos. Others make a distinction between the two. Thus some clinics offer embryo donation but will not create donor embryos, refusing to use both donor sperm and donor eggs in an ART cycle. Other clinics combine donor eggs and donor sperm to create embryos for couples but do not have an embryo donation program.

The Creation of Additional Children

An important ethical issue that arises with embryo adoption is whether it is morally right to create embryos when there are already children awaiting adoption. Those who feel it is not ethical to do so believe that the desires of infertile couples are taking priority over societal good, thereby ignoring the best interests of children. Most programs that will not create embryos for this purpose believe that the advantages that come with being able to gestate are not sufficient justification to create additional children because embryo adoption is genetically identical to adoption after birth. They also do not agree that because adoption is complex embryo adoption may be an easier route to having a child. Many who question the ethics of creating embryos for prebirth adoption believe that families do not have to be either racially or ethnically similar—that the ties necessary for maintaining healthy, loving families transcend racial or ethnic lines.

Elizabeth Bartholet, an author, expert on family law, and an adoptive parent, also questions these assumptions about families. She is an outspoken advocate of the rights of children and an outspoken critic of assisted reproductive technologies. Bartholet, in writing about all reproductive technologies that involve the use of third parties, states:

> Taking children's interests seriously would require us to think about the children we are creating with these new arrangements and about the children who already exist in this world. It would require us to ask whether it is good for children to be deliberately created so they can be spun off from their biologic parents and raised by others. It would require us to ask whether encouraging adults who might provide adoptive homes to produce their own adoptees is good for the existing children in need of such homes.[71]

Those who question the morality of embryo adoption when so many children are in need of homes also object to the way in which resources are being allocated. They cannot justify spending enormous sums of money to create nongenetic children for parents. They do not believe it is right for couples or insurance companies to invest tens of thousands of dollars in this process, especially when the odds are against them. Rather, they argue, the money would be far better spent on reforming the adoption system and helping couples who cannot afford to adopt but would like to do so, find children.

The arguments that it is wrong to create children for adoption when there are living children in need of adoption, and that spending vast amounts of money to do so only accentuates the injustice do not necessarily pertain to embryo donation. When an infertile couple donates surplus cryopreserved embryos to other infertile couples, the recipient couple is not receiving embryos that were created specifically for that purpose. Rather, the embryos were intended to be used by the genetic parents, but due to a change in circumstances—usually the births of their desired number of children—they no longer want to parent them. Because the embryos already exist, the financial cost of adopting them (usually between $3,000 and $4,000, the same as a frozen embryo transfer cycle) is much less than costs to create embryos via ovum donation and donor insemination.

The Commercialization of Embryos

Those who question the ethics of embryo creation are particularly concerned about the potential for commercialization—that donated embryos, as well as gametes used to create additional embryos, will become subject to supply and demand. Will infertile couples in their desperation to have children be willing to pay a high price—whatever the market will bear—for embryos to adopt or for gametes with which to create them? Some fear that the creation of donor embryos will become big business, with entrepreneurs emerging who will serve as embryo brokers, matching couples who can produce embryos to infertile couples who need them.

Bartholet addresses the question of commercialization:

> The IVF process is increasingly used to facilitate full adoptions, whereby one couple's embryos are donated or sold to another for implantation. The advent of embryo freezing can be expected to encourage such arrangements on a large scale. Tens of thousands of frozen embryos are now being stored for future reproductive use; most of them will probably not be used by the contributing couples.[72]

Although her concerns are understandable and the potential for commercialization of embryos exists, as we will see later in this chapter, the number of embryos available for donation is quite small, and there is no reason to believe those numbers will increase appreciably. Furthermore, although we only have anecdotal data to support this, it appears that only a small percentage of couples undergoing IVF procedures are requesting to use both donor eggs and donor sperm. When they do so—and when programs accede to this request—they are using eggs and sperm for which donors have received only modest compensation.

There seems little evidence that existing cryopreserved embryos will be commercialized. Almost all of these embryos are used by their genetic parents, either following a failed IVF cycle or as a means of expanding their family following a successful pregnancy. In addition, most clinics will not allow a couple to store an unlimited number of embryos: once they have accumulated a certain number (often four), they must have them transferred before undergoing a fresh IVF cycle. (This limit does not apply if more than the designated number are obtained in a particular cycle.) Thus, although it is true that ART programs have some "unwanted" frozen embryos, they are only a small percentage of those that were originally frozen. Furthermore we are aware of no programs that allow couples to sell rather than donate their "extra" embryos.

Still, Bartholet's concerns are not irrational. The procurement of eggs and sperm and the "rental" of wombs do have price tags, which many ethicists, attorneys, and some feminists feel are coercively high, while others feel are insultingly low. Hence it must appear to Bartholet and others that embryos, too, have a price, despite the fact that states have laws against such transactions. It is important for this discussion, however, to underscore the distinction between existing, donated embryos, which currently may only be donated, not sold, and created embryos, which might be intentionally conceived from male and female donor gametes. The former do not have a price tag; the latter, particularly because they require donated gametes, may have the potential for commodification and commercialization.

Unfairness to Genetically Related Siblings

Most couples who offer their embryos for donation have completed their families. Another argument by those who object to embryo donation is that the resulting children will have genetic siblings whom they will not know. This situation, they say, is unfair to both the children who were born to their genetic parents as a result of IVF and the children born as a result of embryo adoption. Many who agree in principle with this objection say that the solution is not to prohibit embryo donation but to allow it only if it is done openly, so that the genetic parents and/or siblings can have access to each other should they choose to do so. Others counter this objection by arguing that genetic bonds mean very little in and of themselves—that the bonds formed by kinship and family are the significant ones.

Additional ethical concerns that we have discussed in other chapters apply to embryo adoption as well: the right to have a child (especially so for couples who are older and may be past normal childbearing years);

the separation of the gestational, social and genetic aspects of mother and father (whether it is in a child's best interest to do so); the changing nature of family (whether it is in a child's best interest to be born through such an alternative arrangement to parents whose age and life-style may preclude them from providing an optimal environment for their child); and the potential medical risks to ovum donors in procuring eggs (in the case of created embryos). Because embryo donation is so recent, the long-term emotional and psychosocial effects on a couple (and their children) who have donated their jointly created embryos to another couple, are unknown.

Psychosocial Issues in Embryo Adoption

Traditional adoption has changed drastically in the past decade as we have come to understand the experience of adoption for birthparents, for adoptive parents, and for the children. Much of this understanding and change can and should be applied to embryo adoption.

Searching for Roots: The Need for Information

In the past, most adoption agencies operated on the premise that it was in the best interest of all parties for birthmothers and adoptive parents to have little or no knowledge of each other and for birthparents to have little or no contact at all with their baby. Adoption workers believed that birthmothers would not be able to "cut the emotional cord" if they were permitted to know or to connect in any way with their offspring and that they would have difficulty getting on with their lives if they were to learn information—even nonidentifying information—about the couple who was going to adopt their child. Similarly it was believed that adoptive parents would have trouble bonding with their child or claiming him or her as their own if they met or even had knowledge about the birthparents. The prevailing theory was that attachment and a sense of security would thus come more easily—that it was better not to know and to let genetics unfold in a mysterious fashion.

Mental health professionals who work with adoptive families have come to understand, from listening to adoptees, the yearning that many have to find their genetic roots. As we will discuss in the last chapter, this yearning appears to be of fundamental importance for some adoptees, and seeking their genetic origins may be instrumental in helping them solidify their identity. The information helps them feel complete. The need to know where one comes from in no way seems to be a statement about a lack of bonding with adoptive parents. On the contrary, adoptees who search usually have secure relationships with their families—as do those who choose not to search.

It appears that all parties to adoption have been shortchanged in the past. Birthmothers as well as adoptees have stepped forward to describe the aftermath of having their babies ushered away into what felt like a black hole, having no knowledge of where they were going and who would be raising them. Adoptive parents too craved information, especially as the years unfolded and they had no guideposts, and no facts, to offer their questioning children. As a result of this climate of separation and secrecy and growing awareness of the potentially harmful effects of a genetic void, the open adoption movement emerged.

Open adoption, a process in which birthparents and adoptive parents share information about themselves through letters, telephone calls, and sometimes through personal visits, has gained increasing recognition and acceptance among adoption professionals whose agencies currently practice open adoption to varying degrees. Current policy in the adoption world—even among agencies that practice confidential adoption—is to gather as much information as possible from birthparents about their medical, social, and emotional history. This information is shared with adoptive parents while preserving the privacy and anonymity of all parties. As the children grow, their parents can share information with them about their genetic origins. This information can be extremely helpful in ensuring a feeling of being tied to the past, developing a strong sense of oneself in the present, and having a sense of continuity about the future.

Embryo adoption offers the experience of pregnancy and childbirth—an experience longed for by many women. As soon as a child is born as a result of embryo adoption, however, the family experience is identical to that of other adoptive families, except that the former allows the mother to nurse her baby if she chooses to. (While it is complicated, it is possible for adoptive mothers to nurse babies.) Hence it is important to apply what we have learned from traditional adoption in setting policy regarding embryo adoption, especially the sharing of information between the genetic and the adopting parents. On behalf of their potential child, it is crucial that all adoptive parents—whether the adoption takes place after birth or prior to it—have access to information about their child's genetic parents. Information about their physical, medical, social, psychological, and educational history is likely to help the child's identity formation and self-esteem.

An Existential Conflict

One of the most important psychological differences—perhaps the most important—between offspring born as a result of embryo creation and those born from embryo donation, involves the source of the gametes. Most people born on this earth were conceived as a result of a relationship between two people who chose to be together. At worst that connection might have been a one night stand; at best it is an enduring relationship. An offspring born from embryo donation will know that its genetic parents were in an intimate relationship with each other and that they very consciously decided to become parents. In other words, this child—themselves—was meant to exist. Yet children born from donated embryos will have to deal with the fact that neither of their genetic parents wanted them. Since feelings of rejection are common for adoptees, it is possible that children born from donated embryos will feel rejected by their genetic parents. Some clinicians have speculated, however, that those who were adopted at the four cell stage, because they were not then a real person, might have fewer feelings of rejection by their genetic parents than those who were adopted after birth.

A child born from a created embryo, assuming she learns the truth about her origins (as she has a right to do) will know that the sources of the gametes who produced her did not ever have a human connection or a relationship with each other. Her existence may feel like a *cosmic accident*, like she was not truly meant to exist. Thus children born via embryo creation may have a more difficult time developing a sense of identity and a conviction that they have a place in the world.

Disclosure

As recently as a generation ago many adoptive parents kept adoption a secret from their child, having been advised that it was best for the child not to know the truth about his or her origins. To some extent this rationale was a result of the stigma attached to illegitimate children. According to the theory, if children did not know they were adopted, they would not be subjected to any humiliation. This advice was not only psychologically harmful but impractical; it is impossible to hide adoption unless a couple

328

moves to another part of the country and severs ties with family and friends. As we will see in the last chapter, as long as a secret is known to some people—and in the case of adoption many know—it can always be revealed. In addition, since adoptees often look and act very different from their parents, many guessed the truth. Some who were lied to initially when they asked if they were adopted were told the truth later, only to feel intensely betrayed. Now it is recognized that adopted children must be told the truth—early on—and that they need information about their birthfamily as well.

Although there has been movement toward openness in the use of gamete donation, as we will learn in the last chapter, historically most couples who build their families through DI (we do not yet have hard data about ovum donation) keep the information a secret from their child. Their reasons vary, but the stigma and shame attached to infertility—in particular, male infertility—is probably the underlying reason for secrecy, regardless of whether it is acknowledged as the reason. Because the mother's pregnancy camouflages the couple's method of reproduction, it is tempting not to tell.

In embryo adoption, it is also tempting not to tell; the secret is easily hidden. However, we believe that children who were adopted, regardless of whether the adoption took place at the embryo stage or after birth, deserve to know the truth about themselves. Furthermore they deserve to know facts about their genetic history, facts that will help in their development and maturation.

Availability and Practice of Embryo Adoption

In 1995 The Mental Health Professional Group of the American Society for Reproductive Medicine formed an *Embryo Donation Task Force*, the purpose of which was to survey ART clinics regarding embryo donation and to make recommendations for how it should be practiced. A questionaire was developed the following year and sent out to 315 clinics offering assisted reproductive technology (all the clinics who are members of SART). By the winter of 1997, 108 clinics had completed the survey. As this book goes to press in the fall of 1997, the data is being analyzed, so for the most part we can only give you general impressions based on a preliminary look (not statistical analyses) at the numbers. By the time this book is in print, however, the information should be available from the ASRM.

Dr. Sheryl Kingsberg, a psychologist and Assistant Professor in Reproductive Biology at Case Western Reserve and co-chair of the MHPG's Embryo Donation Task Force, speculates that those who did not return questionaires probably failed to do so because they either got lost in the shuffle (they were sent to the program rather than to a specific person) or because the particular clinic does not do embryo donation and therefore was not interested in the study. Kingsberg believes that clinics offering embryo donation would probably be interested in finding out what other clinics do, and therefore would be more likely to have participated in the study than those that are not offering it. Thus, although we cannot draw any definitive conclusions about the 207 clinics that did not return the questionaire, Dr. Kingsberg speculates (and we would agree) that many of them are not offering embryo donation—at least at this time—and chose not to complete the survey because they were either not interested or felt they had nothing to offer the study.

Of the 108 clinics completing the questionaire, 78 said they offered embryo donation, but only 40 had actually completed cycles. Of those programs completing cycles, a total of 53 births were reported. Because 207—almost two thirds—of the programs surveyed did not respond, can we still draw conclusions about the numbers of births that have resulted from embryo donation? We believe that it is reasonable to assume that few non-respondents are doing embryo donation, so that at the *very most* (assuming the returns did reflect a random sample) we can triple the numbers of cycles and live births. This conservative guestimate would mean that as of the winter of 1997, only about 150 babies—at most—have ever been born from *donated* (not *created*) embryos in this country! Thus the cryopreservation of embryos does not seem to have led to the widespread commercialization that Bartholet and others feared. Fifty-three babies in total is a "drop in the bucket," when compared to the tens of thousands of ART cycles completed yearly in this country (approximately 41,000 in 1993 according to SART data).

The surprisingly low number of births resulting from donated embryos raises the question of why more couples are not electing to donate their extracorporeal embryos to infertile couples, rather than discarding them or donating them to research if the clinic permits. An experience with cryopreserved embryos at Boston's Reproductive Science Center (formerly IVF America) is telling and may be give us clues as to why couples are not opting more frequently to donate embryos.

Prior to undergoing an ART cycle at Reproductive Science Center, couples have an initial consultation with a physician. The consultation includes the signing of consent forms, one of which refers to the future disposition of frozen embryos that they may not want. Although couples are free to change their mind in the future, almost all couples initially state that their intention is to donate their unwanted embryos—should any exist—to an infertile couple.

In April 1993, Reproductive Science Center sent out letters to 107 couples who had had frozen embryos in storage for at least two years. The purpose of the letter was to remind them about their embryos and to inquire about what they wanted to do with them: (1) use their embryos in a cycle within the next six months to try to establish a pregnancy for themselves; (2) leave them in storage; (3) instruct the clinic to discard them; (4) donate them to an infertile couple; (5) remove them from the clinic; or (6) donate them to research. Eighty-five couples responded to the letter (and a subsequent follow-up) by Nov. 1993. The most popular response (48%) was to delay the decision, leaving the embryos in storage; 19% chose to use them in a cycle; 13% indicated they wished to donate them to research; 12% opted to discard; 4% opted to move them to another clinic; and 5%—only four couples of eighty-five—wished to donate them to an infertile couple. Thus of the eighty-five couples who responded to the letter, sixty opted to keep the embryos (i.e. to delay the decision, cycle within six months, or move them to another clinic). And of the twenty-five couples who opted not to keep their embryos, only four couples—16% of them—chose to donate to another couple (later two of those couples changed their minds and decided not to donate). What was surprising was not the low incidence of couples opting for donation to another couple, but rather the dramatic change of heart by almost all couples.

Why do so many couples prior to beginning ART treatment indicate that they want to donate embryos they cannot use and later change their minds? One explanation is that because most couples with frozen embryos that have been stored over two years have children (63% of those who responded to the survey), they have living examples of what an embryo can become and they can no longer imagine giving up a child like the one they see in front of them. Another related explanation involves siblings. Individuals who donate their gametes are aware that their own

331

children will have half-siblings whom they will probably never know nor with whom they will grow up. Although this may be troublesome to some gamete donors, it is usually not an insurmountable obstacle to gamete donation. However, when the picture changes and couples realize that their children will have full genetic siblings they will not know, what was once viewed as an altruistic act may begin to feel emotionally impossible. Finally, couples who have no children but have embryos in storage may not be able to live with the possibility that another couple could raise their genetic child while they themselves remained childless.

Dr. Elaine Gordon, a psychologist in southern California who works with several ART programs, offers an observation that sheds light on the differences between how people regard their gametes and how they regard their embryos. She perceives that far more people seem willing to donate their individual gametes than to donate their joint embryos. From screening numerous women for ovum donation, many of whom have children and are married, we agree with these conclusions. Frequently potential donors say that they do not feel an egg is in any way close to a person. Once it is fertilized with the recipient's husband's sperm, they feel it is a long way from being their child, adding that if it were fertilized with their own husband's sperm it would be a very different story; then it would be their potential child, and they could not give it to someone else. These observations hint at why only a small percentage of couples appear to be willing to donate embryos they created jointly: it feels as if they are giving up their child.

Information and Informed Consent

The issue of informed consent is a difficult and confusing one in the area of reproductive medicine. Informed consent is even more complicated when it comes to procedures involving third parties, as there are additional psychological and social concerns as well as medical concerns. Embryo adoption, because it involves yet a fourth person—a set of genetic parents and (usually) a set of rearing parents—is even more complex.

Donating Couples

An important issue to be decided is whether potential donating couples should be required to meet with a mental health clinician before they can give true informed consent. The clinician is probably the best person to discuss with them the implications of their decision to donate embryos— on their child(ren), on the potential offspring, on his/her parents, and on themselves. The clinician is in a position to propose various scenarios that may develop in the future and to encourage the donating couple to think through them, imagining how they will feel or respond if such an occurrence should come to pass. Data obtained by the Embryo Donation Task Force indicates that only a minority of programs (21 out of 78 respondents) require donor couples to meet with the mental health clinician, and an extremely small minority of programs require legal consultation as part of informed consent.

This information is surprising (and dismaying) to us. Adoption agencies would never allow a birthmother to relinquish her child if she had not had counseling. Adoption practitioners always recommend that birthparents receive counseling before an adoption plan is finalized. Indeed the fact that adequate counseling is much less likely to be available in non-agency adoptions is the most frequently cited criticism of private adoption. Furthermore, increasingly many private adoptions involve varying degrees of openness, so that both birth and adoptive parents learn a great deal of information about each other. If indeed, upon further analysis of the data, the results generated by the Task Force prove to be accurate, it seems fair to say that most donating couples neither receive information about the "adopting" parents, nor have the opportunity to give informed consent, which can only be given after a thorough discussion with a mental health professional regarding the psychological, social, and emotional aspects of embryo donation.

The issue of informed consent raises a related question about whether donating couples should be "screened." Once again, the adoption model is appropriate. Birthparents coming to an adoption agency to make an adoption plan for the child they are expecting are interviewed thoroughly by trained social workers and are prepared, through counseling, for the ramifications of their decision. Birthparents are *counseled*, not *screened* in the manner that gamete donors are screened, because a child is about to be born who will need a home. Essentially that child already exists and therefore must be placed.

An important ethical question is whether a clinic (or society for that matter) has an obligation to find wombs/homes for embryos whose genetic parents decide to donate them. We would argue that if the clinic in question offers embryo donation, and the couple entered into the program knowing that donation was an option if they had extracorporeal embryos, then the clinic is obligated to make their best effort to find suitable parents. The clinic should also disclose whatever information they have to the "adopting couple." If they are unable to find an "adopting couple," (perhaps because the genetic parents have a problematic medical or psychological profile) then the clinic faces a potential conflict: they made a commitment to the genetic parents to offer donation but an appropriate couple cannot be found.

Recipient Couples

Of the 78 programs responding to the survey that offer embryo donation, only 45 require recipients to be screened by a mental health professional. Because we believe strongly that embryo adoption should be practiced as responsibly as traditional adoption is currently being practiced—with the best interests of children and their families in mind—we find it unsettling that close to half of the clinics offering donation do not think it is necessary for recipient couples to meet with a mental health clinician.

Perhaps the traditional adoption model can apply to embryo donation, in that most states require a homestudy before an individual/couple is accepted for adoption. Thus the potential adopters must meet certain criteria before being allowed to adopt a child. Although homestudies may be beyond the scope of services that ART clinics feel they can reasonably provide, a meeting with a mental health professional is not.

We have stressed the need for couples adopting embryos to receive extensive medical, physical, intellectual, and psychosocial information about the genetic parents. This is true regardless of whether the embryos were created with a donated egg and a donated sperm (embryo creation) or whether they were originally created for an ART couple who later decided to donate them. The preliminary findings of the Embryo Donation Task Force appear to indicate that many recipient couples—and ultimately the children who may be born—currently receive little information about their genetic parents.

The MHPG survey also asked questions about what information is given to recipient couples regarding the donor couple. Once again, preliminary numbers indicate that although the vast majority of clinics offer information about the physical characteristics of the donating couple, many clinics do not offer information about educational background, personality traits, skills, or interests.

A set of questions on the survey asked whether clinics would be willing to provide certain information to the offspring when s/he becomes eighteen. Although we cannot report accurate numbers now, it is clear that many clinics at this point in time either do not plan to offer the information to adult children, or they have not clearly thought through this issue (as indicated by the large numbers of clinics who did not respond to the questions). It is quite possible however, that in years to come a significant percentage of adults, adopted as embryos, will seek information about their genetic parents, realizing that they want/need to learn more about the latter's personality as well as their social, educational, occupational, and medical history. If the information is not forthcoming they may even resort to legal means to obtain it if the clinic is not willing to act as an intermediary. Although the numbers are small, embryo adoption is clearly an area where medical and social policy must be established.

Combining Embryos

A related and important issue for programs that have embryos available for donation is whether they will mix embryos from more than one couple in a single ART cycle. Since many couples who might opt to donate their frozen embryos have only one (or two) available and because pregnancy rates are low when just one or two embryos are transferred, it may be tempting to transfer embryos from more than one donating couple, to maximize the couple's chances of becoming pregnant. From a psychological and ethical perspective we feel strongly this practice is a mistake because it fails to take into consideration the best interests of the potential children.

Even if clinics provided extensive information about each couple whose embryos were donated, the adoptive parents would never know—unless they agreed to have their child undergo genetic testing after birth—whose child they were carrying should a pregnancy occur. The confusion in their minds could interfere with the bonding process that normally develops during pregnancy. Couples carrying their genetic child often wonder whether he or she will have the husband's blue eyes, the wife's dark hair, his musical talent, her athletic ability. Many characteristics unfold over time and are part of the mystery of maturation. However, if couples had embryos transferred from more than one donor couple, they would never know—assuming they receive information about each couple—whether couple A, couple B, or couple C were the genetic parents of their child. They might find themselves scrutinizing their child, overly preoccupied with signs that might indicate whether he is destined to become a professional athlete, a mathematical genius, or a jazz musician. Even if they were provided information about each donating couple, they would be likely to have preferences for one couple's embryo over another. Should genetic testing reveal the child came from a couple who was not their first-choice genetic parents, they could be disappointed, and possibly convey, though unintentionally, their feelings to their child.

Knowledge about a child's genetic blueprint can help parents attach only to the child who is theirs. We all understand that genes are a random collection from one's parents and that musical genius in one parent (or even two) for example, does not guarantee that offspring will inherit the desired trait. Although much of the pleasure in parenthood involves the unfolding of a mystery, most parents can turn to genetic history for guidance. Couples who are able to conceive and bear their genetic children are in for fewer surprises and less bewilderment about how their children become who they are. Even more important than parental knowledge, however, is our obligation to the offspring, for children who have no knowledge of their genetic history frequently live with a sense of bafflement about how they came to be and bewilderment about who they are. Our current understanding about human nature and the psychological development of human beings indicates that a genetic void is not in the best psychological interest of a person.

Those who advocate mixing embryos—and they tend to be physicians—argue that because the chances for pregnancy are better when more embryos are placed into the uterus, that should be sufficient reason for mixing. They believe that couples should be informed about their options, including the possibility of transferring embryos from more than one donor couple. Furthermore, they argue, if couples desire to mix embryos, they should be allowed to do so, and to create a policy against such a practice would be not only discriminating but paternalistic. Mental health clinicians counter that argument by reminding physicians that infertility is a major crisis. Infertile couples are often so desperate to have children that they may turn to the most expedient alternative available without thinking through the medical or psychological ramifications of that choice.

Embryo donation seems to be relatively rare among ART programs, confirmed by the recent survey done through the Mental Health Professional Group of the American Society for Reproductive Medicine. Though rare, we cannot ignore the fact that 53 babies have been born over the years through embryo donation in the 108 clinics that responded to the survey, and the actual number could be triple that. We do not know at this point the number of children conceived via the procurement of both donor eggs and donor sperm (*created embryos*), nor the number of clinics willing to provide them for couples. Both methods of embryo adoption, however, produce the same result: a child not genetically connected to the rearing parents but gestated by the mother. And both methods bring with them a host of ethical, social, and psychological implications.

CHAPTER

10

$\mathcal{J}$elling the Truth:
Why, When, and How to Do So

Couples who turn to assisted reproduction—and especially to third party parenting options, inevitably have questions about how they will feel when their long awaited child finally arrives. Will the years and struggle of infertility take a large toll? Or will their experiences in the maze of infertility serve as good preparation for the varied trials of parenting? A full discussion of parenting after assisted reproduction is beyond the scope of this book. However, this chapter will address a central question—perhaps the most essential question—that third party and many ART parents ask: Should we tell our children how they were conceived, and if so, how and when?

As we have noted throughout this book, concerns about privacy and secrecy are central to the experience of infertility and to its resolution. Couples must constantly ask themselves, "Is this something we want or need to keep private or is there a purpose and a value in disclosing it?" They must also grapple with whether maintaining privacy means they are actually fostering a secret which has the potential—because of its hidden nature—to be damaging.

Parents who build their families through assisted reproduction with their own gametes and those who turn to third party parenting options find themselves at different points on the privacy-secrecy continuum. Those who achieve pregnancy with their own gametes generally feel free to decide which parts of their infertility experience they would like to share with their child(ren). Just as fertile couples do not usually tell their children whether they were conceived in a bedroom or in the back of a car, couples using ART are not obliged to tell their children about IVF or GIFT. However, just as many fertile parents eventually do tell their children something about their decision to become parents, couples who have conceived via ART may similarly conclude that they want their children to know how hard they worked, how much they struggled and endured, in order to have them.

Parents whose children came to them with the help of third parties inevitably face larger challenges regarding privacy and secrecy. Today many parents and professionals (we wish it were all) agree that children have a right to know the truth about their origins, but how and when to reveal these truths can be difficult decisions. Moreover, the current appreciation for the importance of truth telling exists against a historical backdrop that was quite different—one that actively promoted secrecy and shame.

In this chapter we will discuss the secrecy that pervaded—and often still pervades—gamete donation, and we will provide explanations for why secrecy can be so damaging. We will discuss some of the questions that arise in talking to young children about their origins, and we will offer some suggestions about how to do so. This chapter is not meant to be a how-to manual—because everyone's family story is different. It is our hope, however, that it will provide third party parents with a solid understanding of why they are committing themselves to truth telling within a framework about how to do so. We hope that it will help parents to stay the course with confidence and with a firm belief in the rightness of their undertaking.

The Historical Context of Secrecy: An Unfortunate Tradition

As we mentioned in "Donor Insemination" (Chapter 5), the tradition of secrecy that until recently dominated the way DI was practiced began approximately one hundred years ago, with the first donor insemination performed by Dr. William Pancoast. He claimed to have told the husband, but not the wife whom he inseminated, about the existence of a donor. Physicians performing the procedure in subsequent years have clearly been more forthcoming with the wives, but the notion of secrecy from everyone else has been built into the process, and it has influenced the practice of all third party options.

Although we feel dismayed that truths have been kept from donor insemination offspring, we believe that this practice probably began with good intentions. Many couples who formed their families via donor insemination in years past report similar versions of their introduction to this option. The physician ushered them into his office, smiled grimly, and said, "Unfortunately, Mr. Smith, you just don't have enough sperm to impregnate your wife. However, you can still have a child. We'll use sperm from a donor—probably a medical student. It's the best treatment for male infertility. Your wife will become pregnant and no one will ever know how. There is no reason to tell anybody, certainly not the child. You will be the father and for all intents and purposes your family will be just like anyone else's. In fact, you should probably have intercourse after the insemination, that way you will never know for sure whose sperm it was and you can always think that it was yours." Because physicians were (and still are) put on pedestals, most couples unquestioningly followed their doctor's direction. It sounded so logical. Many couples never even discussed their feelings— or the implications of donor insemination—with each other, and lived their lives with sealed lips, fearful that their secret would be discovered.

There are several problems with presenting donor insemination (or other third party options) in the above fashion. For one thing, DI is not a treatment for male infertility. Rather, it is an alternative way to form a family for couples with male factor infertility. Presenting donor insemination as a treatment implies that it is a solution or cure, and although DI is a cure for childlessness, it is not a cure for infertility. Although the original intention was probably to minimize the couple's feelings of loss upon learning about their infertility, presenting donor insemination as a solution robs them of the opportunity to grieve the loss of conceiving a child together, to resolve their grief, and then to move on so that they can embrace the child they eventually do parent together. Furthermore, the mandate for secrecy increases a man's sense of shame by implying that there is something inherently wrong with donor insemination, for why else would it be hidden? And since DI involves putting another man's semen inside a wife, to some the act may connote adultery—another explanation for the shame that couples may feel. Finally, the suggestion to have intercourse after the insemination, thereby obscuring the child's true paternity (in some cases physicians actually mix donor and husband semen), unrealistically implies that perhaps the couple will come to feel that the donor conception was "just like having their own biological child," and that they will "forget" the circumstances of its conception.

These messages are damaging as well as misleading. As we acknowledge today, donor insemination is not the same as having a child who is the genetic product of both parents, and couples never forget how their child was conceived, regardless of whether they ever speak about it. Furthermore these statements convey the message that something is wrong with them if they have uncomfortable feelings or nagging questions about donor insemination.

The practice of keeping DI a secret existed for several reasons. Until the last quarter of the 20th century, mental health clinicians were rarely involved in reproductive medicine, and it was solely physicians who discussed DI with the couple. Since physicians were trained neither in family therapy nor in child psychology, they could not know whether openness or secrecy was advisable. Nor could they understand the potential impact of secrecy in years to come—on the child, on the relationship between the child and his/her parents, on the relationship between the parents, and on the family as a whole.

Unfortunately, despite the progress that has been made both in understanding infertility and in eliminating negative male and female stereotyping, there is still much stigma—and therefore shame—associated with male infertility. Since fertility is often equated with virility and masculinity, infertile men are sometimes viewed as impotent and unmasculine. Thus delivering the bad news of male infertility—or worse, sterility—is a difficult and unpleasant task, perhaps more difficult when communicated from man to man. In an informal poll of five doctors in an infertility practice (four of whom were male), all said they had a harder time discussing male infertility than female infertility with their patients.

Although we strongly believe that the primary reasons for promulgating secrecy involve protection against feelings of grief, shame, and loss, it is probably true that medical practitioners promoting secrecy also believe that it is best for the children. In her book, *Having Your Baby By Donor Insemination*, Elizabeth Noble, a nationally recognized childbirth educator, quotes several obstetricians (writing during the 1970s) who strongly believe that couples should tell no one—not even friends or relatives. These physicians felt that if couples were unable to keep the fact of DI confidential, they were not ready to do it. One physician even offered a plan of undoing—deception—to those who had previously discussed donor insemination with others. Proponents of secrecy argued that children could be confused about their identity if they were to learn the truth about their conception. Thus secrecy was seen as a way to shield them as well as their parents. Unfortunately the long term needs and ramifications of donor insemination on both children and their families did not seem to be anticipated nor considered.

Most couples who decide to form their families through either sperm or ovum donation do so using anonymous donors. Research has revealed that as recently as the early 1990s, the majority of couples who formed their families via anonymous donor insemination were deciding to keep the means of conception a secret from their child(ren). A 1993 article by Klock summarized seven studies that addressed this question: three were done in America, two in Australia, one in France, and one in Canada. Couples were asked whether they planned to tell their child about donor insemination. Percentages ranged from one study in which 86% said they would not tell, while 14% said they would, to another study in which 61% said they would not tell while 39% said they would.[73]

Although statistics are not yet available on the percentage of ovum donor couples who plan to tell their children about his/her means of conception, anecdotal research reported by mental health clinicians working with such couples indicates that many accept it as a given that they will tell their children how they became a family. Because we know how tempting secrecy can be, we provide the following sections.

Openness: An Ethically and Psychologically Sound Approach

The importance of telling children the truth about their origins was not always recognized or understood. In the past, parents by both DI and adoption were advised—even instructed—not to tell their children the truth about their origins. In recent years, however, there has been a noticeable shift towards openness. For over a generation adoptive families have been advised about talking to their children about adoption, and more recently increasing numbers of donor families as well as professionals question both the ethics and the wisdom of secrecy. As clinicians our own perspective on this issues has changed dramatically. When we entered this field, almost twenty years ago, we did not have strong opinions about this issue. Our learning and experience over the years has informed us that for ethical as well as for psychological reasons disclosure is the right approach— the one most likely to create psychologically healthy families.

Theories regarding disclosure have been developed primarily from anecdotal research, because DI families are very difficult to identify and study (as they have been so secretive), and ovum donor families are too new to have been researched. Opinions favoring disclosure are based primarily on four categories of information: current knowledge about the importance of genetics; knowledge gained from adoptees and adoption professionals; our growing understanding about the destructive nature of all kinds of family secrets; and reports from donor offspring who found out about their conception "accidentally," usually during unfortunate circumstances.

The Importance of Genetics

Times are changing and the fact that disclosure is now such a central issue in gamete donation reflects how much we have learned about the role of genetics in a person's life. A generation or so ago, couples who adopted children from agencies were cheerfully handed their babies and told to "raise this child exactly as you would had you given birth to it, and other than looking different from you, it will become the same person it would, were it your biological child."

Thus the prevailing belief until relatively recently was that nurture, rather than nature, was primarily responsible for determining how people develop and become who they are. Children who appeared to have happy childhoods, who stayed out of trouble, and who became productive adults, were determined to have been raised properly, by loving parents with good values. Conversely, when children got into trouble, or developed social or psychological problems as teens or adults, the parents tended to be blamed, if not overtly, at least covertly. In fact much of psychoanalytic theory is based on explanations that blame psychopathology on parental (mostly mothers') failures.

In recent years, research from the scientific community has pointed to the increasing importance of genetics in a person's life. Once thought to be almost irrelevant in determining character and destiny, genetics is now understood to be a major player. Although no one yet knows the precise nature/nurture formula, we do know that nature is far from irrelevant. We understand that although discipline, encouragement, and a good education can go a long way when it comes to achievement, it is also true that one's basic abilities—whether mathematical, athletic, artistic, etc—are innately determined. If an individual does not have the requisite genetic make-up s/he cannot become an Olympic athlete despite rigorous training. Many psychological and social traits—extroversion, neatness, a sense of humor, how quickly one walks or talks, for example—once thought to be environmentally determined, are now understood to be in large measure inherited. Furthermore, current research has also determined that certain illnesses—both mental and physical—may be linked to one's heredity. Knowing one's genetic origins, i.e. medical history, can in some instances, play a role in the prevention or amelioration of disease.

The importance of genetics in determining how one's life unfolds does not mean, however, that families or environment are unimportant. Researchers agree that strong and loving families are an important ingredient in children's healthy development, playing a major role not only in the formation of their self-esteem, but also in the actualization of their potential. Loving parents who value their children's uniqueness and do all they can to provide them with the psychological, social, and educational tools to realize their potential are much more likely to see their children develop into happy, well-adjusted adults. Environmental influences thus play an important role in helping (or hindering) one's best (or worst) potential to emerge but they cannot change one's basic genetic blueprint.

The Right to Information about Oneself

Human beings have a basic right to know the truth about their genetic origins. In some respects this statement may seem to be an obvious truth, but professionals in both adoption and donor insemination who advocated secrecy and parents who followed suit did not believe in—or at least did not support—this right. Given our current knowledge about genetics, it is difficult to understand how modern parents of children conceived with donor gametes can justify not telling the truth. Withholding this information means that their children will go through life with an inaccurate medical record. They will in turn pass this false information on to their children, and the lie will go on into perpetuity. In 1987 when Elizabeth Noble wrote a book about donor insemination she declared:

> All persons have a moral right to information that concerns themselves and the circumstances of their birth. The truth does not belong to the parents to withhold—it is the child's birthright. Parents must develop the wisdom and courage to squarely face the whole issue. It is their responsibility to tell the truth, no matter how difficult or painful that task may be.[74]

The ethical question of whether a person has a right to know the truth about his/her genetic origins raises an additional question about whether a person has the right to specific information regarding those origins. Probably all proponents of disclosure would argue that individuals not only need, but deserve as much informaton as possible about themselves. This notion, however, begs the question of whether that individual has a right to know the *identity* of the person who provided the sperm or the egg.

There are currently three sperm banks in the United States that have a pool of identity release donors—men who have agreed to meet their offspring once he or she is at least eighteen. However, all other sperm banks—approximately two hundred—guarantee their donors anonymity. Anonymity though, does not mean absence of information, and most sperm banks in this country, recognizing that the climate is changing, are providing extensive, though non-identifying, information to couples about their potential donors. Similarly, most ovum donor programs seem to be offering extensive information to recipients. This information, however, reflects the donor's psycho-social and medical history up to the point in time of the donation. Updates are neither required nor actively promoted.

Questions about how much information to provide, whether donors should be identified or required to be registered, and whether or not offspring should be told about their donor conception are being debated around the world. It is likely that in the next five or ten years policies regarding gamete donation will change dramatically in many countries. In fact some countries have already enacted legislation or changed their policies in this regard. In 1985 Sweden passed a law (The Swedish Law on Artificial Insemination) regulating donor insemination, and forbidding the use of donated eggs, (although this aspect of the legislation is in the process of being changed). The law gives donor conceived adults the right to obtain the identity of their donor. Although the law does not require the parents to inform the child about the donor-conception (that would be difficult to regulate), couples choosing DI are informed that the offspring will have the right to trace the donor. Clinics are also instructed to confirm that couples plan to tell their child(ren) about the donor conception.[75] A similar law was subsequently passed in Austria as well.

In 1994, as a result of rapidly changing attitudes in New Zealand towards gamete donaton, a two person Ministerial Committee on Assisted Reproductive Technology recommended that a policy of access to information about genetic origins be instituted. This policy was thought to represent "the best interests of offspring," though it was not deemed necessary to institute legislative changes in order to accomplish this end. The Privacy Act, passed in 1993, was thought to cover situations involving the release of information—including the identity—of gamete donors. This information was regarded as "health information" to which offspring were entitled under the law. The committee also recommended some form of counseling for all recipient couples, referring to it as "counseling for openness." Given New Zealand's committment to openness in general, this recommendation can probably be interpreted to mean a directive approach, i.e. encouraging openness, (as contrasted with the non-directive approach used by most counselors in other countries) .[76]

Erica Haimes, a noted sociologist at the University of Newcastle upon Tyne, also argues for donor registries. Haimes states:

> Once it is accepted (as it has been by the Warnock Report) that the child's conception should not remain a secret, and once the legal issue of the child's legitimacy has been resolved, the basis for preserving the donor's anonymity, from the child's point of view, on the face of it seems weak... Therefore, it could be argued that, rather than all parties being protected by the anonymity of the donor, it is, in fact, the donor who is protected, at the child's expense.[77]

Knowledge Gained from Adoption

In recent years there have been many accounts in all facets of the media of adoptees (usually in their twenties and thirties) searching for their birth-parents. The stories are poignant—capturing the most profound of human emotions—lost pasts newly regained, identities reclaimed and futures insured. Sadly, these accounts frequently frighten prospective adoptive parents (and to some extent many potential gamete donation recipients) from building a family created through another's genes. They fear rejection (and replacement) by the child they nurtured so lovingly its whole life. Because we regard gamete donation as a "halfway adoption," at least in a genetic and psycho-social sense (though clearly not in a legal sense), we feel strongly that the knowledge gained from adoptees regarding their struggles for identity can help us understand similar struggles experienced by donor offspring.

Some adoptees describe a sense of confusion that comes from not knowing to whom they belong or from where they came. They describe a feeling of rootlessness—of having sprung from nowhere, leaving their identity in question. Adoptees are therefore more prone to feeling alone or disconnected, despite how emotionally attached they may be to their families. This sense of genetic disconnection is what prompts many adoptees to find their birthparents—in order to find themselves.

Although a search can feel threatening to parents who love and are connected to their child every bit as much as if they had given birth to it, adoptees who search—except in extreme cases—are not doing so to find their "real parents." They are clear that the "real parents" are the ones who raised them—who cared for them on a daily basis, who worried about them when they were sick, tucked them in at night, attended school events, played ball, disciplined them, and gave them love and guidance throughout their lives. A search for birthparents is in reality a search for oneself, not a search for other parents.

Literature on adoption is full of accounts of such searches and reunions. Although most go well and enable the searcher to find closure, occasionally they do not. Some—though not most—birthparents are rejecting, and others are found living in unfortunate and depressing life circumstances. Sometimes adoptees discover that their expectations about "fitting into" their birthfamilies were unrealistic. Whatever the end result, however, adoptees usually report both a sense of closure and of feeling more complete when they encounter the person(s) who created them and learn information about their genetic identity and genealogical heritage.

It is likely that the increased number of adoptees searching for birthparents in recent years is prompted by three phenonmena: recognition of the importance of genetics; greater cooperation and openness from agencies and legal institutions; and greater acceptance by society. In the days when heredity was thought to play a minor role in the unfolding of traits and personality, as well as health, adoptees may have thought less about their genes. Now that we understand the powerful influence of heredity, it stands to reason that a person who does not know the origins of his/her genes, would be curious to find out. Adoption agencies, courts, and hospitals that hold records are also cooperating (to greater or lesser extents) with adults who wish to trace their origins, aware that times are changing and that openness—rather than secrecy and dead ends—is in a person's best interest. Furthermore, these factors have made it more acceptable for adoptees to want information about their birthfamilies.

Despite these changes in knowledge and social climate, many adoptees do not seem to be curious about their origins. Although they may recognize genetic influence as being important, some hold the view that there is a *humankind gene pool* —that no one person or family has a monopoly on a particular gene. In other words, all traits, characteristics, and abilities exist in multiple forms, in multiple people. Therefore they are not interested in meeting the person who provided the egg or the sperm that created them. Those who hold that perspective reason that they know who they are, and that knowing the person(s) from whom they sprang will make no difference in their identity. Other adoptees less interested in connecting with their families of origin feel comfortable and complete with the importance of nurture in their lives, explaining that they have always felt a sense of psychological "fit" with their adoptive families.

Adoptees who search for their birthparents do so for many reasons. Some may want to learn more about their cultural or religious family heritage; others may want to understand why they were given up. Still others describe a sense of not fitting into the psychological framework of their family. They may be optimists among pessimists or athletes among couch potatoes.

Adoptees who search may belong to what might be called the *unique gene pool* school. Recognizing that no one else exists in the world who is exactly like them, and that their particular genetic make-up is unique, they are intent on discovering the source of their existence. Furthermore, some people are naturally curious about all facets of life, including themselves, while others who may be more easy going, are not necessarily interested in probing life's depths—including their own.

The parallel to gamete donation is hopefully obvious at this point. The concept of genetic disconnection or confusion may apply to donor offspring as well as to adoptees. Knowing half of one's genetic identity may not be enough for some to feel secure about how s/he came to be. Donor offspring, especially if they are dissimilar to both parents (and may have inherited many of their dominant traits from the donor), may be especially vulnerable to feeling different or out of place in their families. It is likely they will be curious about the donor and want to know as much as possible about him or her. Hence it is important that parents through gamete donation obtain as much information as possible about the donor, understanding that only identity -release donors can be traced. Although it is possible the law will change over the next few decades, it will be difficult—if not impossible—for most donor offspring born today to find their donor parent. Prospective parents, however, can acknowledge their children's needs by choosing sperm banks and ovum donation programs that are forthcoming in providing information—information that may be essential in helping their child fit the pieces of his/her life together.

The Impact of Secrecy

In the winter of 1997, Madeleine Albright, the Secretary of State was the recipient of a startling revelation. Raised as a devout Catholic by her parents, who emigrated to the United States from Czechoslavakia when she was a young child, Albright learned that in fact all four of her grandparents had been Jewish and three had perished in the Nazi death camps. Her parents, having fled from Hitler, took on a new identity, erasing their heritage, keeping it a secret from everyone—including their own children—and fabricating a past that never existed. Whether Albright had actually known or suspected the truth about her heritage prior to her admission of it in 1997 is not clear. What is most important is that she eventually learned the truth as a mature adult, long after her parents had died. We can speculate that the discovery of their deception and of her own unacknowledged roots must have wrought far more emotional havoc than it would have had they been forthcoming all along.

The February 24, 1997 edition of *Newsweek Magazine* ran a feature article (alongside a story about Albright's discovery) entitled "Family Secrets." The article described several instances—many involving celebrities—of family secrets spilled out of the closet. Some of these secrets involved revelations regarding previously unknown biological parentage. Next to the article was a powerful quote by the authors that reflects its primary message: "From hidden adoptions to hushed-up romances, that which you don't know still has the power to hurt you."[78] Hence we see that the perspective—that secrets are destructive forces within a family constellation—extends far beyond experiences in adoption and third party parenting.

The history of adoption practice provides an important lesson about origin-related family secrets. For much of the first half of this century most adoption professionals advised parents never to tell their children that they had not been born to them. Adoptive parents often constructed elaborate ruses involving feigned pregnancies to lay the framework for this deception. But these secrets were too often revealed by other relatives, or on parents' deathbeds, or in clearing up an estate, leaving adoptees feeling betrayed by the parents they had loved. It was professionals' acknowledging the magnitude of their professional error, and the impact on the families they helped to create, that provided much of the impetus to change the way adoption was practiced from the 1960s forward.

Increasing numbers of mental health professionals are speaking and writing about family secrets. Their message is the same as the *Newsweek* article. Most of their conclusions are based on their experience working with families who are in trouble and are seeking professional help. The secret, whatever it is, is usually thought to be the basis of much of the difficulty. It must be acknowledged that relying only on anecdotal evidence has its flaws. By definition there is no control group available—i.e. families with well-kept secrets with whom to compare the troubled families. That does not mean, though, that we should ignore the experiences of those who are speaking up and urging others not to promote secrecy in families. On the contrary, we must listen carefully to those whose personal or professional experience has caused them to be spokespeople for openness.

Because families formed via gamete donation have almost uniformly kept it a secret from their children, in the past decade many mental health professionals in reproductive medicine have been speaking up about the potentially destructive impact such a secret can have. Patricia Mahlstedt and Dorothy Greenfeld, experienced clinicians and researchers, recognize that certain situations, generally involving cultural or religious traditions, may prompt a desire for secrecy. However, in a 1989 article in *Fertility and Sterility*, "Assisted Reproductive Technology with Donor Gametes: The Need for Patient Preparation," they present cogent arguments for being open with donor offspring about the origins of their conception, including the following:

> There is a growing body of research documenting the
> negative effects of family secrets and their unique power
> in the family. Since there is no psychological theory which
> supports secrecy in any situation, secrecy about one's begin-
> nings is particularly difficult to justify, as it places a lie at the
> center of the most basic of relationships, the one between
> parent and child.[79]

Annette Baran and Reuben Pannor, social workers who have been involved for decades in the field of adoption and more recently have written about donor insemination, are known for their strong stand against secrecy in DI. Their book, *Lethal Secrets*, published in 1989, created a stir among many professionals in the field of infertility, for whom the notions of donor insemination and secrecy had gone hand in hand. Baran and Pannor studied DI—the effects on offspring and on their families—after being involved in a number of situations in which donor families sought help. Their research spanned six years and included 171 self-selected subjects: donor offspring, donor couples, sperm donors, single women, and lesbian women.[80]

These authors have chilling stories to tell: of adult children who learned they were conceived by donor sperm after a parent had died and the remaining parent could no longer tolerate the burden of the secret; of families in which the father could never get close to his children—presumably because he feared that if he got too close, the secret might be revealed; of couples who decided to adopt a second child, rather than conceive another through donor insemination, because the father's negative feelings about his infertility had begun to surface and to feel overwhelming. In some cases divorce precipitated the telling; one mother felt that if her children knew the truth, they would understand why their father was abandoning them and might not feel so rejected. The authors point out that although initially in all these situations the parents had every intention of keeping DI a secret forever, in most cases the truth came out, and often in a punitive way.

Like adoptees before them, many donor offspring interviewed described the confusion they felt upon learning about their conception, and the feelings of anger and betrayal that resulted from not having been told the truth all along. For many, learning the truth was an enormous relief; it explained some of the strangeness they experienced in their family. The consensus of most of the donor offspring, however, is that it is not the fact of DI to which they are objecting—they would not exist without it—but rather the secrecy in which it is practiced that creates the problem.

In *Having Your Baby by Donor Insemination*, author Elizabeth Noble refers to Suzanne Ariel, an activist in the adoption reform and donor insemination movement, who is herself a donor offspring. Ariel learned about the origins of her conception when she was 31, shortly after her mother died. Her father, who could no longer keep the secret, told her the truth in the presence of his therapist. She speaks out about the deception involved in the practice of DI.

> The lies and deceptions upon which DI families are built,
> warp and poison family relationships. No healthy family can

be built upon such lies and deception; and in the DI family, deception is at the very core of the relationship. It is a cruel hoax to play on a trusting child.

Candace Turner is another donor offspring who devotes much time to speaking out and educating others about what she feels are the evils in the practice of donor insemination. She learned about her DI status when she was 13 in the midst of a family fight. Although she cares for and respects her father, she believes that her parents made serious mistakes in how they handled donor insemination in the family. Turner, who experienced six years of infertility herself before conceiving her four children, identifies strongly with the plight of infertile couples. She is not against donor insemination as much as she is against the secrecy that typically surrounds it.

The March 7, 1994, edition of *Newsweek Magazine* contains a first person article, "Whose Eyes are These, Whose Nose?" written by Margaret Brown, a nineteen-year-old college freshman who was conceived via donor insemination. She learned the truth when she was 16 after her parents had been divorced for several years. In the article Brown, who openly shares her confusion about her identity, urges DI parents to find out who their donors are, to keep records, and to give the information to their child. Her words are poignant:

> This is my nightmare—I'm a person created by donor insemination, someone who will never know half of her identity. I feel anger and confusion, and I'm filled with questions. Whose eyes do I have? Why the big secret?.... The news has affected my sense of identity and belonging. 'Who am I? is a hard question to answer when I don't know where I came from... I have a more difficult obstacle since the secret's been out: trust. I've wondered if there are other secrets being kept from me... Parents must realize that all the love and attention in the world can't mask that underlying almost subconscious feeling that something is askew.

Some couples choose openness because they are uncomfortable with the notion of keeping a secret and fear that someone will guess the truth, catching them off guard. One DI couple came to meet with a psychologist because the mother, although having agreed initially to keep DI a secret, wanted to change their agreement. She was tired of having to monitor herself. The father was hurt and appalled, not only by her strong feelings, but also by what he felt to be a betrayal of trust. His wife's change of heart had been precipitated by various conversations with friends. On numerous occasions people asked questions that made her feel uncomfortable and forced her to lie, such as "Who did Jimmy get his curly hair from?" or "Was his father that big when he was two?" One woman who knew the couple had gone through infertility treatment asked, "How did you ever get Jimmy?" Although others who do not know the truth rarely guess, the point is that the fear of someone guessing is the real threat. Being open means that they no longer have to live with this fear.

Being open allows family members to be close to one another without having to erect emotional boundaries. Keeping a secret means that there must be some distance between those who hold the secret and those who are not supposed to find it out. The closer one person gets to another— whether husband to wife, or parent to child—the more likely it is that she or he will see something that has not been previously revealed. Being open means that parent and child and husband and wife need have no barriers to intimacy between them.

Family therapists claim that even when secrets do not come out in the open, their very existence creates an atmosphere of uneasiness. Children pick up on nonverbal cues and sense that something is odd within the family. The exact nature or the source of the problem may not be known, yet children surmise that something or some piece of information is being withheld from them, and that they are not supposed to ask about it. Secrecy also breeds shame, and children who grow up in such families may turn that shame inward, feeling that there must be something fundamentally bad about themselves.

The negative effects of keeping a secret and the emotional burden of it may be felt long past childhood, and parents can be anguished for years about whether to reveal the truth to their adult children. A case example illustrates this point well. A woman in her mid-fifties was seriously considering telling her two DI-conceived children, now in their twenties, the truth about their origins. She had been divorced from their father since the children were very little, and over the years, although he moved hundreds of miles away, she had done her best to help them maintain a relationship. Her ex-husband, however, barely kept in touch with the children, and years would go by without contact. Her daughter, currently in graduate school, had struggled for years with feelings of rejection from her father. She could not understand why he abandoned her and kept blaming herself for their lack of a relationship. Her mother believed that her daughter's low self-esteem was attributable, at least in part, to these feelings of abandonment. The mother sought out a psychologist familiar with these issues because she needed help with her dilemma.

Although years before she had vowed to keep the secret, she was no longer dealing with an abstract idea, but rather with a person whose mental health seemed at stake. She believed that if her daughter knew the truth about her DI origins, she would not experience her father's abandonment of her so personally. The mother hoped her daughter would understand that her father's actions were most likely connected to his unresolved feelings about infertility, and that she would then be able to move on in her own life, free from her unresolved feelings toward her father. The mother had no illusions that her daughter's problems would be solved merely by revealing the secret. She understood that telling the truth would likely result in other emotional dilemmas for her daughter, yet her hope was that ultimately the positive effects of telling would far outweigh the negative ones. The psychologist helped her client explore the ramifications of telling versus not telling. She also agreed to meet with the mother and her children in the future, should she decide to tell, and should the latter desire a meeting.

Almost two years later the therapist heard from the daughter. Although she mentioned having learned about her DI origins, she stated that her purpose in setting up the appointment was to discuss the troubling relationship in which she was currently involved. The daughter came in for several sessions, but unfortunately ended treatment because she was having financial trouble. Although the focus was on ending the troubled relationship, it was understood that her relationship with her father—and the implications of her DI origins—may have contributed to her current problem. During one session she stated that she wished she had learned sooner about her conception, but understood why her mother had not told her. She surmised that perhaps her relationship with her father would have been better had she been told when she was very young; that way she could have let her father know that she loved him, even though she didn't come from his genes.

Openness allows trust to develop between parent and child. If there is a secret, and the secret is revealed under unfortunate circumstances, or is sensed or guessed by the offspring, the bond of trust is harmed, and it is extremely difficult to repair. When children have been deceived once, they fear they cannot trust their parents again. They point to adoption's lessons for confirmation. George Annas, an attorney and ethicist, agrees with this notion. In writing several years ago about donor insemination (before ovum donation began) he stated:

> It seems to me a similar argument can be made for consistently lying to the child—i.e., that it is a violation of parental-child confidence. There is evidence that AID [artificial insemination by donor] children do learn the truth... If AID is seen as a loving act for the child's benefit, there seems no reason to taint the procedure with a lie that could prove extremely destructive to the child.[81]

Another advantage to being open is that should a medical emergency arise in which locating the genetic father could mean life or death, the child does not have to deal with the emotional trauma, in addition to the medical trauma, that would surface upon learning the origins of his or her conception. Such circumstances are rare, yet many couples have decided to be open just in case an emergency does arise. Although they realize that the odds of such an occurrence are remote, they do not want even the possibility of such a traumatic event to be made even more traumatic because the secret might be at the root of the solution.

A more likely occurrence than the child's developing a life or death medical condition is that the non-genetic parent because s/he is older and illness happens more frequently as people age, will develop a medical condition that could possibly be hereditary. A donor offspring whose parent has a serious heart attack at a young age may worry about a similar fate unless he or she knows that the genetic parent is a different person. Furthermore, physicians routinely take family medical histories of their patients in order to ascertain whether the individual is at risk for any health problems. A donor offspring who does not know the truth will give inaccurate medical information all his/her life and possibly may receive unnecessary precautionary treatment. It is difficult for loving, concerned parents to justify allowing their child to go through life presenting a false medical history.

A more practical reason for openness relates to the changing nature of the legal system, another situation in which adoption serves as an example. Although the practice of gamete donation is commonly done anonymously and both donors and recipients are protected from any knowledge of or claims by the other, there is no guarantee that this situation will always prevail. Those touched by adoption were once promised absolute and permanently sealed records, yet states are now changing those "rules." As we mentioned earlier in this chapter, three countries—Sweden, Austria, and New Zealand—handle gamete donation (legally and psychologically) differently from the United States. In 1997 the Mental Health Professional Group of the American Society for Reproductive Medicine set up a task force whose mandate was to look into forming a donor registry in the United States. Due to the fact that the climate is changing in favor of openness, it may very well happen that the United States will also rethink policies regarding both sperm and ovum donation. Thus couples opting for gamete donation today cannot be completely assured that a mandate requiring sperm banks and clinics to open their records will not occur in their child's lifetime. Given this possibility, many couples are choosing to tell their child(ren) about gamete donation rather than face even the remote chance of a request several years hence by the donor wanting to meet his/her genetic offspring.

Keeping any secret can be difficult, but keeping a lifelong secret that is so fundamental to their child's existence can feel like a tremendous weight. Secrets that are unspeakable become more potent and despite physician's assurances that couples will forget about the donor conception, they cannot. Some parents through gamete donation have reported feeling as if there is a "scarlet D' on their chest, visible to the entire world. In fact Baran and Pannor found that most of the donor parents they interviewed were generally open people who do not lie well. Keeping the secret had been a tremendous burden because it forced them to behave differently from their natural inclinations. Having been instructed by their physicians never to tell, they unquestioningly obeyed and paid a heavy emotional price.

Fears Regarding Disclosure

Couples who choose to keep third party origins a secret from their children probably believe that they are doing what is best for them. They may have a list of "logical" reasons why they are choosing this approach. On further scrutiny, however, it is often apparent that they are motivated primarily by fear. When these fears are brought out in the open and viewed rationally, many such couples come to see the value of disclosure.

Identity Confusion

One reason frequently articulated for secrecy is a fear that children/ adults would feel confused about their identity if they were to learn of their donor origins. A study by Klock and Maier investigated the attitudes of thirty-five DI parents toward openness and secrecy and found that the most common reason given for not telling the child was their fear that it would unnecessarily complicate his or her life and that the child would be confused about who s/he was.[82] Accounts from donor offspring conceived over a decade ago (who were informed about their origins), give some credence to this argument. Until recently—in particular before the spread of HIV made physicians turn to sperm banks where semen could be frozen and quarantined for six months—doctors performing inseminations used fresh sperm from donors, frequently medical students or graduate students at a local university. In order to protect their identities, minimal records were kept, and they were often thrown out after a short period of time. Couples received almost no information at all about their donor. They may have been told his height, coloring, and educational status, but probably not much more. Much like children adopted in the early part of this century, children conceived under such circumstances—especially if they had no way to ever trace the donor—might well be confused about half of their genetic origins. As we mentioned earlier in this chapter, however, couples building families through gamete donation today, even if they doing so anonymously, can choose sperm banks or clinics that provide extensive information about donors. Although information is not a substitute for a relationship or a face to face meeting, it can go a long way in helping a donor offspring understand his/her genetic make-up. Attempting to protect children from confusion can hardly justify secrecy.

Lack of Acceptance from Relatives

Another fear frequently articulated by parents through donor gametes is their concern that if the child's relatives knew, they would not be able to completely accept the child. Since they do not want their offspring to be subjected to any form of discriminaton within their family, keeping the secret seems to be the best assurance that s/he will be loved and accepted to the same degree as the other (biological) relatives. It is the case, sadly, that in some cultures and within certain ethnic groups, lineage is crucial and children who are adopted into their families may in fact have lower status and be treated differently. If potential parents are worried about this possibility, they may want to discuss their fears with family members. Rarely do relatives feel that the couple should remain childless rather than adopt or chose gamete donation. If the topic is so charged that they are unable to discuss it, then keeping the secret would be an even greater burden than it might otherwise be—a good reason to choose openness, or if that feels impossible, to reject gamete donation in favor of adoption or childfree living.

Stigmatization

Another fear of parents through donor gametes is societal stigmatization. The extent to which a donor offspring is stigmatized depends to a great extent on the community in which s/he lives and the values espoused by the community. No matter how open or accepting an environment, however, there is no way to control for narrow mindedness or the individual expression of feelings. Once parents tell their child, the information belongs to him or her. The child may decide to tell no one, or conversely, to make an announcement in grade school on a day when the class is planting its spring garden. Classmates may go home and tell their parents that "Jessica's daddy did not have enough seeds and her mommy had to go to the doctor to get some seeds from a donor." Depending on how the parents react, Jessica may or may not be the recipient of a hurtful comment on a future occasion. The point is that telling the child about how s/he was conceived leaves open the possibility of being stigmatized. Parents naturally feel protective of their children, and many see the potential hurt that openness could cause as an argument in favor of secrecy.

Children are vulnerable, yet no matter how well parents protect them, there is no way possible that they can protect them from hurt—from the knocks and bruises of life. Good parents can give their children the emotional tools to help them deal with difficult situations, including hurtful comments from others, but they cannot prevent the scars that result from being human. Just as adoptive parents have learned to do, donor parents of donor-conceived children can teach their children how to respond to ignorant or painful comments about their origins, they can create an environment in which their children are free to be open with them about the circumstances of their life, and they can be supportive and helpful when their children need them.

Rejection of the Non-genetic Parent

Probably the biggest fear that lies beneath the desire for secrecy is that a donor-conceived child will reject the non-genetic parent should s/he learn the truth. Those contemplating adoption frequently express this same worry: that their child will be psychologically connected to his biological parents and never truly bond with his adoptive parents. They fear that someday their child will decide to search for his birthparents and reject them, leaving them bereft and childless. The fear of rejection is often based on an underlying assumption that love between parents and their children comes primarily from genetic ties rather than from the daily nurturing and gradual unfolding of their relationship. Rarely are children who were adopted into their families rejecting of their parents—it probably occurs far less often than it does with biological children who may have been unplanned, and therefore unwanted. There is no logical reason to think that a donor offspring would reject a parent who loved, nurtured and raised him to adulthood, simply because s/he was not the genetic parent.

Although couples planning to keep gamete donation a secret from their child(ren) believe that this would be in the child's best interest, the truth is that the intended secret usually is being kept for the sake of the parents. At the root of their reasons and justifications for secrecy may be a host of fears involving personal shame, humiliation and rejection. A recent study of families created by donor insemination found a relationship between stigma and the father's parental warmth and fostering of independence. Fathers who felt greater stigma about their infertility exhibited less warmth and fostered less independence in their children than did those who did not feel such stigma, leading the researchers to conclude that:

> It is possible that fathers who feel greater overall stigma may psychologically distance themselves from their DI offspring or have concerns about stigma affecting their child that differ in degree from the mothers' concerns.[83]

In discussing donor insemination, Kyle Pruett, a well known psychologist at the Yale University Child Study Center, who has a special interest in families built by reproductive technology, writes about the psychological impact of male infertility on the ability to parent.

> One of the deeply personal questions for the man is whether he has the potency to be a father *psychologically* and a functioning adult male in the world, even though he is infertile. The failure to grieve adequately his biological generativity may interfere significantly with his ability to interact appropriately with a child who so desperately seeks his love, commitment, and sense of belonging.[84]

Many clinics, recognizing the necessity of grieving the loss of one's biological child before turning to alternatives, now require a waiting period before couples can attempt pregnancy via gamete donation. The wait does not guarantee the couple will use the time to adequately grieve, but it does give a powerful message to couples about the nature of their loss and the need to mourn before they can truly accept a "donor child" as their own.

$\mathcal{T}$alking to Children about their Origins

As we mentioned in the beginning of this chapter, our focus here is solely on third party parenting. Parents of children conceived via assisted reproductive technology with their own gametes are free to discuss the circumstances of their child(ren)'s conception or not to discuss it, depending on their own need for privacy. Our one caveat is that if infertility and ART feels like a secret from which parents are hoping to "protect" their child, then it is best to discuss their infertility, and the measures they took to conceive, with their child.

Like so many issues involving child development, there are many opinions—among both professionals and parents—about how and when to tell children born through collaborative (third party) reproduction about their genetic origins. Although we are not experts in child development, we have worked for many years with individuals/couples who have become parents via assisted reproduction, and have collaborated extensively with colleagues in the field. Hence we have some ideas about how best to share this information with one's children. And because we regard gamete donation and traditional surrogacy as "half an adoption" (genetically speaking), we have drawn extensively upon knowledge learned from the field of adoption. Since we view children born via gestational care as having much more in common with ART children who are genetically connected to their parents, than to children born via traditional surrogacy, we will devote our discussion of this option to what it might mean to a child to be carried by a woman other than its mother. Similarly, since we regard embryo adoption as having much more in common with traditional adoption—and there are many resources for adoptive parents (resources which we encourage embryo adoptive families to use)—we will only introduce a brief discussion about this alternative as well. At the same time we recognize the unique features of third party arrangements, including the fact that the mother (in situations involving gamete donation) gives birth to her child, which may mitigate feelings of rejection in the offspring. In this section we present a framework for discussing third party parenting with one's children.

Adoption as a Model

Prior to the industrial revolution, adoptions tended to be informal arrangements, usually between relatives or friends, frequently involving childless couples. Consequently, most adoptees knew their family background. Legalized adoption, as we know it today, has only existed for about one hundred years, as a consequence of an increasingly mobilized society. The need thus arose for "stranger adoptions," and with it came laws sealing birth certificates and adoption records. Because of the stigma and shame associated with illegitimacy and with infertility, as adoption became more and more a transaction between professionals and would-be parents, and more and more institutionalized, the pervasive opinion became "what children don't know won't hurt them." Thus parents were advised not to tell their children they were adopted; the secret was thought necessary to protect them from this shame. A guiding principle was that love would be enough, and the fact that they did not spring biologically from the parents who raised them was thought to be unimportant, almost irrelevant.

Over subsequent years, adoptive parents and professionals in the field changed their viewpoint because the "old" approach (love is enough) was not working. Since adoption is a public event and cannot be hidden unless the parents go to great lengths to move and/or create an elaborate cover-up, many adoptees learned about their origins from others. Some found out from relatives who deliberately made a decision to tell, some overheard conversations, and still others learned unwittingly from people who knew but were unaware that the adoptee had not been told. The discovery of a secret, whenever it occurred, was almost always traumatic, leaving children (often adult children) with feelings of confusion—or worse, betrayal—wondering why their parents had hidden such an important piece of information from them. One story we heard involved a woman who was the only adopted child in a family of four daughters. While in church with her sisters one morning she overheard an older woman, a few pews behind her, whisper to a friend, "They're all so beautiful, which one was adopted?" Instantly the woman knew it was she, and in the midst of being stunned, she began to understand why it was that she had felt a constant sense of secretiveness in her family; a kind of evasiveness and indirectness had seemed to permeate her family's relationships.

Since the late 1930's and early '40s, adoption professionals have advised parents of the eventual need to tell their children about their origins. The age at which they were encouraged to do so has changed over time and has become increasingly younger; today most children are learning about their adoption by the time they enter pre-school. The younger they are when they learn the facts of their lives, goes the current thinking, the less surprised they are, and the easier it is to integrate the information into their self-concept. Through the experience of adoption both parents and professionals began to learn that telling children at a very young age helped them to feel comfortable with the information and to integrate it over time into their identity. It became one other fact about them—like the fact that they were tall, or had brown hair, or were good at math. Later when they were older and could understand the complexities of adoption more fully, it was likely to become a fact that was also laden with feelings, questions, and confusion. By the 1970s, though adoption was still almost always confidential, adoptive parents were encouraged to be forthcoming with information about their children's birthparents and to the circumstances that led to the adoption. It also seemed that the more resolved the parents were about their infertility (which led them to adoption), the more comfortable they were with adoption. Logically, the more comfortable the parents, the better able they were to discuss adoption with their children, who in turn felt a greater sense of security and a stronger sense of self. Research seemed to bear this out—the most successful adoptive families (free from pathology) were those in which the parents had resolved their infertility.[85] This information corroborates Pruett's sentiments relative to donor insemination: "When that grief is more completely resolved, the father is much more likely to be free to make a vigorous emotional commitment to the well-being of (what he'll more likely feel) is *his* child."[86]

How and When to Tell

In *Flight of the Stork: What Children Think (and when) about Sex and Family Building* (Perspectives Press 1994), Anne Bernstein, a psychologist and family therapist who has worked extensively with children, provides valuable information for parents about how to discuss sex and family building with their children. Focusing on reproduction, Bernstein explains in detail how children develop cognitively. She discusses six levels of understanding leading to cognitive maturation, and informs the reader how to recognize on what level children are functioning and when they are able to comprehend increasingly complicated concepts. Although much of her book is written for parents whose children were conceived and born in the usual way, she devotes a lot of space to providing information about how to discuss collaborative reproduction with children and we refer the reader to her book for a more extensive discussion.

Bernstein makes many important points in her book, including the necessity of always telling the truth—a point we too have been emphasizing throughout this chapter. Bernstein states that children ask sincere questions and therefore deserve sincere answers. She is clear to point out that it is not necessary, especially with very young children, to explain the process of reproduction in precise medical detail, if they are unable to absorb it. Rather, parents can provide the information they are requesting in a straightforward way that satisfies their curiosity and does not evade important truths.

Bernstein also stresses the importance—in situations of gamete donation and surrogacy—of parenting partners feeling psychologically equal as parents, although they are genetically unequal. Although collaborative reproduction has the potential to stir up feelings of illegitimacy or inferiority, it is important that both parents feel like the real legitimate parents of their child. She writes:

> The greatest challenge for families formed by these means is to create a sense of equal psychological relatedness between the child and each of his parents, even though only one of them contributed genetically to his creation. It is vital that the adults maintain a commitment to deal with each other directly about differences between them in feeling empowered and responsible as parents rather than involve their child in their conflicts.[87]

The last part of this book has focussed on the five kinds of third party parenting for which many ART couples have opted (excluding adoption which is beyond the scope of this book). Bernstein's principles, together with our own understanding of child development and our discussions with third party parents and professionals who work with such families, have enabled us to form ideas about how to discuss these various options with the resulting children. Because each option is different, each has unique emotional implications for the offspring. We are not attempting to present a thorough discussion of this complicated issue, but we wish to present some basic ideas about how children may be able to think about—and hence to understand—the way in which they came into the world.

Gestational Care

Gestational care is the only third party parenting option in which the child is conceived and raised by its genetic parents. Yet in gestational care a baby spends its entire pre-natal existence in the womb of another woman. Many couples who turn to gestational carriers regard them as prenatal nannies or gestational daycare providers. As we mentioned earlier in this chapter, although there is no compelling genetic (i.e. medical) reason to tell the child, keeping it a secret is likely to pose a great burden on the parents, affecting the child in ways that may only be determined in retrospect.

Children born to gestational carriers, like many other young children, will surely ask their mother, "Did I grow in your tummy?" And when they do, it is important to answer truthfully—and the truthful answer begins with a statement like, "No, but I wish you had." That statement can be followed by a simple explanation, which can be elaborated upon depending on the child's ability to understand. Since most people are curious about any unique aspect of their beginnings—including, for example, a premature birth, Caesarean section, or medical complication—it is likely they would be curious about the woman who nurtured them *in utero*.

Since gestational care has not been available as a parenting alternative long enough for the children and their families to have been observed over time, we can only speculate about its impact on the child's/adult's identity. It is our belief that the importance of the gestating mother will most likely recede into the background as a child matures, probably not re-surfacing until much later in life—perhaps, if she is a female, around the time of her first pregnancy. We suspect that from the child's perspective, especially as she grows and matures, the fact that she was gestated by another woman will probably have less impact on her identity than it would if she was born via gamete donation. Her growing understanding of herself will enable her to view herself as a combination of her heredity (which she inherited from both parents) and her environment. Since she was raised by her genetic parents she will not have to wonder about them or about what of them she inherited. Discovering her identity will be an experience similar to most people's.

A child born to a gestational carrier will most likely be curious about the woman who played such a unique and important role in his life. If the carrier lives close by the child may have already been introduced to her; if not, he may want to meet her, regardless of where she lives. He may want to know why she agreed to the arrangement, or whether it was difficult to give him to his parents. But he will not look to her for clues about his own identity.

Gamete Donation

Much of what we will say in this section applies to children conceived by surrogacy as well as to those conceived with donated sperm or ova. Later we will discuss the unique issues that apply to surrogacy. Since the notion of discussing gamete donation is a relatively new one, there is not much theory written about how and when to tell donor offspring of their origins. In addition to Anne Bernstein, mentioned previously, Annette Baran and Reuben Pannor, referred to earlier in this chapter, expressed their viewpoint in their book, *Lethal Secrets*. Unlike the advice given about children who were adopted and are generally told when they are quite young, Baran and Pannor recommend waiting until children conceived with donated gametes are nine or ten, until they can understand the basic facts of conception and reproduction. Bernstein, on the other hand, does not state a specific age at which she feels children can be told about gamete donation; she stresses their developmental readiness. Like Bernstein, and others, Baran and Pannor stress the importance of telling the truth, even to young children, about how babies are born—without lying about the circumstances of *their* conception.

Baran and Pannor stress that the initial explanation of donor insemination (and we would add ovum donation as well) should affirm three important facts: the father (or mother) was infertile (or had a genetic disease); the existence of a donor (genetic parent) who is a human being and wanted to provide the sperm or ova; the child was deeply wanted and is deeply loved. However the telling unfolds, it is essential that the child be left with a feeling that he or she is normal, having been conceived in the same way as everyone else—through the joining of egg and sperm.[88]

Kyle Pruett has similar notions about talking to donor offspring. He feels that the decision to tell a child about his or her origins should be guided by the psychological readiness of that child, and not by the parent's anxiety. Pruett believes that only basic information is appropriate when the child is very young—information about where babies grow inside mothers' bodies and how they come out. When children are a little older he suggests telling them about sperm and eggs and that they can be put together inside or outside the mother's body. Finally when children are even older (he is not specific about the age) Pruett recommends talking about infertility, mentioning that the seed can come from another man or the egg can come from a different woman. Pruett stresses that in telling children about their DI origins parents must distinguish between a *birth father* and a *life father*, emphasizing the importance of the latter rather than the former.[89] We actually prefer the term *genetic father* to *birth father* because it more accurately describes the role of the donor. Certainly with ovum donation, where women give birth to their children, the term *birthmother* is a misnomer.

Other professionals who advocate openness believe in telling children the salient facts at a very young age. Several have written books discussing donor insemination all of which offer straightforward information in a loving context. One such book, *How I Began: The Story of Donor Insemination*, was written by a group of social workers in Australia. The book is geared for children between the ages of four and eight, depending on the developmental level of the particular child. The book includes simple illustrations of male and female anatomy, as well as diagrams of sperm attempting to fertilize an egg. It offers a simple but truthful explanation of sexual intercourse, conception, and childbirth, and then discusses infertility by introducing a couple who is very sad because they cannot have children. The book explains simple facts about male infertility and the process of donor insemination in a careful way that emphasizes how much the child was wanted and how grateful the parents are to have him or her. Another book, *My Story*, published in England, is geared towards even younger children, and offers very basic information about conception, male infertility, and donor insemination. Its purpose is to convey information about the child's conception in a factual and loving way.

A third book, *Let Me Explain: A Story about Donor Insemination* (Perspectives Press, 1995), written by Jane Schnitter, is for slightly older children (between seven and ten). The book, which discusses donor insemination in a more sophisticated way, is a story about a girl who adores her Dad and has a wonderful relationship with him. She talks about how much they have in common and how they share so many things together despite the fact that she does not have his genes. The girl explains to the reader—in a very understandable way—what genes are and how they are responsible for so many traits. The most important message the story conveys, however, is that although genes are very important because they form the building blocks of who we are, loving relationships between family members have nothing to do with genetic ties.

Although books can be excellent tools in facilitating a discussion of the ways in which children join their families, it is important that they not replace conversations between parents and their children. Parents' openness and the mutual dialogue this openness engenders are what enable children to integrate the information they receive into a positive self concept.

Surrogacy

The major difference between gamete donation and surrogacy is that in traditional surrogacy the genetic mother is also the gestational mother. Although we stressed earlier that in gestational care arrangements we believe the gestational component will have minimal impact on the child's identity, we suspect that the combination of genetic and gestational components in surrogacy might actually have greater emotional significance to the child than the sum of both factors. This speculation is based on knowledge gained from adoption, from research (mostly anecdotal) on children conceived from donor sperm, and from our understanding of developmental psychology. Research with children/adults born via surrogacy is non-existent, as it is a relatively new third party parenting alternative.

Surrogacy is the only situation in which a woman deliberately conceives and gestates her genetic child with the intention of giving it to another woman who will be its legal and psychological parent. The key word is deliberate, as women who make adoption plans for the children they bear do so because they unintentionally became pregnant and determine that adoption is the best solution for them. Adoptees, struggling to make sense of who they are and to whom they are biologically connected, frequently express feelings of having been rejected by their birthparents. They wonder why their birthmother did not choose to parent them, fearing—perhaps assuming—that there was something undesirable about them that caused the rejection. Most often the truth is that adoption is usually a wrenching experience for a birthmother and if she were in a position to parent her baby and provide a good home for him/her, she would. As adoptees mature most can eventually accept this explanation and understand that their birthmother was not rejecting them—the adoption plan was underway before she gave birth—and their feelings of rejection will hopefully be mitigated, though perhaps never completely erased.

Children born to surrogates may also feel rejected by their birthmothers, but the reason for their (planned) placement is very different from birthmothers who make adoption plans, and it is difficult to know what

368

the impact of this difference will be on the child. The common (and usually truthful) adoption explanation is something like the following: "Your birthmother/birthparents loved you and cared about your well being. They realized they were not in a position to be good parents and could not give a baby the kind of life they wanted their baby to have, so they made an adoption plan." An explanation for becoming a surrogate would be more like the following: "The surrogate/birthmother's family was complete. She was so happy with her children, and enjoyed being pregnant, that she wanted to help us have a baby of our own."

It is impossible to know the effect of one explanation vs. another on a child's self-esteem, or whether a deliberate conception for adoption is easier or more difficult to accept than unplanned pregnancy. In the adoption scenario the message to the child is that his/her best interest was the primary consideration. In the surrogacy situation the message is that the best interest of the intended parents was the primary consideration. Children born to traditional surrogates will have to make sense of this arrangement and of their birthmother's willingness—probably even eagerness—to participate.

Hilary Hanafin, a psychologist at the Center for Surrogate Parenting and Egg Donation, who has been practicing in the field for fourteen years, anticipates that children born to surrogates (the oldest surrogacy child she knows is twelve) will probably experience feelings of rejection to a lesser degree than adoptees. According to Hanafin, a major difference between adoption and surrogacy is that the child a surrogate bears for a couple was always meant to be the child of that couple; there was never a moment when it was meant to be otherwise. She stresses that parents and surrogates must be clear with the child that s/he exists solely because the parents wanted him/her—that they planned and worked hard to have him.

Because of its similarity to adoption—its obvious difference is that the genetic father, unlike adoption, is the father who raises the child—we expect that parents through surrogacy will discuss their child's origins with him/her at an early age, and that disclosure will not be an issue to be debated. As with gamete donation, each situation is unique and it is not possible to predict to what extent knowing the source of half his/her genes will mitigate possible feelings of identity confusion in the child.

Since the surrogates and parents will be known to each other, and will most likely have had extensive contact prior to (and sometimes after) the birth of their child, it is likely that the child will meet her or ask to meet her. This situation might be similar to an open adoption which is so recent a phenomena that to date there is not adequate research on the psycho-loical effects on the children involved. It is our belief that if a child wants to meet the woman who bore her—whether it be in an adoption or a surrogacy situation—that the parents should enable her to do so as soon as they feel she is ready. According to Hanafin, parents through surrogacy who have not revealed the circumstances of their child's birth to him/her prior to age nine tend to feel awkward and uncomfortable, wishing they had previously done so. By the time the child is nine, they feel like they have already betrayed him and frequently feel stuck about how to then introduce the information.

Hanafin says that the biggest challenge for most couples embarking on surrogacy is how to regard and treat the surrogate's children, who will be genetic half siblings to their child. Some surrogates and couples seem to downplay the sibling issue and do not consider the children to be related, at least not in a family sense. Others refer to "your half sister in Chicago," clearly giving the child(ren) permission to regard half siblings as part of their family if they choose to do so. Although, according to Hanafin, most parents by surrogacy have, or plan to have other children, many couples parenting only children are pleased that their child has extended family, believing that s/he has everything to gain from having more relatives.

Regardless of whether half siblings are played up or down, the concept of genetic "kin" is confusing and not comprehensible to very young children. Their notion of family involves the people who live in their house, or extended family like grandparents, aunts, uncles, and cousins—people who visit each other and frequently spend holidays together. We know from adoption that until a child reaches early adolescence s/he is unable to understand that people can be related to each other in a genetic sense and not just through social groupings.

We also know from adoption that it's impossible to predict whether or not children will have strong feelings about or a desire for connection to their genetic families. Even within the same families children often react differently. We can assume then that children from surrogates may have similarly unpredictable reactions. Children born from a surrogate may experience feelings of loss about not being raised with their half siblings, but those feelings will probably not emerge until adolescence or adult-hood. It is also possible—once they comprehend that genetic connections also link people to each other—that they will be pleased to have siblings and will experience this knowledge as a *gain* rather than as a loss. On the other hand, as among some adoptees, some children born from surrogates may feel little interest in their genetic half siblings and other relatives, preferring to limit their sibling relationships to the children with whom they were raised.

Embryo adoption

As we mentioned in Chapter 9, embryo adoption can be accomplished in two ways: couples who have extracorporeal embryos they do not want for themselves may elect to donate them to an infertile couple (*embryo donation*); or a clinic may use donated eggs and sperm to create embryos for a couple who need both male and female gametes (*embryo creation*). One of the tenets of this book is that the way a person is created will undoubtedly have both a psychological and medical impact on him. We believe that it is incumbent on parents to understand what this impact is likely to be, and to discuss their child's origins openly and honestly, in age appropriate ways throughout his childhood and adolescence. Again, as we have stressed throughout this chapter, many of these alternative parenting options are very new, and the resulting offspring are too young to have been studied, so we can only speculate on the effects these new technologies will have on the children created. Because embryo adoption is so similar to traditional adoption—once the child is born—we will devote only a small space here to this alternative, referring the reader to the extensive literature on adoption that is available, including many of the books in our reference notes.

Unlike adoption, in which a child was probably not intended to be conceived by a particular man and woman, embryos donated by couples (or by single women using donor sperm) were very much deliberately conceived, and intended for use by the genetic parents. Like adoption, embryo donation is a solution to a problem—in this case embryos that were created but are no longer wanted, probably because the couple has completed their family, and for moral reasons will not discard them. And, like adoption, such couples are usually pleased that other infertile couples may be able to become parents in this way. Although the genetic mother did not gestate and give birth to the child, the child may still later experience feelings of rejection and confusion about why her genetic parents could not/did not raise her. The explanation may or may not be sufficient to mitigate her feelings of loss and bewilderment.

We feel it is essential for clinics performing "donated embryo" transfers to treat this parenting alternative as if it were an adoption, at least in a medical and psycho-social sense. Both the donating parents and the recipient parents need to understand the potential for residual feelings of loss in their lives and in the life of the child-to-be. The donating parents ideally should agree to make themselves known to the offspring someday if s/he desires to meet them. They should provide extensive medical and psycho-social information about themselves that can be passed on to the parents and child.

Embryo creation is different from embryo donation in two major ways: the resulting child was intended from the very beginning to be the child of the woman (and her partner if she has one) who carried it; and the man and woman who provided the sperm and egg will have never known each other (unless the gametes both come from known donors). Again, we can only speculate on the impact of this difference on the offspring. The fact that the child was intentionally created for its parents may minimize feelings of rejection, though the child may feel very confused about its identity. Embryo creation (providing the donors were anonymous) is the only deliberate family building option in which neither of the genetic parents ever had a relationship with each other or with the child. It is possible that the child will feel a great sense of rootlessness and frustration, especially if s/he would like to meet the donor(s) and is unable to.

We have serious reservations about "embryo creation" (see Chapter 9), but understand that many clinics are offering it to couples. We hope that individuals/couples opting to create embryos will think long and hard about this alternative, which aside from gestation, is akin to adoption—as there are already existing children in the world who need homes. Those who decide to create embryos with anonymous gametes should ideally go through clinics that provide extensive information about their ovum donors, and similarly they should order sperm from banks that are also forthcoming with information.

Always Knowing: An Integrative Approach

Today's adoptive parents have been advised to begin to talk about adoption from the very beginning, sometimes even before their children understand language. They can do this in the same way that they talk to their babies about all sorts of things. When parents change diapers, feed their babies, or take them out in their strollers, they tend to babble about various issues or observations, knowing perfectly well that their offspring under a year or two, cannot understand their words. This chatter is important in the development of language skills: babies and toddlers who are spoken to frequently develop language skills faster than those whose parents or caretakers exchange little verbal communication with them.

Adoption is a concept that children will understand only over time, but they can be introduced to it from the moment they are born. For example, when a parent kisses her baby or toddler goodnight, and feels herself filling with love, she can say, "I love you so much, I'm so happy we could adopt you." Or the parent might say at a different moment, "You are wonderful, I'm so glad your birthmother chose us to be your parents." Although they won't understand the meaning of the words, the children will become familiar with them and gradually they will comprehend the concept of adoption. By introducing adoption terminology from the beginning of their life, parents do not have to figure out when to sit down and tell their children they were adopted. This understanding gradually unfolds as adoption becomes a part of their story—something they always knew— like how much they weighed, or what hospital they were born in, or whether they had colic. This approach has other advantages. Adoptees will not look back as teenagers or adults, and recall the dramatic (or traumatic) moment when their parents sat them down and told them the truth about their origins—a truth that may be more charged than it needs to be because it was hidden for their early years. This kind of early use of an adoption vocabularly and casual talk also gives parents "practice" in talking about adoption—practice that can help them feel more comfortable later when their older children ask more complex questions.

This concept of always knowing can be applied to gamete donation, gestational care, and surrogacy as well. Although it may seem more awkward, parents can find opportunities to use words that relate to their children's origins. For example, upon kissing his child goodnight, a parent might say, " I love you so much, I'm so glad a doctor could help us have you," or, perhaps at a slightly older age, "You are so wonderful, the donor must have been a wonderful person," or "We are so glad that we could get ova (or eggs) to make you grow." For surrogacy situations a parent might say, "I am so glad that Gail agreed to help us make you because I love you so much." These simple statements will not be understood by a toddler, and maybe not even by a pre-schooler, but the words will be remembered and eventually the meaning will be understood.

Telling: A Process that Occurs over Time

Probably the most important guideline that anyone can offer to parents through collaborative reproduction is that being open is a process that happens over time, it is not a one-time event. If parents do not explain gamete donation or gestational care or surrogacy exactly as they had hoped to the first time, there will be other chances. In fact, parents should look for and welcome opportunities to discuss their children's origins with them, perhaps after seeing a movie about adoption, or reading a newspaper article about reproductive technology, for example. At the same time parents should not put so much emphasis on the means of conception that it overshadows other vital aspects of a child's life—play, friends, family events, outings, and most importantly, the child's emerging, wonderous self. The point is to be able to convey the information in a straightforward, confident, and loving way that enables the child to feel loved and wanted, and secure about who s/he is. As their child grows older it is certainly appropriate for parents to acknowledge sadness that their wonderful child did not come from both of his parents' genes; that although they would wish for no other child than the one they have, it is a loss for them not to have created him/her together.

As children grow and develop, gamete donation (or surrogacy) will take on new meaning. A four or five year old probably does not care which grocery store the egg came from that was used to create her; at that age one egg is the same as another. However, she has heard a story which she will hear again—and again—and understand in different ways as she grows.

All young children enjoy having their parents read to them. Children between the ages of four and eight are especially receptive to stories—including stories about how they were born. Earlier we mentioned books that apply solely to donor insemination; however, another book, *Mommy, Did I Grow In Your Tummy?* by psychologist, Elaine Gordon, is about all the new reproductive options and alternatives, including ovum and sperm donation, surrogacy, and adoption. The story describes a happy couple who have a wonderful life, but something is missing—a child with whom they can share their lives. As hard as they try, they cannot make a baby. They go to a doctor because doctors understand a lot about how people's bodies work and can often help people have babies. The story describes how most babies are created and then explains that some people need even more help than a doctor can give. The book then discusses the various third party options, including adoption, that enable couples to build families. The message is very clear—that all family building options result in normal, healthy, families, and that the means of becoming a family is far less important than the bonds that are created between parents and children, however the latter arrive.

By pre-adolescence children appreciate the fact that ova and sperm are all unique and that is why people are different from one another. A latency age or pre-adolescent child may ask, after a discussion about gamete donation, "Does that mean that Daddy's not my real father?"—a question many prospective donor parents fear. Bernstein has a simple and loving response to such a question. She advises parents to say, "Daddy (or Mommy) will always be your dad. It's just that Daddy's sperm (or Mommy's ovum) didn't make you. The donor is your biological [we prefer "genetic"] father (mother)."[90] The point is that a donor is not a parent in a psychological sense, only in a biological sense, and attachments are not based on biology. In adolescence a child conceived with donated gametes will grapple in a more intense way with her identity and sense of self, possibly wondering to what extent genetic influences have shaped her life. She may feel a sense of loss about not knowing the donor, and may experience feelings of anger, frustration, and sadness.

It is especially important that parents give their children permission to express the range of feelings, questions, and concerns they have about the way in which they came into the world. It may be difficult—particularly during adolesence—for parents who struggled long and hard with infertility to listen to their child's negative reactions about gamete donation. Getting angry at one's parents, however, is a normal part of adolescence. Children born through third party assistance just have one more "weapon" they can use against their parents if they choose to. Thus if a mother tells her fourteen-year-old son to be home at midnight, the son (in an effort to truly make his mother feel badly and change her mind) might say, "I don't have to listen to you, you're not even my real mother." If the mother has been prepared for this moment, and is able to reassure herself that her (normal) rebellious son is merely giving her a hard time because he is angry rather than seeking to replace her, she may be able to muster her sense of humor. The mother might then reply, "Let's try to find the donor and see what time she thinks you should be back. You better hope she doesn't say 11:00 o'clock."

It is important to remember that arguments and outbursts are a normal part of growing up, and on a positive note, they can indicate that the child feels secure enough to know that s/he will not be rejected, no matter how intense his/her feelings. Such an outburst can also indicate an awareness on the child's part that the parent is secure enough in his/her role as parent that s/he will not be permanently wounded by the hurtful remark. Parents must have faith that just as they were able to move beyond their sadness, anger and frustration about infertility, their children —with their parents' help—can move beyond theirs.

We have attempted to present in this chapter a rationale about why we feel strongly that children born via third party arrangements must be told the truth about their origins; we have also presented a framework for doing so. Although adequate research has not been done—and can probably never be—that would demonstrate without a doubt whether secrecy or disclosure is psychologically best for children, we feel there is adequate "evidence" from which to draw these conclusions. We also feel that there are legitimate ethical arguments for openness. Our strong defense of a child's right to the truth—and of a parent's mandate to tell it—does not mean that we fail to appreciate how daunting this task feels to many would-be and expectant parents. We recognize that the temptation not to tell is there and that at times it seems compelling. However, all of us have learned that there are truths better confronted than avoided. We agree with Kyle Pruett when he says:

> Until the essential prospective, longitudinal studies are done on these children and their families, it is my best clinical judgment that we should err on the side of disclosure over secrecy, as it is less damaging to the child's inner emotional world than the gap in the narrative of the self. Knowing the circumstances of one's origins is less psychologically malignant than not knowing, assuming the content of the knowledge is not especially nefarious or emotionally charged for a particular family or parent. By knowing the facts of one's conception, these children have a better chance of feeling and understanding that they were conceived in love (if not *in situ*), a knowledge reassuring to all young beings pondering the mystery of their origins and its human connection.[91]

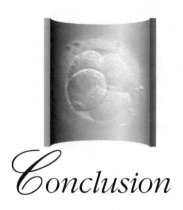

Conclusion

The assisted reproductive technologies have brought profound changes in reproduction, permanently altering the definitions of mother, of father, of family. Humbled—and somewhat startled by these changes—we arrive at the end of this book with neither conclusions nor predictions. Rather, we bring to this final page two perspectives which we hope have infused our book: caution and optimism.

Our optimism comes from the fact that these new technologies are nothing short of miraculous, bringing lives into the world that otherwise would never have been born, and bringing joy to countless infertile people. Our caution, however, comes from an understanding that although the creation of life is a highly regarded value, there may be instances when the pursuit of that goal comes with too high a price tag.

In Chapter One we discussed the psychological and ethical issues that lay at the heart of assisted reproduction. Many of these issues raise questions regarding the best interest and emotional well being of children not yet conceived, or of "willing" third parties. For example, there are many who argue that it is never in a child's interest to be intentionally created in order to be given away, or for a healthy fertile woman to unnecessarily undergo invasive and potentially damaging medical procedures. Others feel just as strongly that technological advances, including third party parenthood, will have minimal, if any, effect on a person's life; and furthermore that the gift of life itself will be a mitigating force if hardship prevails. Each perspective forms the endpoint of a long continuum—one that has many possible stops along the way.

And so we end our book, leaving you, the reader—whether clinician or consumer—with the task of searching your own minds and hearts and consciences regarding the psycho-social and ethical issues of assisted reproduction. We hope that this book has provided you with a foundation with which to do so. May caution guide you in your search and may optimism sustain you in your pursuit—whatever it is.

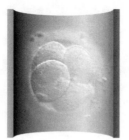

$\mathscr{R}$esources and $\mathscr{F}$ootnotes

American Society for Reproductive Medicine
1209 Montgomery Highway
Birmingham, Alabama 35216-2809
205-978-5000
http://www.asrm.org

American Surrogacy Center
http://www.surrogacy.com
E-mail:joan@surrrogacy.com.

Center For Loss in Multiple Birth
c/o Jean Kollantai
P.O. Box 1064
Palmer, AK. 99645-1064
907-746-6123
E-mail:climb@pobox.alaska.net.

Childfree Network
6966 Sunrise Blvd. Suite 111
Citrus Heights, California 95610
916-773-7178

INCIID (The International Council on
Infertility Information Dissemination)
P.O. Box 6836
Arlington VA 22206 ·
520-544-9548
http://www.inciid.org

Infertility Awareness Association of Canada (IAAC)
201-396 Cooper St.
Ottawa, Ontario K2P 2H7, CANADA
613-234-8585
e-mail: iaac@fox.nstn.ca

Organization of Parents Through Surrogacy (OPTS)
P.O. Box 213
Wheeling, Illinois
847-394-4116
http://www.opts.com

RESOLVE
1310 Broadway
Somerville, Mass. 02144-1731
617-623-0744 (helpline)
617-623-1156 (business line)
http://www.resolve.org

$\mathcal{F}$ootnotes

1 R. Nachtigall, G. Becker and M. Wozny, "The Effects of Gender Specific Diagnosis on Men's and Women's Responses to Infertility," *Fertility and Sterility*, 57:113-21, 1992.

2 M. Mahowold, "Medically Assisted Reproductive Technology: Variables, Verities and Rules of Them," a talk given at the *Ethics of Reproductive Medicine: Responsibilities and Challenges* conference, U.C. Irvine, April, 1996.

3 J. Robertson, *Children of Choice: Freedom and the New Reproductive Technologies* (New Jersey: Princeton University Press, 1994) 39.

4 M. Sandelowski, et al; "Pregnant Moments: The Process of Conception in Infertile Couples," *Research in Nursing and Health*, 13:273-282, 1990.

5 Ibid

6 A. Whittemore, et al, "Characteristics Relating to Ovarian Cancer Risk: Collaborative Analysis of 12 U.S. Case-Control Studies. Invasive Epithelial Ovarian Cancers in White Women;" *American Journal of Epidemiology*, 136:1184-1203, 1993.

7 M.A. Rossing, et al, "Ovarian Tumors in a Cohort of Infertile Women," *New England Journal of Medicine*, 331:771-6, October, 1994.

8 R. Bristow and B. Karlan, "Ovulation Induction, Infertility and Ovarian Cancer Risk," *Fertility and Sterility*, 66:499-507, October, 1996.

9 A. Domar, "Stress and Infertility in Women," *Infertility: Psychological Issues and Treatment Strategies*, ed. Sandra Leiblum, (New York: John Wiley, 1996) 67-82.

10 Ibid

11 M. Sandelowski, B.G. Harris and D. Holditch-Davis, "Pregnant Moments: The Process of Conception in Infertile Couples," *Research in Nursing and Health*, 13:273-282, 1990.

12 B.K. Rothman, *The Tentative Pregnancy: Prenatal Diagnosis and the Future of Motherhood* (New York: Viking Press, 1988.)

13 M. Sandelowski, B.G. Harris, and D. Holditch-Davis, "Amniocentesis in the Context of Infertility," *Health Care for Women International*, 12:167-178, 1991.

14 D. Holditch-Davis, B.P. Black, B.G. Harris, M. Sandelowski and L. Edwards, "Beyond Couvade: Pregnancy Symptoms in Couples with a History of Infertility," *Health Care for Women International* 15:537-548, 1994.

15 J.L Ecker, M.R. Laufer, and J.A. Hill, "Measurement of Embryo Toxic Factor Is Predictive of Pregnancy Outcome in Women with a History of Recurrent Abortion," *Obstetrics and Gynecology*, 81:84-87, 1993.

16 K.E. Smith and R.P. Byalos, "The Profound Impact of Patient Age on Pregnancy Outcome after Early Detection of Fetal Cardiac Activity," *Fertility and Sterility*, 65:35-40, January 1, 1996.

17 H. Deutsch, *The Psychology of Women II* (New York: Bantam Books, 1945) 152.

18 S. Lee, *Our Newsletter: A Multiple Birth Loss Support Network*, VI,1:8-9.

19 *Vital and Health Statistics*, National Center for Health Statistics, U.S. Department of Health and Human Services, Hyattsville, MD.

20 Office of the American Society for Reproductive Medicine, July, 1997.

21 Office of the American Society for Reproductive Medicine, July, 1997.

22 D. Berger, et al, "Psychological Patterns in Donor Insemination Couples," *Canadian Journal of Psychiatry*, 31:814-823, December, 1986.

23 A. Braverman, "Survey Results on the Current Practice of Ovum Donation," *Fertility and Sterility*, 54:1216-1220, June, 1993.

24 E. Sherman and G. Annas, "Social Policy Considerations in Noncoital Reproduction," *Journal of the American Medical Association*, 255:62-68, January 3, 1986.

25 "Guidelines for Donor Insemination," American Society for Reproductive Medicine, 1993.

26 A. Baran and R Pannor, *Lethal Secrets* (New York: Warner Books, 1989.)

27 K. Daniels, "Semen Donors in New Zealand: Their Characteristics and Attitudes," *Clinical Reproductive Fertility*, 5:177-190, August, 1987.

28 "Guidelines for Donor Insemination," American Society for Reproductive Medicine, 1993.

29 K. Daniels, "Semen Donors in New Zealand: Their Characteristics and Attitudes," *Clinical Reproductive Fertility*, 5:177-190, August, 1987.

30 P. Mahlstedt and K. Probasco, "Sperm Donors: Their Attitudes toward Providing Medical Psychological Information for Recipient Couples and Donor Offspring," *Fertility and Sterility*, 56:747-753, October, 1991.

31 S. Elias and G. Annas, "Social Policy Considerations in Noncoital Reproduction," *Journal of the American Medical Association*, 255:62-68, January 3, 1986.

32 K. Daniels, "Semen Donors in New Zealand: Their Characteristics and Attitudes," *Clinical Reproductive Fertility*, 5:177-190, August, 1987.

33 Authors note: The chapter on ovum donation in our earlier book, *Beyond Infertility: The New Paths to Parenthood* (Boston: Lexington Books, 1994,) was originally co-authored with Susan Levin, LICSW, BCD; Jeane U. Springer, LICSW, BCD; and Sharon Steinberg, RN, MS, CS. We acknowledge with gratitude that substantial portions of that original material serve as the basis for this chapter.

34 Lutjen et al, "The Establishment and Maintenance of a Pregnancy Using In Vitro Fertilization and Embryo Donation in a Patient with Ovarian Failure," *Nature*, 207:174-76, 1994.

35 "Guidelines for Donor Insemination," American Society for Reproductive Medicine, 1993.

36 A.M. Braverman, et al, "Survey Results on the Current Practice of Ovum Donation," *Fertility and Sterility*, 59:1216-1220, June, 1993.

37 B. Raboy, et al, "Mental Health among Families with Children Conceived by D.I.," research paper presented at the Mental Health Professional Group meeting of the American Society for Reproductive Medicine, November 6, 1997, Cincinnati, OH.

38 R. J. Paulson, M.H. Thornton, M.M. Francis and H.S. Salvador, "Successful Pregnancy in a 63-year-old Woman," *Fertility and Sterility*, 67:949-951, May, 1997.

39 A.M. Braverman, et al, "Survey Results on the Current Practice of Ovum Donation," *Fertility and Sterility*, 59:1216-1220, June, 1993.

40 Ibid

41 Ibid

42 Ibid

43 Ibid

44 M. Grodin, "Surrogate Motherhood and the Best Interests of the Child," *Women's Health Institute Journal*, 1,3:135-137, Summer, 1991.

45 P.I. Johnston, "Speaking Positively: Using Respectful Adoption Language," article on the web site of Perspectives Press: The Infertility and Adoption Publisher, http://www.perspectivespress.com.

46 G. Corea, *The Mother Machine*, (New York: Harper and Row, 1985) 217.

47 *People Magazine*, September, 1993:69-75.

48 M. Harrison, "Financial Incentives for Surrogacy," *Women's Health Institute Journal*, I.3:145, 1991.

49 G. Corea, *The Mother Machine*, (New York: Harper and Row, 1985) 243.

50 G. Corea, *The Mother Machine*, (New York: Harper and Row, 1985) 229.

51 *Newsletter*, Center for Surrogate Parenting, May, 1993.

52 Ibid

53 "Opinion 88" American College of Obstetrics and Gynecology (November, 1990) as referenced in Women's Health Institute Journal, 3:133, Summer, 1991.

54 F. Chervenak and L. McCullough, "Respect for the Autonomy of the Pregnant Woman in Surrogacy Agreements: An Elaboration of A Fundamental Ethical Concern," *Women's Health Institute Journal*, 1:143-147, 1991.

55 "Opinion 88" American College of Obstetrics and Gynecology (November, 1990)

56 "Opinion 88" American College of Obstetrics and Gynecology (November, 1990.)

57 M. Grodin, "Surrogate Motherhood and the Best Interests of the Child," *Women's Health Institute Journal*, 1,3:135-137, Summer, 1991.

58 Cristie Montgomery, personal conversation

59 P.J. Parker, "Motivation of Surrogate Mothers: Initial Findings," *American Journal of Psychiatry*, 140:117-118, 1983.

60 K. Forest, "Surrogate Mothers' Experiences and Social Support Networks," unpublished Master's thesis, Colorado State University, 1989) 2.

61 Ibid

62 *Newsletter* of Organization of Parents through Surrogacy, Winter-Spring, 1990.

63 M. English, A. Mechanick-Braverman, and S. Corson, "Semantics and Science: The Distinction between Gestational Carrier and Traditional Surrogacy Options," *Women's Health Institute Journal*, I,3:155-157, Summer, 1991.

64 "Opinion 88" American College of Obstetrics and Gynecology (November, 1990.)

65 G. Annas, "Determining the Fate of Gestational Mothers," *Women's Health Institute Journal*, I,3:158, Summer, 1991.

66 N. Reame, "The Surrogate Mother as a High-Risk Obstetric Patient," *Women's Health Institute Journal*, I,3:151-154, Summer, 1991.

67 "Weekly Speaking" column, ASRM *Fertility News*, June, 1993:10.

68 *Johnson vs Calvert, Daily Appellate Report*, California Supreme Court, May 27, 1993 Case #SO23721.

69 L. Capone, letter to the editor, *Sacramento Bee*, March 11, 1992.

70 "Sart Report-1994 Statistics," *Society for Assisted Reproductive Technology*, ASRM.

71 E. Bartholet, *Family Bonds: Adoption and the Politics of Parenting* (Boston: Houghton-Mifflin, 1993,) 225.

72 Ibid

73 S. Klock, "Psychological Aspects of Donor Insemination," Infertility and Reproductive Clinics of North America, IV,3:455-471, July, 1993.

74 E. Noble, *Having Your Baby by Donor Insemination* (Boston: Houghton-Mifflin, 1987.)

75 K. Daniels and G. Lewis, "Openness of Information in the Use of Donor Gametes: Developments in New Zealand," *Journal of Reproductive and Infant Psychology*, 14:57-68, 1996.

76 Ibid

77 E. Haimes, "Recreating the Family? Policy Considerations Relating to the 'New' Reproductive Technologies," *The New Reproductive Technologies* (London: Macmillan, 1990) 160.

78 D. Gelman and D. Rosenberg, "Family Secrets," Newsweek, February 24, 1997:24-30.

79 P. Mahlstedt and D. Greenfield, "Assisted Reproductive Technology with Donor Gametes: The Need for Patient Preparation," *Fertility and Sterility*, 52:908-914, December, 1989.

80 A. Baran and R. Pannor, *Lethal Secrets* (New York: Warner Books, 1989.)

81 G. Annas, "Beyond the Best Interests of the Sperm Donor," *Family Law Quarterly*, 14:1-13, November 1, 1980.

82 S. Klock and D. Maier, "Psychological Factors Related to Donor Insemination," *Fertility and Sterility*, 56:484-495, 1991.

83 R. Nachtigall et al, "Stigma, Disclosure, and Family Functioning among Parents of Children Conceived through Donor Insemination," *Fertility and Sterility*, 68:83-91, July, 1997.

84 K. Pruett, "Strange Bedfellows? Reproductive Technology and Child Development," *Infant Mental Health Journal*, 13,4:312-317, Winter, 1992.

85 H. D. Kirk, *Shared Fate: A Theory and Method of Adoptive Relationships* (New York: The Free Press, 1964) 156-67 and E. Lawder, et al, "A Follow-up Study of Adoptions, Vol I" (New York: Child Welfare League of America, 1969) 66.

86 K. Pruett, "Strange Bedfellows? Reproductive Technology and Child Development," *Infant Mental Health Journal*, 13,4:312-317, Winter, 1992.

87 A. C. Bernstein, *Flight of the Stork: What Children Think (and When) about Sex and Family Building* (Indianapolis: Perspectives Press, 1994) 198.

88 A. Baran and R. Pannor, *Lethal Secrets* (New York: Warner Books, 1989.)

89 K. Pruett, "Strange Bedfellows? Reproductive Technology and Child Development," *Infant Mental Health Journal*, 13,4:312-317, Winter, 1992.

90 A. C. Bernstein, *Flight of the Stork: What Children Think (and When) about Sex and Family Building* (Indianapolis: Perspectives Press, 1994) 173.

91 K. Pruett, "Strange Bedfellows? Reproductive Technology and Child Development," *Infant Mental Health Journal*, 13,4: 316, Winter, 1992.

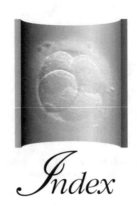

Index

adultery, and donor insemination, 164-65, 239, 341

AFT testing. *See* alpha-fetoprotein testing

aging eggs, 249

Albright, Madeleine, 350

alpha-fetoprotein testing, 90

American Association of Tissue Banks, 180

American College of Obstetricians and Gynecologists, 258, 260, 265, 293

American Fertility Society, 178

American Society for Reproductive Medicine, 54, 161, 180, 185-86, 201-2

   Mental Health Professional Group, 329, 336, 356

   Ovum Donation Task Force, 234

   Psychological Special Interest Group, 213-14

   and semen donation, 178-79

amniocentesis, 85, 90-91

   and genetic disorders, 158

   and gestational care, 303

   and ovum donation, 202, 223

   and surrogacy, 273, 277

"Amniocentesis in the Context of Infertility", 90

anesthesia, 43, 71, 98

Annas, George, 169, 188, 293, 355

anticardiolipin antibody syndrome, 115

antiphospholipid antibody syndrome, 115

Ariel, Suzanne, 352

ART. *See* assisted reproductive technology

artificial insemination. *See* donor insemination

Asherman's syndrome, 102, 300

aspirin, 115

ASRM. *See* American Society for Reproductive Medicine

assisted reproductive technology, 14, 40, 81, 137-38. *See also* donor insemination; gestational care; *in vitro* fertilization, surrogacy

   access to, 35-38, 47, 137

   age restrictions in, 35-38, 137

   alternatives to, 23, 138, 142-47

   counseling in, 26, 334

   criticism of, 216, 323

   decision to end treatment, 79-81, 133ff., 141-42

   and depression, 50

   and disclosure, 339-40

   and donor insemination, 191-92

   and ectopic pregnancy, 116-17, 120

   and embryo adoption, 322, 330

   and embryo donation, 329, 331-32, 336

   ethical considerations of, 15-16, 21-26, 206

   explaining to child, 361, 373

   and gestational care, 291, 298

   initiation of process, 60-63

   insurance coverage for, 79, 137

   legal issues, 21-22, 30

   and loss of control, 65-68

   and loss of intimacy, 27

   medication in, 47, 64-66, 68-71, 77-79

   mixing embryos, 335-36

   negative results with, 77-79, 306

   openness in, 339ff.

   optimism in, 62-63

   options in, 16-17, 40, 78-79, 134-38

   and ovum donation, 200, 211, 217, 224-25, 229, 241

   physical demands of, 50-51

   physical discomfort in, 27, 71

   and pregnancy loss, 129-31

   and privacy, 361

   religious issues in, 39

   restrictions, 137-38

   risks associated with, 25-26, 33

   side effects of, 48-50

   statistics associated with, 54-60

   and storage of embryos, 325

   time demands of, 46-47, 61

   treatment history, 134

   women's issues in, 25-26, 39

"Assisted Reproductive Technology with Donor Gametes: The Need for Patient Preparation", 351

attachment

   and adoption, 326

   and donor insemination, 163, 193

   to fetus, 92, 104, 110, 123

   and gestational care, 292

   and ovum donation, 221

   in surrogacy, 277

attorneys, 220, 295. *See also* legal considerations

Austria

   donor conception in, 346

   and gamete donation, 356

autoimmune conditions, 103, 197. *See also* human immunodeficiency virus

autonomy, 15-16, 22, 37

   concerns about, 26

   and ethics, 15-16, 25

   of gestational carrier, 293-94

   and surrogacy, 259, 261-62

azoospermia, 44, 155, 157, 342

B

Baby M, 256-59

baby showers, 97-98

baby, preparation for, 96-98

Baran, Annette, 351, 357, 365

Bartholet, Elizabeth, 23, 323-25, 330

Beck Depression Inventory, 65

Behavioral Medicine Program, 64

beneficence, 22, 37

   concerns about, 267

   and ethics, 15-16

   and surrogacy, 261-62

Bernstein, Anne, 363-65, 374

beta subunits, 58, 75, 103, 108
Beth Israel Deaconness Hospital, 64-65
Bible, infertility in, 13-14, 152, 245-46
bio-ethics, 37
biological equality, 165, 195
birth, preparation for, 96-98
birth certificate, 284
birth control, and adoption, 250
birth defects, 91, 123, 198
  and gestational care, 294
  and miscarriage, 102
  and ovum donation, 197
  and surrogacy, 266
birthfamily, 329, 348. *See also* family
Birthmother, 252
birthmother, 205, 372. *See also* birthparents;
  mother
  and adoption, 255, 327
  advocacy for, 257
  anonymity of, 326
  counseling for, 333
  and ovum donation, 366
  rejection by, 368
  and surrogacy, 247, 255, 258, 270
birthparents, 250-51. *See also* birthmother;
  father; mother; parents
  and adoption, 253, 327
  counseling for, 333
  information about, 327, 363
  rejection by, 368
  rights of, 21
  search for, 347-49, 359
bleeding, during pregnancy, 118
blood clots, in placenta, 115
blood donation, 229, 232
blood tests, 50, 66, 69-71, 80
  and gestational care, 312
  and multiple gestation, 121
  in ovum donation, 225
  for pregnancy, 75, 85, 92, 108
bonding
  and adoption, 327
  and embryo adoption, 321
  and ovum donation, 220-21
  and pregnancy, 92-93, 335
  and surrogacy, 270, 276, 284
bone marrow registry, 229
Braverman, Andrea, M. D., 209, 211, 217, 231,
  233, 306
Brown, Louise, 39, 81
Brown Margaret, 353

C

Caesarean section, 307, 309, 365
California Cryobank, 181-82
Calvert, Crispina and Mark, 258, 296
cancer
  cervical, 48
  and infertility, 48-49, 207-8

  ovarian, 48
  survivors, 157, 299-300
Capone, Lori, 306-7
capsule, intravaginal, 42-43
caregivers, 191-31, 142
Carter, Jean and Michael, 147
Catholic Church. *See* Roman Catholic Church
Center for Loss in Multiple Birth, 123-24
Center for Surrogate Parenting and Egg
  Donation, Inc., 247, 256, 285, 294-95,
  305, 369
cerclage, 111
cervix, 111, 116, 153
chemotherapy, 129
  for cancer, 197
  for ectopic pregnancy, 119, 121
  and gestational care, 299
  and ovarian function, 210, 216
Chervenak, Frank, 259
child free living, 142-43, 146-47, 165, 194, 292,
  358
  and donor insemination, 192
childbirth, 18-19, 303, 327
childbirth class, 98, 110
children
  cognitive development of, 363
  of surrogate, 278-79, 369-70
chorionic villus sampling, 202
chromosomal abnormalities, 102, 109, 111-12,
  201
  and surrogacy, 258
circumcision, 284
CLIMB. *See* Center for Loss in Multiple Birth
Clomid, 48
Clomid challenge test, 56
clomiphene citrate, 48, 56
collaborative reproduction. *See* embryo
  adoption; gestational care; ovum donation;
  parenting, third party; semen donation;
  surrogacy
conception, 339
  right to know, 24-25, 352
  unnatural, 16, 26-31
Concerned United Birthparents, 257
control, loss of, 65-68
Corea, Gena, 253
cryopreservation
  of embryos, 27-29, 39, 41, 51-53, 81, 201-2,
  292, 309, 312, 319, 323-25, 330
  for second pregnancy, 29
  and gestational care, 299-300
  legal implications of, 52-54
  options in, 21
  of ova, 51, 195, 200, 211-12
  of sperm, 45, 177-78, 358
  and surrogacy, 280-81
cystic fibrosis, 30, 159
cytomegalovirus, 178

D

D & C. *See* dilatation and curettage
Daniels, Ken, 184-85, 187
Davis v. Davis, 29-30, 54
DeBoers, Jessica, 284
DES. *See* diethylstilbestrol
Deutsch, Helene, 114
DI. *See* donor insemination
diabetes, 89, 103, 127
diaphragmatic breathing, 64
diethylstilbestrol, 48, 300
dilatation and curettage, 102
divorce, 32, 204, 352
    and infertile couples, 144
    and surrogacy, 258, 277
Domar, Alice, Ph.D., 64-65
donation, gamete. *See* donor gametes; donor
    insemination; embryo donation; gamete
    donation; ovum donation; sperm donation
donor couples, 352
donor gametes, 21
    and attachment, 164
    ethical considerations, 23
donor insemination. 24, 98-100, 140, 145,
    151ff., 324. *See also* assisted
    reproductive technology; gamete
    donation; parenting, third party;
    sperm donation
    with anonymous donor, 25, 175-79, 343
    attempting pregnancy by, 191-92
    candidates for, 156-59
    compared to ovum donation, 243
    compensation for, 253
    counseling for, 161, 174-75
    explaining to child, 374
    fear of error in, 192-93
    and fertile men, 158-59
    financial considerations, 167-68
    and gestational care, 250
    and grief, 363
    history of, 151-55
    and identity confusion, 357-58
    with known donor, 168-75, 191
    and legitimacy, 167
    and lesbian couples, 204
    and male infertility, 43, 154, 341
    need for genetic information in, 170-71, 358
    need for medical history in, 173
    negative view of, 353
    and openness, 343, 353-55
    as option, 134, 160, 165
    and privacy, 166
    record keeping in, 186-90, 353, 358
    with relatives, 171-73, 176
    and secrecy, 154, 329, 340-41, 343, 345,
        351-52, 355-56, 360
    selection of donor, 170-73, 181-83, 189-91

    simplicity of, 196
    and single women, 204
    statistics regarding, 155, 167
    and surrogacy, 307
    in Sweden, 346
    unsuccessful, 194
donor insemination reform, 352
donor offspring, 352
    rejection by, 359-60
donor registries, 347, 356-57

E

ectopic pregnancy. *See* pregnancy, ectopic
egg. *See* ovum
egg donation. *See* ovum donation
egg retrieval, 40, 42, 45, 50, 57, 66-68, 70-72,
    119, 199, 200-202, 225
    anesthesia during, 71
    avoidance of, 78
    and insemination, 72
    and ovum donation, 208, 235
    problems with, 302
    time allotment, 47
Einwohner, Joan, M. D., 256
electroejaculation, 158
Elias, Sherman, 169, 188
embryo adoption, 18, 53, 146, 319ff.
    See also embryo creation; embryo
        donation; parenting, third party
    combining embryos in, 335-36
    and donating couples, 332-34
    ethical issues in, 322-26
    explaining to child, 370-72
    financial considerations, 324
    and informed consent, 332-35
    practice of, 329-332
    psychosocial issues in, 326-28
    reasons for selecting, 321-22
    and recipient couples, 334-35
    and traditional adoption, 323, 327, 361, 371
embryo creation, 320-322, 326, 328, 334, 337,
    370-72.
    See also embryo adoption
embryo donation, 19, 23, 29, 39, 53-54, 98-100,
    320-22, 330, 334, 370-71. *See also* embryo
    adoption
    estimated occurrence, 330, 336
    and genetic siblings, 325, 331
    informed consent for, 332-34
    for research, 29
Embryo Donation Task Force, 329-30, 333-34
embryo toxic factor, 103, 114
embryo transfer, 40-42, 51-53, 57, 66-67, 71, 73,
    85, 107
    chances of pregnancy with, 79
    and ectopic pregnancy, 117
    and embryo adoption, 319
    financial considerations, 324
    and gestational care, 290, 307, 312-13

and decision to continue treatment, 78-79
of donor insemination, 167
of embryo donation, 324
of gestational care, 298-99, 304, 313
incentives to donor participants, 26, 199
of ovum donation, 195-96, 210
and surrogacy, 146, 252-54, 264, 298
Flight of the Stork: What Children Think (and when) about Sex and Family Building, 353
folic acid, 84
follicle stimulating hormone, 55-56, 63, 68-70, 197
follicles, 66
    attachment to, 70
    and egg retrieval, 71
    growth of, 68-69
    stimulation of, 201
    ultrasound monitoring of, 70
follicular fluid, 202
Follisti, 69
Forest, Kathy, 277, 286
frozen embryo transfer cycle, 51-52
FSH. *See* follicle stimulating hormone
funeral
    for baby, 113
    for stillborn child, 128-29

G
gamete donation, 24, 168, 195, 215, 250, 331-32, 369, 373-74. *See also* donor insemination; ovum donation; sperm donation
    and adoption, 239-40, 347-49, 361
    anonymous, 99-100, 347, 356-60, 372
    changes in, 357
    and coersion, 26
    and embryo adoption, 321
    and embryo creation, 371
    ethical implications, 24, 204, 241
    explaining to child, 365-67, 373-74
    and grief, 360
    history of, 23
    and identity, 365
    and information about donor, 100, 349, 356
    negative perceptions of, 358-59
    in New Zealand, 346
    openness in, 329
    policies concerning, 346
    pregnancy after, 98-100
    psychological equality of parents, 364
    and privacy, 98-99
    and rejection by non-genetic parent, 359-60
    and role of genetics, 344-47
    screening of donors, 236
    and secrecy, 23-25, 340-343, 345, 351, 360
    and surrogacy, 367

gamete intrafallopian transfer, 40-43, 68, 77, 113
    as alternative to *in vitro* fertilization, 78
    and donor insemination, 191
    and ectopic pregnancy, 117-18, 121
    and egg retrieval, 51, 71
    and laparoscopy, 51, 120
    medication protocols in, 69
    openness about, 339
    and ovum donation, 201
    and privacy, 91
    success rates for, 56-57, 133
gametes, 232, 235, 332, 328
gender discrimination, 35
genealogical confusion, 171
genetic connection, 18-20, 139-40, 143-44, 200, 374. *See also* parents, genetic
    and bonding, 220
    and donor insemination, 161-63
    and embryo adoption, 320
    and extended family, 233
    and gestational care, 291-92, 297-98
    and *in vitro* fertilization, 19, 249
    and ovum donation, 211, 214, 227, 230
    significance of, 142, 238
    and surrogacy, 246
genetic defects. *See* birth defects
genetic disease, 30-31
genetic disorders, 158-59, 178
genetic equality, 165, 193
genetic history, 250, 326-28, 344-49
    and donor insemination, 186, 188
    and embryo adoption, 336
    explaining to child, 361-76
    and gamete donation, 349, 358
    and identity, 327
    and illness, 345
    and prenatal testing, 91
    right to information about, 23-25, 204, 213, 329, 340, 345-47
genetic selection, 31
gestation, multiple. *See* multiple gestation
gestational care, 139-40, 146, 249, 258, 289ff. *See also* assisted reproductive technology; gestational carrier; surrogacy
    and assisted reproductive technology, 361
    availability of, 298
    and birth, 314-15
    and birth defects, 294
    and bonding, 310
    compensation for, 294
    contract for, 204, 294
    coordination of cycles, 312
    counseling for participants, 311
    couples in, 297-98, 302-5
    emotional considerations, 313
    ethical considerations, 291-94
    explaining to child, 304, 364-65, 373

Ministerial Committee on Assisted
  Reproductive Technology, 346
miscarriage, 75, 77, 80, 135. *See also* loss, of
    pregnancy; pregnancy, loss of
  contributing factors, 102-3, 111-12, 114-15
  and diethylstilbestrol, 48
  emotional reaction to, 104-7, 112, 115-16
  and gestational care, 302, 313
  and HCG levels, 118
  and maternal age, 136
  and multiple gestation, 121-26
  partial, 122
  repeated, 111, 114-16, 301, 308
  statistics concerning, 101
  and surrogacy, 267, 276, 278, 282
  symptoms of, 122
  unexplained, 112
MMPI-2, 274
Mommy, Did I Grow In Your Tummy?, 374
Montgomery, Cristie, 271, 273
moral considerations, 24
mother. *See also* parents
  adoptive, 257, 284
  biological. *See* mother, genetic
  defined, 205-6
  genetic, 205, 208, 219-20, 227-28, 237, 249,
    255, 262, 274, 295, 326, 367-68, 371
  and gestational care, 304, 307, 312
  gestational, 205, 208, 215, 219, 221, 249,
    274, 310, 326, 367
  legal, 205, 257, 293
  rearing (social), 205, 215, 219, 326
motherhood
  and age, 23, 36-38, 138.
    See also maternal age
  expectations about, 18-19
  single, 35-36, 250
multifetal reduction, 86-89, 101
  and gestational care, 303, 309, 312, 314
  and ovum donation, 223
  and privacy, 91-92
multiple birth. *See* multiple gestation;
    pregnancy, multiple
multiple gestation, 28, 41, 51, 53, 73, 75,
    85-86, 126. *See also* pregnancy, multiple
  and gestational care, 307, 309-10, 312-13
  loss in, 101, 12
  and multifetal reduction, 87-89
  and ovum donation, 223
  and privacy, 99
  risks in, 86-89
  and surrogacy, 278
multiple pregnancy. *See* multiple gestation;
    pregnancy, multiple
multiple sclerosis, 256, 301
mumps, and infertility, 158
My Story, 367
myomectomy, 111

N
Nachtigall, Robert, 19
National Association of Surrogate Mothers, 254
National Institute of Mental Health, 64
natural cycle IVF, 42, 68
natural oocyte retrieval and intravaginal
    fertilization, 43
needles
  becoming accustomed to, 80
  fear of, 70, 234
  and stress, 68
neonatal intensive care, 124
neonatal problems, 209
neural tube defects, 84
New Zealand
  donor conception in, 346-47
  amd gamete donation, 356
Newsweek Magazine, 350-51, 353
Noble, Elizabeth, 342, 345, 352
NORIE. *See* Natural oocyte retrieval and
    intravaginal fertilization
nursing, 327
nutrition, in pregnancy, 84-85

O
obstetrical care, 76, 89, 99, 249.
    See also prenatal care
obstetrician, 85, 89
oligospermic men, 155
oocyte donation. *See* ovum donation
oocytes, 40. *See also* embryos; ovum
openness
  fears about, 357-60
  and third party parenting, 343-347
OPTS. *See* Organization of Parents
    through Surrogacy
organ donation, 229
Organization of Parents through Surrogacy,
    247, 254-55, 261-64
Organon, 69
ovarian tumors, 48
ovaries, 40, 63-64, 66
  and ectopic pregnancy, 116
  failure of, 216, 197
  and follicle production, 50
  function of, 201
  hyperstimulation of, 50, 69-71, 77, 202, 208
  and ovum donation, 201
  removal of, 197
  and surrogacy, 289-90
ovulation, 63-64
  and assisted reproductive technology, 47, 50
  drugs to induce, 47-49, 69
  and gestational care, 309
  and *in vitro* fertilization, 42
  and ovum donation, 235
  and stress, 63

393

ovum
   cryopreservation of, 195, 200
   handling in laboratory, 66-67
   retrieval of. *See* egg retrieval
   and surrogacy, 295
   transfer of, 195
ovum donation, 18-19, 21, 23-24, 35, 39,
      98-100, 140, 145, 195ff., 200-202, 320, 322,
      324. *See also* gamete donation; ovum
      donor; parenting, third party
   age as factor in, 36-37, 137, 207
   and attachment, 163
   and birth defects, 219-20
   changes in, 357
   claiming in, 222
   commercialization of, 209-210
   compared to donor insemination, 243
   considerations for recipients, 221-23, 235-36
   and control, 212
   and embryo adoption, 319, 322, 332
   and embryo creation, 324, 371
   emotional considerations, 217-221
   and endometrium, 200-1
   ethical considerations, 198-99, 201-4, 209-10,
      236-37
   explaining to child, 223-24, 228, 237, 346,
      349, 374
   financial compensation for, 199, 209-10, 223,
      228-29, 324
   financial considerations, 195-96, 249
   genetic screening in, 202
   and gestational care, 205, 250, 312
   and health insurance, 210
   history of, 249
   and human immunodeficiency virus, 202
   and identity confusion, 223
   and *in vitro* fertilization, 249, 289
   inter-generational, 213-14
   lack of consent for, 67
   and menopause, 210
   and mental illness, 232
   offering, 216-17
   openness in, 224, 237, 239-41, 346, 349
   and ovulation, 235
   and privacy, 223-24, 228, 249
   readiness for, 237
   recipient couples and, 235-38
   requesting, 216-17
   resistance to, 217
   risks involved in, 25, 198-99, 203, 207-9, 326
   and scarcity of ova, 196, 198, 211-12, 237
   screening of recipients, 217-18, 235
   secrecy in, 239-40, 329, 343-44
   and semen donation, 205, 211
   side effects of, 26
   and surrogacy, 205
   in Sweden, 346

ovum donor. *See also* ovum donation
   anonymous, 198, 211-12, 215, 226-30,
      242-23, 343
   concern for, 222
   counseling for, 183, 202-3, 217-18, 223,
      230-36
   exit interview with, 235
   expectations about, 237-38
   experience of, 222-23, 234-35
   friend as, 200, 214
   identification of recipient, 346
   information about, 202, 212-13, 233, 372
   known, 168, 211-26
   matching with recipient, 240-41
   motivation of, 198, 214-16, 229
   recruitment of, 198-200, 228-29
   relationship with offspring, 220, 224, 232,
      237
   relationship with recipient, 224-25
   relative as, 171, 200, 213-15, 223, 227
   and reproductive loss, 232
   screening of, 201-3, 217-18, 228, 230-34
   selection of, 213-14
ovum retrieval. *See* egg retrieval

P
pain, tolerance to, 51
PAL. *See* Positive Adoption Language
Pancoast, William, M. D., 23, 154, 340
Pannor, Reuben, 351, 357, 366
parenthood, 19, 32, 81
   adjustment to, 286
   alternative routes to, 18
   alternatives to, 18, 142
   components of, 16-18, 21-26
   expectations about, 18-19
   experience of, 20-21
   insecurity about, 228
   posthumous, 21
   social, 142, 169, 251
parenting
   third party, 14, 18, 21, 140, 316, 323, 357-61.
      See also donor insemination; embryo
      adoption; gestational care; ovum
      donation; semen donation; surrogacy
   coersion in, 26
   counseling in, 26
   explaining to child, 361-76
   and openness, 339ff., 375-76
   secrecy about, 350, 376
   through surrogacy, 287-88
parents. *See also* birthparents; father; mother
   adoptive, 21-23, 251, 326-29, 347, 359,
      361-62, 372
   and bonding, 326
   and embryo adoption, 332, 337
   and open adoption, 327
   biological. *See* parents, genetic
   deception by, 350

progressive muscle relaxation, 64
prostaglandins, 159
Pruett, Kyle, 360, 363, 366, 376

R
Raboy, Barbara, 182-83
Ranoux, Claude, M. D., 43
rape, 70
Reame, Nancy, 293
regret, 32-33
    and assisted reproductive technology,
        61-62, 80
    avoidance of, 80, 139
    and ectopic pregnancy, 120
    ethical considerations, 33-34
    in gestational carrier, 308
    and multifetal reduction, 87-88
    and ovum donation, 221, 232
    and surrogacy, 276-77
Reiki therapy, 65
rejection, fear of, 359-60
relaxation techniques, 64, 70
religious considerations, 13-14, 26-28, 39,
        105, 107, 113, 128
    ceremonies, 113, 128-29, 148
    in donor insemination, 152, 165, 193
    in surrogacy, 245-46
reproductive endocrinologists, 117, 154, 291
reproductive freedom, 18, 21-24
    and surrogacy, 254, 258-59, 261
Reproductive Science Center, 331
reproductive technology.
    See assisted reproductive technology
RESOLVE, Inc., 147, 179, 263
Robertson, John, 21-22
Roe v. Wade, 250
Roman Catholic Church, 27-28, 30
Rorsharch, 274
Rossing, M.A., 48
Rothman, Barbara Katz, 90
rubella screening, 60

S
Sandelowski, Margarete, 27, 32, 85, 90
SART. See Society for Assisted Reproductive
    Technology
Schmidt, Anna, 284
Schnitter, Jane, 367
secrecy
    and adoption, 362
    and artificial insemination, 154
    and assisted reproduction, 340-43
    and gamete donation, 25, 211
    impact of, 350-57
    and third-party parenting, 340-43, 376
semen. See also sperm
    analysis of, 60, 159, 266
    collection of, 72
Serono, 69
Serophene, 48

sexual abuse, 70
siblings
    competition between, 172
    and embryo adoption, 332
    and embryo donation, 331
    genetic, 325-26, 332
single motherhood, 35-36, 250
single women, 138, 170, 204, 352, 371
    and embryo adoption, 319
Skolnick, Julia, 66, 192-93
Society for Advanced Reproductive
    Technology, 55, 137, 178
Society of Reproductive Endocrinologists, 178
Society of Reproductive Surgeons, 178
Sorkow, Judge, 257
Spencer, Marietta, 251
sperm, 40-45, 66-67, 71, 152. See also semen
    cryopreservation of, 21, 211-12, 358
    quality of, 55-56, 153
    quantity of, 153
    washing of, 159
sperm bank, 168, 180-83
    and anonymity, 189, 346
    and artificial insemination, 154
    and cancer treatment, 157
    differences between, 180-83
    and donor information, 178
    and embryo adoption, 321
    error by, 192-93
    and HIV, 202
    matching donors with recipients, 240
    and openness, 346, 349, 357
    and ovum donation, 230
    and RESOLVE, 179
    role of in conception, 155
    and surrogacy, 278
Sperm Bank of California, 182-83
sperm donation, 18, 21, 23-24, 98-100, 173-75,
        320, 322, 368. See also donor insemina-
        tion; gamete donation; sperm donor
    changes in, 357
    and embryo adoption, 319, 322, 371
    and embryo creation, 324, 371
    explaining to child, 374
    first use of, 23, 154, 340
    guidelines for, 178-79
    lack of consent for, 67
    and lesbians, 36
    openness in, 346
    and ovum donation, 198, 205, 211
    psychosocial issues in, 184-85
    and secrecy, 239, 241
    simplicity of, 211
    and surrogacy, 253
sperm donor, 352. See also sperm donation
    advertisement for, 176
    anonymous, 24-25, 168, 175-79, 180-83,
        185-86, 343, 346
    compensation of, 209, 324

counseling for, 174-75, 183-85
and embryo adoption, 321
identification of, 346
information about, 179, 189-90, 372
motivations of, 173-74
parameters for, 178-79
screening of, 230
selection of, 181-82
spina bifida, 84
spinal cord injury, 158
spontaneous abortion. *See* loss, of pregnancy;
   miscarriage; pregnancy, loss of
stem cell storage, 181-82
sterility. *See* azoospermia
Stern, Betsy, M. D., and Bill, 256-58
steroids, 115
stillbirth, 101, 127-28
stress, 63-65, 76-78
stretch marks, 98
substance abuse, 232, 266
Subzonal Insemination, 44
superovulation, 40-42, 159, 199
surrogacy, 266, 268, 373-74. *See also* assisted
      reproductive technology; gestational care;
      surrogate and adoption, 250, 252, 255,
      260, 263-65, 280, 361, 369
   advocates for, 254
   and aging eggs, 247
   candidates for, 261-62
   contact between participants, 252, 283,
      285-86
   contract for, 252-56, 258-59, 279-80, 294
   criticism of, 247-48, 254-55, 266
   different practices of, 263-64
   ethical concerns, 255-59
   explaining to child, 367-70, 373-74
   and fetal defects, 266, 273
   financial considerations of, 264, 298
   and gamete donation, 365, 367
   gestational. *See* gestational care
   and gestational care, 250-52, 258, 291-2, 298,
      304, 306-7, 310, 361
   history of, 248-49
   host-uterus. *See* gestational care
   and identity, 251
   implications of, 262, 288
   and *in vitro* fertilization, 249-50, 290
   and insemination, 280-81
   and interest of child, 254-55
   internet sites, 247, 263
   language of, 251
   legal considerations of, 249, 255-60, 263,
      265, 279-80, 284, 296
   and ovum donation, 205, 216
   postpartum, 285-88
   practical aspects of, 262-65
   pregnancy and, 280-83
   preparation for, 266-68, 275-79
   and privacy, 288

psychological considerations of, 264-68,
   271, 274-79, 281
psychological equality of parents in, 364
reasons for choosing, 246-48
relationship between participants, 272-73
and reproductive freedom, 254, 258-29, 261
risks in, 26
screening of parents, 265
second experience, 286-87
surrogate, 260-62, 268-71. *See also* surrogacy
   autonomy of, 250
   and the birth experience, 284-85
   changing, 281-82
   children of, 278-79, 369-70
   coersion of, 26
   compensation of, 252-54, 259, 261, 269-70,
      294
   locating, 248, 265, 272-73
   medical evaluation of, 264-65, 273
   motivation of, 305
   psychological evaluation of, 265-68, 271
   rights of, 253
   screening of, 273-80
   support network for, 283
Surrogate Mothers, Inc., 295
Sweden
   donor conception in, 346
   and gamete donation, 356
Swedish Law on Artificial Insemination, 346
*Sweet Grapes: How to Stop Being Infertile
   and Start Living Again*, 147
syphilis, 178, 202

T

TASC. *See* The American Surrogacy Center
Tay-Sachs disease, 30, 159
technology, reproductive. *See* assisted
   reproductive technology
testicles, 44-45, 157-58
TET, 40
The American Surrogacy Center, 247, 263
The Mother Machine, 253
The Psychology of Women II, 114
The Tentative Pregnancy, 90
thyroid disease, 103, 197
toxemia, 127
trans-vaginal follicular aspiration, 202
triplets. *See* multiple gestation;
   pregnancy, multiple
tubal ligation, 198-99
tubal spasm, 64
Turner, Candace, 352-53
twins. *See* multiple gestation;
   pregnancy, multiple

U

ultrasonography, 58, 70-71, 86
   and attachment to fetus, 104
   to confirm pregnancy, 92, 103, 112

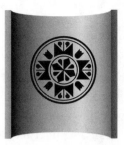

$\mathscr{P}$erspectives Press

The Infertility and Adoption Publisher
http://www.perspectivespress.com

Since 1982 Perspectives Press has focused exclusively on infertility, adoption, and related reproductive health and child welfare issues. Our purpose is to promote understanding of these issues and to educate and sensitize those personally experiencing these life situations, professionals who work in these fields, and the public at large. Our titles are never duplicative or competitive with material already available through other publishers. We seek to find and fill only niches which are empty. In addition to this book, our current titles include:

For Adults

Perspectives on a Grafted Tree
Understanding Infertility: Insights for Family and Friends
Sweet Grapes: How to Stop Being Infertile and Start Living Again
Residential Treatment: A Tapestry of Many Therapies
A Child's Journey through Placement
Adopting after Infertility
Flight of the Stork: What Children Think (and When) about Sex and Family Building
Taking Charge of Infertility
Looking Back, Looking Forward
Launching a Baby's Adoption: Practical Strategies for Parents and Professionals
Toddler Adoption: The Weaver's Craft
Choosing Assisted Reproduction: Social, Emotional and Ethical Considerations

For Children

The Mulberry Bird: An Adoption Story (Revised)
Our Baby: A Birth and Adoption Story
Filling in the Blanks: A Guided Look at Growing Up Adopted
William Is My Brother
Lucy's Feet
Two Birthdays for Beth
Let Me Explain: A Story about Donor Insemination

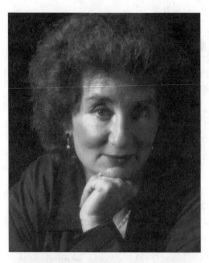

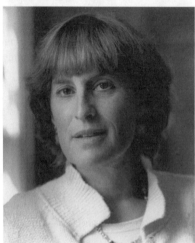

About the Authors

Susan Lewis Cooper is a psychologist with over twenty years of private practice experience specializing in infertility, adoption, and third party reproductive options. In addition, she is a psychologist at the Reproductive Science Center-Boston and at Focus Counseling and Consultation, Inc., in Cambridge, where she is also a co-director.

Ellen Sarasohn Glazer is a clinical social worker with over twenty years' experience. For the past ten years her private practice has focused on infertility, pregnancy loss, adoption, and related issues. She is also program counselor at the Boston Regional Center for Reproductive Medicine in Stoneham, MA. She is the author of *The Long-Awaited Stork: A Guide to Parenting after Infertility*.

Together, Cooper and Glazer co-authored two previous books. *Without Child: Experiencing and Resolving Infertility* and *Beyond Infertility: The New Paths to Parenthood* are now out of print. Both women are members of the American Society for Reproductive Medicine and its Mental Health Professional Group and each served for several years on RESOLVE, Inc.'s national board of directors.